Y. Honda   T. Juji   (Eds.)

HLA in Narcolepsy

With 50 Figures and 63 Tables

Springer-Verlag Berlin Heidelberg New York
London Paris Tokyo

Yutaka Honda, MD, DMedSc
Seiwa Hospital, Neuropsychiatric Research Institute
91 Bentencho, Shinjuku-ku, Tokyo 162, Japan

Takeo Juji, Prof., MD, DMedSc
Blood Transfusion Service
Tokyo University Hospital, 7-3-1 Hongo
Bunkyo-ku, Tokyo 113, Japan

ISBN-13: 978-3-642-83389-2 e-ISBN-13: 978-3-642-83387-8
DOI: 10.1007/978-3-642-83387-8

Library of Congress Cataloging-in-Publication Data
HLA in narcolepsy / Y. Honda, T. Juji (eds.). p. cm. Based on papers from the Second International Symposium on Narcolepsy held in Fairchild Auditorium, Stanford University, 6-7 July 1985. Includes bibliographies and index.
1. Narcolepsy-Genetic aspects-Congresses. 2. HLA histocompatibility antigens-Congresses. I. Honda, Y. (Yutaka), 1929- . II. Juji, T. (Takeo), 1935- . III. International Symposium on Narcolepsy (2nd : 1985 : Stanford University) [DNLM: 1. HLA Antigens-immunology-congresses. 2. Narcolepsy-immunology-congresses. WM 188 H677 1985] RC549.H57 1988 616.8'49-dc 19 88-12312

Softcove reprint of the hardcover 1st edition 1988

2123/3145-543210

Preface

The Second International Symposium on Narcolepsy was held at Fairchild Auditorium, Stanford University, on 6–7 July 1985 under the presidency of Drs. William C. Dement and Christian Guilleminault. It succeeded the First International Symposium on Narcolepsy held in La Grande Motte, France, organized by Pierre Passouant in July 1975 in commemoration of the 100th anniversary of the publication of Jean B. E. Gelineau's paper which proposed the naming of narcolepsy.

At the second narcolepsy symposium, many important research reports on both basic and clinical aspects of narcolepsy were given by investigators from many countries of the world. Audience interest was particularly attracted by the section on the relationship between HLA and narcolepsy, in which recent evidence that almost all narcoleptic patients are HLA-DR2 positive was reported by investigators from Japan, England, France, Canada, and the United States. The close relationship between the HLA antigens, hitherto considered as immune-related genetic markers encoded by genes on human chromosome 6, and narcolepsy appeared to open a new approach not only for the research of narcolepsy but also for the mechanism of sleep in general.

Publication of all these new findings on the association of HLA and narcolepsy was considered; an outline was worked out and all the groups agreed to prepare a contribution covering the various aspects of this topic.

It will fill us with great happiness if this project contributes to the development of further molecular biological research on the true cause of narcolepsy and leads to the true cure for and prevention of narcolepsy.

March 1988

Y. Honda
T. Juji

Table of Contents

Introduction
Y. HONDA 1

1. An Overview of the HLA System
T. JUJI 10

2. Clinical features of Narcolepsy: Japanese Experiences
Y. HONDA 24

3. HLA in Narcolepsy in Japan
K. MATSUKI, Y. HONDA, M. SATAKE, and T. JUJI 58

4. HLA in Narcolepsy/Cataplexy in the United Kingdom
C. B. LOCK, K. I. WELSH, J. D. PARKES, A. SO, D. C. BRIGGS, R. W. VAUGHAN, and M. VAN DAMM 76

5. HLA in Narcolepsy in France
M. BILLIARD, J. SEIGNALET, H. BETUEL, A. MARCADET, L. GEBUHREL, A. C. FREIDEL, C. CONFAVREUX, A. BESSET, and J. CADILHAC 89

6. HLA in Narcolepsy in Canada
J. MONTPLAISIR and G. POIRIER 97

7. HLA-DR2 and the Narcolepsy Syndrome: The Stanford Experience
C. GUILLEMINAULT, J. HOLLOMAN, C. GRUMET, T. KILDUFF, H. O. MCDEVITT, W. C. DEMENT, and M. M. MITLER 108

8. Narcolepsy and HLA in the Federal Republic of Germany: Population and Family Data
K. MEIER-EWERT, G. MUELLER-ECKHARDT, and D. J. SCHENDEL 114

9. Positive HLA-Dw2 in Narcolepsy
T. NAOHARA, Y. HONDA, and T. JUJI 121

10. HLA-Linked Complement Markers in Narcolepsy
K. Tokunaga, K. Matsuki, T. Juji, and Y. Honda 130

11. DNA Typing in Narcolepsy
H. Inoko 137

12. Immunological Features of Narcolepsy in Japan
K. Matsuki, T. Juji, and Y. Honda 150

13. Immune Factors in Narcolepsy in the United Kingdom
J. D. Parkes, K. Welsh, N. Langdon, and C. Lock 158

14. Disorders of Excessive Daytime Sleepiness Without Cataplexy, and Their Relationship with HLA in Japan
S. Harada, K. Matsuki, Y. Honda, and T. Someya 172

15. HLA in Disorders of Excessive Daytime Sleepiness Without Cataplexy in Canada
J. Montplaisir and G. Poirier 186

16. Genetic Markers Other than HLA in Narcolepsy
Part 1: Findings on 16 Genetic Markers
A. Asaka 191
Part 2: Red Blood Cell Antigens in Narcolepsy
K. Matsuki, M. Uchikawa, T. Juji, and Y. Honda . 199

Subject Index 203

List of Contributors

ASAKA, Akio, MD
Department of Mental Health, School of Health Sciences, Faculty of Medicine, The University of Tokyo, Hongo 7-3-1, Bunkyo-ku, Tokyo 113, Japan

BESSET, Alain, PhD
Unité des Troubles du Sommeil, Centre Médical Gui de Chauliac, 34059 Montpellier, Cedex, France

BETUEL, H., MD
Laboratoire d'Histocompatibilité, Centre de Transfusion Sanguine, 69007 Lyon, Cedex, France

BILLIARD, Michel, MD
Unité des Troubles du Sommeil, Centre Médical Gui de Chauliac, 34059 Montpellier, Cedex, France

BRIGGS, David, C., MSc
Tissue Typing, Guy's Hospital, St. Thomas' Street, London, SE1 9RT, UK

CADILHAC, Jean, MD
Service de Physiopathologie des Maladies Nerveuses et Musculaires, Centre Médical Gui de Chauliac, 34059 Montpellier, Cedex, France

CONFAVREUX, C., MD
Département de Neurologie, Hôpital Neurologique, 69003 Lyon, Cedex, France

DEMENT, WiliamC., MD PhD
Stanford University School of Medicine, Sleep Research Center, Building TD, Room 114, Stanford, CA 94305, USA

FREIDEL, A.C., MD
Laboratoire d'Histocompatibilité, Centre de Transfusion Sanguine, 69007 Lyon, Cedex, France

GEBUHREL, L., MD
Laboratoire d'Histocompatibilité, Centre de Transfusion Sanguine, 69007 Lyon, Cedex, France

GRUMET, Carl, MD
Stanford University School of Medicine, Department of Pathology, Stanford, CA 94305, USA

GUILLEMINAULT, Christian MD
Stanford University School of Medicine, Sleep Research Center, Building TD, Room 114, Stanford, CA 94305, USA

HARADA, Seiichi, MD
Comprehensive Mental Health Center of Tokyo Metropolitan Central District, 2-1-7 Kamikitazawa, Setagaya-ku, Tokyo 156, Japan

HOLLOMAN, John D., MD
Stanford University School of Medicine, Sleep Research Center, Building TD, Room 114, Stanford, CA 94305, USA

HONDA, Yutaka, MD
Seiwa Hospital, Neuropsychiatric Research Institute, 91 Bentencho, Shinjuku-ku, Tokyo 162, Japan

INOKO, Hidetoshi, PhD
Department of Transplantation, Tokai University School of Medicine, Bohseidai, Isehara, Kanagawa-Pref. 259-11, Japan

JUJI, Takeo, MD
Blood Transfusion Service, Tokyo University Hospital, Hongo 7-3-1, Bunkyo-ku, Tokyo 113, Japan

KILDUFF, Thomas, Dr.
Stanford University School of Medicine, Sleep Research Center, Building TD, Room 114, Stanford, CA 94305, USA

LANGDON, Nicola, Dr.
Department of Neurology, King's College Hospital, Denmark Hill, London SE5 9RS, UK

LOCK, Christopher B., MB BChir
Department of Neurology, King's College Hospital, Denmark Hill, London SE5 9RS, UK

MARCADET, A., PhD
Centre d'Etude du Polymorphisme Humain, Annexe du College de France, 75005 Paris, France

MATSUKI, Kazumasa, MD
Blood Transfusion Service, Tokyo University Hospital, Hongo 7-3-1, Bunkyo-ku, Tokyo 113, Japan

McDEVITT, Hugh O., MD
Stanford University School of Medicine, Department of Medical Microbiology, Stanford, CA 94305, USA

MEIER-EWERT, Karlheinz, Prof. Dr.
Neurological Hospital and Sleep Disorder Unit, Heinrich-Wiegand-Straße 57, 3578 Schwalmstadt 1, FRG

MITLER, Merrill M., Dr.
Scripps Clinic and Research Foundation, La Jolla, CA 92037, USA

MONTPLAISIR, Jaques, Dr.
Centre d'Étude du Sommeil, Hôpital de Sacré-Coeur de Montréal, 5400, Boulevard Gouin Ouest, Montréal, Québec H4J 1C5, Canada

MUELLER-ECKHARDT, G., Dr.
Institut für klinische Immunologie und Transfusionsmedizin, Justus-Liebig-Universität, Langhansstraße 7, 6300 Gießen, FRG

NAOHARA, Tohru, MD
Central Blood Center, The Japanese Red Cross, 4-1-31, Hiroo, Shibuya-ku, Tokyo 150, Japan

PARKES, J. David, MA MD FRCP
Department of Neurology, King's College Hospital, Denmark Hill, London, SE5 9RS, UK

POIRIER, Gaétan
Centre d'Étude du Sommeil, Hôpital de Sacré-Coeur de Montréal, 5400, Boulevard Gouin Ouest, Montréal, Québec H4J 1C5, Canada

SATAKE, Masahiro, MD
Second Department of Surgery, Tohoku University School of Medicine, Sendai, Japan

SCHENDEL, D.J., Prof. Dr.
Institut für Immunologie, Maximilians-Universität, Goethestraße 31, 8000 München 2, FRG

SEIGNALET, J., MD
Institut d'Hématologie, Centre de Transfusion Sanguine,
34059 Montpellier, Cedex, France

SO, Alex K.L., MA MRCP
Imperial Cancer Research Fund, Lincoln's Inn Fields,
London WC2A 3PX, UK

SOMEYA, Toshiyuki, MD
Department of Psychiatry, Shiga University of Medical Sciences,
Otsu, Japan

TOKUNAGA, Katsushi, PhD
Department of Anthropology, Faculty of Science, Tokyo
University, 7-3-1 Hongo, Bunkyo-ku, Tokyo 113, Japan

UCHIKAWA, Makoto, PhD
Blood Transfusion Service, Tokyo University Hospital,
Hongo 7-3-1, Bunkyo-ku, Tokyo 113, Japan

VAN DAM, Mieke G.
Tissue Typing, Guy's Hospital, St. Thomas' Street,
London SE1 9RT, UK

VAUGHAN, Robert W., MA MSc
Tissue Typing, Guy's Hospital, St. Thomas' Street,
London SE1 9RT, UK

WELSH, Ken I., PhD
Tissue Typing, Guy's Hospital, St. Thomas' Street,
London SE1 9RT, UK

Introduction

Y. HONDA

Recent findings that all, or almost all, narcoleptic patients typed for human leukocyte antigen (HLA) are DR2 and DQw1 positive indicate that of all HLA-associated diseases, narcolepsy has by far the strongest association with HLA. Thus narcolepsy must be considered a special disease from the molecular biologist's point of view. In addition, the fact that narcolepsy has a close relationship with HLA genes provides promising clues for molecular biological research on sleep and arousal disorders.

This volume begins with an overview of the HLA system (Chap. 1) and clinical features of narcolepsy (Chap. 2) to explain the backgrounds of these two hitherto unrelated fields. Then specialists in narcolepsy research from various countries of the world contribute to the discussion on the relations between HLA and narcolepsy (Chaps. 3-8). HLA-D specificities (Chap. 9), HLA-linked complement markers (Chap. 10), and DNA typings (Chap. 11) are described by researchers of HLA and immunogenetics. Immunological features (Chaps. 12, 13) and genetic markers other than HLA (Chap. 16) in narcolepsy are also described by specialists of each field. HLA in disorders of excessive daytime sleepiness without cataplexy is further added to clarify the differences and similarities between narcolepsy and other sleep disorders with excessive daytime sleepiness (Chaps. 14, 15). The concept of narcolepsy differs slightly for each investigator. Although these differences are not large, they may have serious implications for HLA findings. These discrepancies reflect the present status of narcolepsy research.

The HLA System

The HLA system is composed of a set of closely linked genes on the short arm of chromosome 6 and the proteins encoded by these genes. One of the important characteristics of the HLA system is that the HLA genes exhibit a very high level of polymorphism; for example, nearly 50 alleles are known at present at the HLA-B locus. For the seven HLA loci, a total of 124 different antigens have been identified. The HLA system is also important for organ transplantations and immunogenetics. The HLA antigens show strong association with various diseases, especially with those for which autoimmune mechanisms are postulated. It is natural to speculate that some immunological mechanisms are involved in the development of narcolepsy (Chaps. 12, 13). But so far there is little actual evidence for this speculation. At present, HLA typing is very useful for detecting at-risk subjects in the families of narcoleptic patients. Future development of techniques that detect HLA-DR2 and Dw2 accurately and more quickly will provide a helpful measure for the clinical practice of sleep disorders.

A Story Behind the HLA Finding

At this point let me present an episode in the discovery of the strong association between HLA-DR2 and narcolepsy. In 1980 Akio Asaka, a psychiatrist and geneticist at the Department of Mental Hygiene, University of Tokyo, proposed that we joint them and investigate narcolepsy as a part of their joint research program on the host factors of intractable diseases. They were then analyzing genetic markers for various disorders such as systemic lupus erythematosus and parkinsonism (Asaka et al. 1981). After the analysis of 51 phenotypes of 16 genetic markers on 118 narcoleptic patients, 5 markers showed significant differences in frequency as compared with normal subjects in Japan (Asaka 1981). In addition to these 16 genetic markers, HLA antigens were also typed at the Blood Transfusion Service, Tokyo University Hospital. As the result of the HLA analysis of A, B, and C loci on 58 narcoleptic patients, significant increase in Bw35 ($\chi^2 = 15.6$) and significant decrease in Bw52 ($\chi^2 = -10.5$) were observed. (Juji et al. 1981, Honda et al. 1983a). Two years later, in March 1983, at a casual occasion, I recalled this unfinished HLA study, and contacted Dr. Takeo Juji, Professor of Blood Transfusion at Tokyo Women's Medical College at the time. Dr. Juji kindly accepted my proposal to determine the HLA-DR antigens in narcolepsy. Since it was a continuation of a previous study, he indicated that 20-30 cases would be needed in order to obtain statistically significant differences.

Thus we started typing of HLA for narcolepsy again in May of 1983. It was not long before Dr. Juji and his group noticed that every narcoleptic patient typed for HLA was DR2 positive and that this was an extraordinary finding. The proposal to press on then came from Dr. Juji's side. We reported our finding at the 6th Annual Meeting of the Japanese Society of Biological Psychiatry held in Tokyo on 24 March 1984, and at the 9th Annual Meeting of the Japanese Society of Sleep Research held in Kanazawa on 11 May 1984. The proceedings of these meetings were later published in English in *Folia Psychiatria et Neurologica Japonica* in September 1984, and in June 1985.

In August 1984, I visited the headquarters of the American Narcolepsy Association (ANA) in San Carlos, California. The officers of the ANA were very interested in the significance of our HLA findings. Later *The Eye Opener,* a bulletin of the ANA, reported the issue of HLA in September 1984, and explained very clearly in easy terms the significance of the finding on HLA. It runs as follows:

> **Japanese Studies Shared**
> Most recently, when he (Honda and his group) tested 102 of his narcoleptic patients, every single one of them had a specific human leukocyte antigen (HLA) that is usually only found in about 30% of the population in Japan.

> This is something like the finding that everyone who had cataplexy had red hair. While it might not cause narcolepsy, it might indicate who could develop it. That is, if every person who was known to have cataplexy had red hair, then a child who did not have red hair would not be likely to develop cataplexy!

This was the first English publication outside Japan on the finding of HLA-DR2 to be read by the general public.

Our findings were also published in *Tissue Antigens* in November 1984 (Juji et al. 1984); at the same time British colleagues reported very similar findings in the *Lancet* (Langdon et al. 1984), followed by French colleagues (Billiard and Seignalet 1985) and Canadian colleagues (Poirier et al. 1986).

Narcolepsy as a Disease or Syndrome: A History of Controversy

Historically there have been controversies on the concept and definition of narcolepsy. Even today full international agreement on the definition of narcolepsy has not yet been reached. Before we consider the definition, however, it is necessary to settle the dispute whether or not narcolepsy is a disease entity. The historical background of these controversies may be worthy of brief comment here.

The medical description of excessive daytime sleepiness (EDS) dates back to 1672 when Thomas Willis (see Lennox 1939) described a case of morbid somnolence. There have been further descriptions of similar clinical cases by Schindler (1829), Graves (1851), Caffé (1862) cited by Passouant (1976), Westphal (1877), and Fischer (1878).

In 1880 Jean Baptiste Edouard Gelineau, a French practitioner of the nervous system disorders, described two cases of EDS. He considered them as "neurosis," an independent neural disorder different from epilepsy, and named the disorder *narcolepsie* in his paper, *"De la narcolepsie,"* which appeared serially in *Gazette d'Hopitaux*. The first case was a citation of a case reported by Caffé: a 47-year-old male who had frequent and intractable daytime sleepiness persisting for 4 years. Cataplexy was not noted, but hallucinations were described. The second case was a 38-year-old male, a wine barrel retailer. From the age of 36, the patient fell asleep often in the daytime and in unusual situations, such as in the middle of a meal and in front of a physician in the consultation room. Intense emotions were correlated with these attacks of sleep and with the falls or muscle weakness, which Gelineau called "astasia." The patient also had sudden numbness of his legs and whole body when he laughed aloud or when he had a good hand while playing cards. His legs would buckle, and he appeared inebriated.

In 1881, Gelineau then published a monograph, *De la narcolepsie* describing 14 cases, in which he discriminated essential and secondary narcolepsies. Since then the term narcolepsy has been used to describe a disorder of morbid somnolence.

In the early twentieth century, clinical studies of the symptomatology of narcolepsy were performed extensively in Germany (Redlich 1915, 1931, Thiele and Bernhardt 1933, Wilder 1935). The major symptoms of narcolepsy became settled as the narcoleptic tetrad (Yoss and Daly 1957), which included sleep attacks, cataplexy (Loewenfeld 1902, Henneberg 1916), sleep paralysis (Levin 1933), and hypnagogic hallucinations (Moyer 1898, Wenderowic 1924). Other symptoms often associated with narcolepsy were obesity, disturbed nocturnal sleep, automatic behaviors, and characteristic personality traits.

Symonds (1926) and Spiller (1926) examined patients who developed narcoleptic symptoms after lethargic encephalitis and used the term symptomatic narcolepsy. They considered these patients etiologically different from those of idiopathic narcolepsy. Wilson (1928) stressed similarities in clinical features between epilepsy and narcolepsy. He studied exogenous factors involved in the development of narcolepsy, and classified 13 types of symptomatic narcolepsies. Secondary narcolepsy was described by Roth (1962) in his elaborate monograph on narcolepsy and hypersomnia.

Psychological factors have also been studied. The psychogenic origin of narcolepsy was advocated by some investigators from the psychoanalytic tradition (Missriegler and Karpman 1941, Spiegel and Oberndorf 1946, Coodley 1948).

In 1960 Vogel discovered the appearance of a REM period at the onset of nocturnal sleep of one narcoleptic patient. Vogel interpreted this finding as the projection of fantasy which is gratified in a dream in a way unacceptable during the waking life of the narcoleptic patient. The frequent appearance of sleep-onset REM periods in narcoleptic patients was confirmed by Rechtschaffen et al. and Takahashi and Jimbo in 1963. Through this new finding, the recognition that narcolepsy is not a simple symptom but an independent disorder with a unique pathophysiology of sleep mechanism, especially REM sleep, gained ascendancy.

Genetic studies of narcolepsy provided supporting evidence. A weak familial loading was demonstrated as the result of family studies of narcolepsy (Nevsimalova-Bruhova and Roth 1972, Kessler 1976, Baraitser and Parkes 1978, Honda et al. 1983b). In addition to characteristic clinical symptomatology, uniform treatment responses to psychostimulants and tricyclic antidepressants (Akimoto et al. 1960, 1961) have also been noted. These findings are in favor of the concept that narcolepsy is a disease entity.

The recent findings that all or almost all narcoleptic patients are HLA-DR2 positive irrespective of the preceding history of serious disturbances of the brain function due to external stressors (Honda et al. 1984, 1985, 1986), and that all narcoleptic patients have specific DNA fragments in common (Marcadet et al. 1985, Inoko 1986), can be considered as persuasive evidence in establishing narcolepsy as an independent disease entity.

Use of the Term Narcolepsy and the Need for Diagnostic Criteria

Although Gelineau explained the meaning of the term *"narcolepsie"* by *"narco"*=somnolence and *"lepsy"*=seizure, the original Greek meaning of *"narke"* is numbness or loss of power. Thus the term narcolepsy literally means attacks of numbness. In view of today's recognition of the special importance of cataplexy (*"kata"*=down, *"plexis"*=striking) as an essential symptom of narcolepsy, the choice of the term narcolepsy with its emphasis on numbness was somewhat appropriate, but to represent the most important symptom, recurrent daytime somnolence, the term seemed inadequate. Because of this lack of fit, Gowers (1907) proposed the term "somnosis" (*"somnos"*=somnolence), and Curschmann and Prange (1925) proposed *"Einschlafsucht"*, meaning morbid inclination to fall asleep. Singer (1917) and Wenderowic (1924) proposed the term "hypnolepsy" (*"hypnos"*=sleep). Other expressions of narcolepsy have included "Gelineau's syndrome", "Westphal-Gelineau's syndrome", and "Gelineau-Redlich's syndrome". In Japan the colloquial term for narcolepsy is *"Inemuribyo"* or "napping disease". However, these terms have not been used widely, and the term narcolepsy is used internationally today.

Currently the actual use of the term narcolepsy differs for individual investigator. Some investigators use it to denote simply the symptom of sudden daytime somnolence or sleep attacks. Others use it to indicate a syndrome consisting of narcoleptic tetrads. Another standpoint in the use of the term narcolepsy is to represent a prototype of a disease with only the symptom of excessive daytime sleepiness, like "independent narcolepsy" (Roth 1980).

The classification of sleep and arousal disorders adopted by the Association of Sleep Disorders Centers and the Association of Psychophysiological Study of Sleep described the essential features of narcolepsy in 1979 as a syndrome consisting of excessive daytime sleepiness and abnormal manifestations of REM sleep.

The group of investigators at Stanford University defined narcolepsy on the basis of pathophysiology. They stressed the significance of short sleep latency and more than two sleep onset REM periods on the Multiple Sleep Latency Test (MSLT) as indicators of narcolepsy (Carskadon and Dement 1977, Richardson et al. 1978, Mitler et al. 1979).

Further efforts to reach an international consensus concerning the concept and the use of the term narcolepsy are needed. Establishment of clear and operational diagnostic criteria for narcolepsy is very important in order to obtain a high level of diagnostic reliability, clinical validity, and usefulness in exchanging research and treatment results.

DR2-Negative Narcolepsy

In recent years the presence of DR2-negative narcolepsy has been reported. Two such cases were reported by Guilleminault and Grumet (1986), one by Langdon et al. (1986), and two by Andreas-Zietz et al. (1986), including one of the two cases that Müller-Eckhardt et al. reported (1986). Theoretically the presence of DR2-negative narcolepsy is within the realm of consideration if the liability gene to narcolepsy is located outside but very close to the HLA-DR2 gene. However, clinical examination of every DR2-negative case will be very important to ascertain the presence and types of difference in clinical symptoms. For example, we think that precise examination of the nature of cataplexy in DR2-negative cases is extremely important. If we do not use a common definition of cataplexy, it is quite possible that nonnarcoleptic attacks of muscle weakness might be considered as cataplexy.

In Japan all of the 190 narcoleptic patients diagnosed clinically by ourselves before HLA-typing were DR2 positive, and we still have no exception (Chap. 3). This may be due to the general homogeneity of the Japanese population, although there was a short report of a DR2-negative "narcoleptic" patient in Japan from Tokai University among 12 narcoleptic patients they reported (Nezu et al. 1985). The clinical picture of this DR2-negative case was not described in the report, but the history and clinical picture subsequently provided by the psychiatrist in charge indicated that the patient was an alcoholic who had an irregular sleep life. Her attacks of powerlessness were unclear, and treatment response to imipramine or clomipramine was not examined (personal communication). Thus, presence of cataplexy and diagnosis of narcolepsy for this case were dubious.

Narcolepsy Associations of the World

Societies of narcoleptic patients are now established in many countries of the world, such as Canada, England, Japan, Netherlands, Switzerland, and the United States. Among them, the American Narcolepsy Association is the largest and most active. They distribute information on their self-help activities, and raise funds for research on narcolepsy. The narcolepsy associations in other countries are also actively pursuing self-help activities and endeavor to exchange information on research and treatment of narcolepsy. The Japan Narcolepsy Association (JNA) is the oldest of these societies and will celebrate its 20th anniversary in 1987. It is composed only of narcoleptic and hypersomniac patients and is run autonomously by the patients themselves. It has contributed greatly to the facilitation of mutual friendship and self-help activities, to the exchange of information, to the assurance of continued availability of necessary medicines, and to the coverage of such medicines by the public health insurance system (Honda 1983c). The willing cooperation of the members of the JNA with the research activities is highly appreciated.

Narcolepsy Clinic in Tokyo

In Japan, I have seen and treated several hundred narcoleptic patients and a smaller number of patients with excessive daytime sleepiness without cataplexy. This clinical activity in collaboration with Dr. Yasuro Takahashi and others has continued without intermission for almost 30 years at the Department of Neuropsychiatry, University of Tokyo, every Tuesday afternoon since 1957. After April 1985, this narcolepsy clinic moved to Seiwa Hospital, Neuropsychiatric Research Institute, where more than 200 narcoleptic patients are now regularly treated.

My clinical experiences with narcoleptic patients in Japan are summarized from a personal point of view in Chap. 2.

Future Prospects

It will fill me with great happiness if this publication becomes a step forward in the elucidation of the etiology of narcolepsy. The true cause of narcolepsy is still surrounded by a thick mist of riddles. It is my sincere hope that the results of this publication will be utilized for the better lives of the patients who suffer from narcolepsy. It is further hoped that early diagnosis and early treatment will be more easily made by using the HLA-DR2 and DNA analysis, and that prevention of the development of narcolepsy will be achieved, especially in at-risk children of narcoleptic patients. I wish that this book will be useful not only for specialists in the field of sleep pathology, HLA, neuropsychiatry, and neurology, but also for a wider range of clinicians and researchers in other fields of medicine and related areas and will facilitate the understanding and improvement of the social life of narcoleptic patients.

References

Akimoto H, Honda Y, Takahashi Y (1960) Pharmacotherapy in nacrolepsy. Dis Nerv Syst 21: 704-706

Akimoto H, Nakakuki M, Honda Y, Takahashi Y, Toyoda J, Sasaki K, Machiyama T (1961) Clinical evaluation of the effect of central stimulants, MAO inhibitors, and imipramine in the treatment of affective disorders. Proceedings of the third world congress of psychiatry, Montreal, pp 958-963

American Narcolepsy Association (1984) Japanese studies shared. The Eye Opener, fall: 3

Andreas-Zietz A, Keller E, Scholz S, Albert ED, Roth B, Nevsimolova S, Sonka K et al. (1986) DR2 negative narcolepsy. Lancet ii: 686-685

Asaka A (1981) Genetic markers and neuropsychiatric disorders (in Japanese). Jpn J Clin Psychiatr [Rinsho Seishin Igaku] 10: 401-414

Asaka A, Park K, Honda Y, Kuroiwa Y, Tsuji S, Hamaguchi H, Akizuki M, Matsumoto H, Omoto K (1981) Studies on genetic markers in intractable diseases. In: Watanabe I (ed) Annual report of Research Committee on Host Factors of Intractable Diseases, for the year 1980 (in Japanese). Ministry of Health and Welfare, Tokyo, pp 123-131

Association of Sleep Disorders Centers and Association for the Psychophysiological Study of Sleep (1979) Diagnostic classification of sleep and arousal disorders. Sleep 2: 1-137

Baraitser M, Parkes JD (1978) Genetic study of narcoleptic syndrome. J Med Genet 15: 254-259

Billiard M, Seignalet J (1985) Extraordinary association between HLA-DR2 and narcolepsy. Lancet i: 226-227

Carskadon MA, Dement WC (1977) Sleep tendency: an objective measure of sleep loss. Sleep Res 6: 200

Coodley A (1948) Psychodynamic factors in narcolepsy and cataplexy. Psychiatr Q 22: 696-717

Curschmann H, Prange F (1925) Über Einschlafsucht (Narkolepsie und Verwandtes). Dtsch Rev Neurol 104: 242-245

Fischer F (1878) Epileptoide Schlafzustände. Arch Psychiatr Nervenkr 8: 200-203

Gelineau JBE (1880) De la narcolepsie. Gaz Hop (Paris) 53: 626-628, 54: 635-637

Gelineau JBE (1881) De la narcolepsie. Tessier et Tessier, Imprimerie de Surgeres, Paris

Gowers WR (1907) Borderland of epilepsy. Blakiston's, Philadelphia

Graves (1851) Observations on the nature and treatment of various diseases. Dubl J Med Sci 11: 1

Guilleminault C, Grumet C (1986) HLA-DR2 and narcolepsy: not all narcoleptic-cataplectic patients are DR2. Hum Immunol 17: 1-2

Henneberg R (1916) Über genuine Narkolepsie. Neurol Zentralbl 30: 282-290

Honda Y, Asaka A, Tanaka Y, Juji T (1983a) Discrimination of narcoleptic patients by using genetic markers and HLA. Sleep Res 12: 254
Honda Y, Asaka A, Tanimura M, Furusho T (1983b) A genetic study of narcolepsy and excessive daytime sleepiness in 308 families with a narcolepsy or hypersomnia proband. In: Guilleminault C, Lugaresi E (eds) Sleep/wake disorders; natural history, epidemiology and long-term evolution. Raven, New York, pp 187-199
Honda Y (1983c) Activities of the Japan Narcolepsy Association (in Japanese). Jpn J Clin Psychiatr [Rinsho-seishin Igaku] 12: 1525-1530
Honda Y, Doi Y, Juji T, Satake M (1984) Narcolepsy and HLA: positive DR2 as a prerequisite for the development of narcolepsy. Folia Psychiatr Neurol Jpn 38: 360
Honda Y, Doi Y, Juji T, Satake M (1985) Positive HLA-DR2 findings as a prerequisite for the development of narcolepsy. Folia Psychiatr Neurol Jpn 39: 203-204
Honda Y, Juji T, Matsuki K, Naohara T, Statake M, Inoko H, Someya T, Harada S, Doi Y (1986) HLA-DR2 and Dw2 in narcolepsy and in other disorders of excessive somnolence without cataplexy. Sleep 9: 133-142
Inoko H, Ando A, Tsuji K, Matsuki K, Juji T, Honda Y (1986) HLA-DQ beta chain DNA restriction fragments can differentiate between healthy and narcoleptic individuals with HLA-DR2. Immunogenetics 23: 126-128
Juji T, Maeda H, Honda Y, Asaka A, Akizuki M, Kashiwagi H, Horiuchi T (1981) An analysis of human B lymphocyte antigen system other than HLA-DR locus, and HLA typing for narcolepsy and SLE. In: Watanabe I (ed) Annual report of Research Committee on Host Factors of Intractable Diseases, for the year 1980 (in Japanese). Ministry of Health and Welfare, Tokyo, pp 141-147
Juji T, Satake M, Honda Y, Doi Y (1984) HLA antigens in Japanese patients with narcolepsy - all the patients were DR2 positive. Tissue Antigens 24: 316-319
Kessler S (1976) Genetic factors in narcolepsy. In: Guilleminault WC, Dement C, Passouant P (eds) Narcolepsy. Spectrum, New York, pp 285-302
Langdon N, Lock C, Welsh K, Vergoni D, Dorow R, Wachtel H, Palenschat D, Parkes JD (1986) Immune factors in narcolepsy. Sleep 9: 143-148
Langdon N, Welsh KI, Dam MV, Vaughan RW, Parkes D (1984) Genetic markers in narcolepsy. Lancet ii: 226-227
Lennox WC (1939) Thomas Willis on narcolepsy. Arch Gen Psychiatry (Chicago) 41: 348-351
Levin M (1933) The pathogenesis of narcolepsy with a consideration of sleep paralysis and localized sleep. J Neurol Psychopathol 14: 1-15
Loewenfeld L (1902) Über Narkolepsie. Münch Med Wochenschr 49: 1041-1045
Marcadet A, Gebuhrer L, Betuel H, Seignalet J, Freidel AC, Confabreux C, Billiard M, Dausset J, Cohen D (1985) DNA polymorphism related to HLA-DR2 Dw2 in patients with narcolepsy. Immunogenetics 22: 679-683
Missriegler A, Karpmann B (1941) On the psychogenesis of narcolepsy. Report of a case cured by psychoanalysis. J Nerv Ment Dis 93: 141-162
Mitler MM, van den Hoed J, Carskadon MA et al. (1979) REM sleep episodes during the multiple sleep test in narcoleptic patients. Electroencephalogr Clin Neurophysiol 46: 479-481
Moyer HN (1898) A case of paroxysmal sleep, sleep epilepsy or narcolepsy. Med Res 54: 750-751
Müller-Eckhardt G, Meier-Ewert KA, Schendel DJ, Reinecker FB, Müller-Eckhardt C (1986) HLA and narcolepsy in a German population. Tissue Antigens 28: 163-169
Nevsimalova-Bruhova S, Roth B (1972) Heredofamilial aspects of narcolepsy and hypersomnia. Arch Suisses Neurol Neurochir Psychiatr 110: 45-54
Nezu S, Noji K, Tsutsumi Y, Sato N, Iga T, Shirakura K, Inoko H, Sato K, Tsuji K, Hoshi A, Kaiho M (1985) An interim report about correlation of HLA antigens with narcolepsy. J Psychiatr Soc Kanagawa Prefecture 35: 81-86
Passouant P (1976) The history of narcolepsy. In: Guilleminault C, Dement WC, Passouant P (eds) Narcolepsy. Spectrum, New York, pp 3-14
Poirier G, Montplaisir J, Decary F, Momege D, Lebrun A (1986) HLA antigens in narcolepsy and idiopathic central nervous system hypersomnolence. Sleep 9: 153-158
Rechtschaffen A, Wolpert W, Dement W, Mitchell S, Fischer C (1963) Nocturnal sleep of narcoleptics. Electroencephalogr Clin Neurophysiol 15: 599-609
Redlich E (1915) Zur Narkolepsie-Frage. Monatsschr Psychiatr Neurol 37: 85-95

Redlich E (1931) Epilegomena zur Narkolepsie-Frage. Z Ges Neurol Psychiatr 136: 129-173
Richardson GS, Carskadon MA, Flagg W, van den Hoed J, Dement WC, Mitler MM (1978) Excessive daytime sleepiness in man: multiple sleep latency measurement in narcoleptic and control subjects. Electroencephalogr Clin Neurophysiol 45: 621-627
Roth B (1962) Narkolepsie und Hypersomnie vom Standpunkt der Physiologie des Schlafes. VEB Verlag Volk und Gesundheit, Berlin
Roth B (1980) Narcolepsy and hypersomnia. Karger, Basel
Schindler HB (1829) Die idiopathische, chronische Schlafsucht. Krahn, Kirschberg, p 8
Singer K (1917) Echte und Pseudo-narkolepsie. Z Gesamte Neurol Psychiatrie 36: 278-291
Spiegel LA, Oberndorf CP (1946) Narcolepsy as a psychogenic symptom. Psychosom Med 8: 28-35
Spiller WG (1926) Narcolepsy occasionally a postencephalitic syndrome. J Am Med Assoc 86: 673-674
Symonds CP (1926) Narcolepsy as a symptom of encephalitis lethargica. Lancet 2: 1214-1215
Takahashi Y, Jimbo M (1963) Polygraphic study of narcoleptic syndrome with special reference to hypnagogic hallucinations and cataplexy. Folia Psychiatr Neurol Jpn [Suppl] 7: 343-347
Thiele R, Bernhardt H (1933) Beiträge zur Kenntnis der Narkolepsie. Karger, Berlin, pp 1-187
Vogel G (1960) Studies in psychophysiology of dreams. III. The dream of narcolepsy. Arch Gen Psychiatry 3: 421-428
Wenderowic E (1924) Hypnolepsie ("Narcolepsia Gelineau") und ihre Behandlung. Arch Psychiatr Nervenkr 72: 459-472
Westphal C (1877) Eigentümliche mit Einschlafen verbundene Anfälle. Arch Psychiatr Nervenkr 7: 631-635
Wilder J (1935) Narkolepsie. In: Bumke O, Förster O (eds) Handbuch der Neurologie, vol 17. Springer, Berlin, pp 87-141
Wilson SAK (1928) The narcolepsies. Brain 51: 63-109
Yoss RE and Daly DD (1957) Criteria for the diagnosis of the narcoleptic syndrome. Proc Staff Meet Mayo Clinic 32: 320-328

Chapter 1

An Overview of the HLA System

T. Juji

Introduction

In this chapter, a review of the history, typing methods, genetic and molecular backgrounds, and clinical applications of HLA (human leukocyte antigen system A) will be presented.

In the 1930s, a series of experiments on skin transplantations between different strains of mice revealed the presence of several histocompatibility antigen systems, in which H-2 was confirmed to be the major system because it constituted the strongest barrier for allografts. A number of genes were subsequently identified in the same chromosomal region of the H-2 gene which play important roles in the immune responses. The gene complex in this region was designated as the major histocompatibility complex (MHC). Comparative studies in chemistry and genetics indicated that the HLA in man is homologous with the H-2 in mice and is genetically encoded in human MHC. Recent advances in cellular immunology and DNA technology have expedited an explosive increase in our knowledge of the genes and their products in human MHC.

History of the HLA System

Doan described antibodies reactive with human leukocytes as early as 1926. However, his findings were not extended any further. In 1952, Dausset and Nenna found a leukoagglutinin in the serum of a patient with agranulocytosis. Serological analyses of the leukoagglutinin and studies of monozygotic and dizygotic twins revealed the presence of an alloantigen system on human leukocytes. This was a milestone for the remarkable developments in research of the HLA system. Payne and Rolfs (1958) and van Rood et al. (1958) independently found potent leukoagglutinins in multiparous women's sera. These leukoagglutinins were rather monospecific when compared with those from multitransfused patients, because the mothers had been immunized by their children's leukocyte antigens derived from paternal haplotypes. Hereafter multiparous women's sera were screened for reagents for HLA typing.

The next major breakthrough was the development of a microlymphocytotoxicity test (LCT) by Terasaki and McClelland in 1964. Since leukoagglutination was disadvantageous because of its low reproducibility, LCT could provide a means to bypass the problems of reproducibility and to obtain clear results with an extremely small volume of reagents such as 1 μl. This technique has made it possible to obtain enormous amounts of data with limited volumes of antisera and blood samples.

Current findings of the HLA system and its genetic backgrounds are mainly obtained through a unique system of international collaborative studies, namely a series of International Histocompatibility Workshops. LCT and computerized data processing made these large-scale studies possible. At the 3rd and the 4th Workshops (1967 and 1970), the basic framework of HLA-A and HLA-B antigens was established. HLA-C antigens and HLA-D antigens were officially accepted at the 5th and 6th Workshops (1972 and 1975) respectively. HLA-D antigens were typed by mixed lymphocyte culture (MLC) using specific homozygous typing cells (HTCs). At the 7th Workshop (1977), another antigen system was first examined. These antigens were serologically identified on human B lymphocytes but not on T lymphocytes, and were named HLA-DR (D related) antigens because their specificities were closely related to HLA-D specificities. This antigen system was more clearly defined by an improved technique proposed at the 8th Workshop (1980). At the 9th Workshop (1984), two additional groups (HLA-DQ and HLA-DP) of HLA antigens were described.

HLA Antigen Specificities

The major histocompatibility complex has been identified in all vertebrates studied to date. It is a complex of closely linked genes and encodes self/nonself recognition systems which regulate various aspects of the immune responses. The human MHC is mapped on the short arm of the sixth chromosome. The HLA antigens are encoded by closely linked three loci (HLA-A, B, and C locus) and one region (HLA-D region). By the different characteristics of the antigen molecules and their biological functions, HLA antigens are divided into two categories, namely class I (HLA-A, B, C antigens) and class II (HLA-D, DR, DQ, DP antigens). As shown in Fig. 1, HLA loci are very tightly linked to each other. The region which codes for class II molecules is called the HLA-D region.

The HLA system is also the most polymorphic alloantigen system known in man. The number of officially recognized alleles in each locus increased after each of the International Histocompatibility Workshops. Table 1 lists the HLA specificities which have been identified and officially accepted by the World Health Organization (WHO) HLA Nomenclature Committee after the 10th International Histocompatibility Workshop in 1987.

There are two types of designation: those with a "w" and without a "w". The retention of a "w" in the designation indicates that the antigen specificities is not always clearly or easily defined. If an antigen is confirmed to be defined without difficulty and upgraded to full status, the "w" designation is omitted. For example, the following antigens lost the "w" in 1984: A23, A24, A30, A31, A32, B16, B21, B35, B38, B39, B44, B45, B49, and B51.

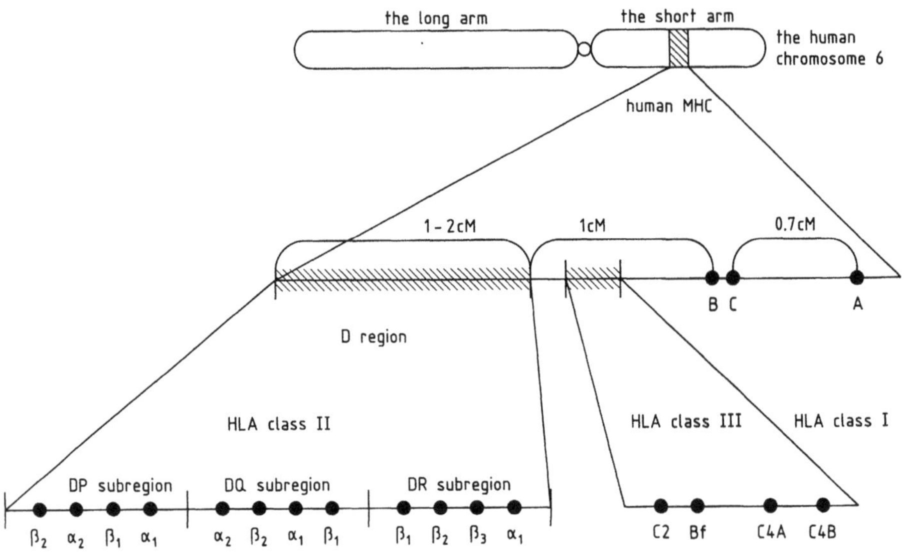

Fig. 1. Map of the HLA region on the short arm of the human chromosome 6

Table 1. A list of HLA specificities (1987)

HLA							
A	B		C	D	DR	DQ	DP
A1	B5	B51(5)	Cw1	Dw1	DR1	DQw1	DPw1
A2	B7	Bw52(5)	Cw2	Dw2	DR2	DQw2	DPw2
A3	B8	Bw53	Cw3	Dw3	DR3	DQw3	DPw3
A9	B12	Bw54(w22)	Cw4	Dw4	DR4	DQw4	DPw4
A10	B13	Bw55(w22)	Cw5	Dw5	DR5	DQw5(w1)	DPw5
A11	B14	Bw56(w22)	Cw6	Dw6	DRw6	DQw6(w1)	DPw6
Aw19	B15	Bw57(17)	Cw7	Dw7	DR7	DQw7(w3)	
A23(9)	B16	Bw58(17)	Cw8	Dw8	DRw8	DQw8(w3)	
A24(9)	B17	Bw59	Cw9(w3)	Dw9	DR9	DQw9(w3)	
A25(10)	B18	Bw60(40)	Cw10(w3)	Dw10	DRw10		
A26(10)	B21	Bw61(40)	Cw11	Dw11(w7)	DRw11(5)		
A28	Bw22	Bw62(15)		Dw12	DRw12(5)		
A29(w19)	B27	Bw63(15)		Dw13	DRw13(w6)		
A30(w19)	B35	Bw64(14)		Dw14	DRw14(w6)		
A31(w19)	B37	Bw65(14)		Dw15	DRw15(2)		
A32(w19)	B38(16)	Bw67		Dw16	DRw16(2)		
Aw33(w19)	B39(16)	Bw70		Dw17(w7)	DRw17(3)		
Aw34(10)	B40	Bw71(w70)		Dw18(w6)	DRw18(3)		
Aw36	Bw41	Bw72(w70)		Dw19(w6)	DRw52		
Aw43	Bw42	Bw73		Dw20	DRw53		
Aw66(10)	B44(12)	Bw75(15)		Dw21			
Aw68(28)	B45(12)	Bw76(15)		Dw22			
Aw69(28)	Bw46	Bw77(15)		Dw23			
Aw74(w19)	Bw47	Bw4		Dw24			
	Bw48	Bw6		Dw25			
	B49(21)			Dw26			
	Bw50(21)						

Table 2. Relationship between the original broad specificities and their split antigens

Original broad specificities	Splits
A9	A23, A24
A10	A25, A26, Aw34, Aw66
Aw19	A29, A30, A31, A32, Aw33, Aw74
A28	Aw68, Aw69
B5	B51, Bw52
B12	B44, B45
B14	Bw64, Bw65
B15	Bw62, Bw63, Bw75, Bw76, Bw77
B16	B38, B39
B17	Bw57, Bw58
B21	B49, Bw50
Bw22	Bw54, Bw55, Bw56
B40	Bw60, Bw61
Bw70	Bw71, Bw72
Cw3	Cw9, Cw10
Dw6	Dw18, Dw19
Dw7	Dw11, Dw17
DR2	DRw15, DRw16
DR3	DRw17, DRw18
DR5	DRw11, DRw12
DRw6	DRw13, DRw14
DQw1	DQw5, DQw6
DQw3	DQw7, DQw8, DQw9

Table 3. Inclusion of HLA-B specificities into Bw4 and Bw6

Bw4:	B5, B13, B17, B27, B37, B38(16), B44(12), Bw47, B49(21), B51(5), Bw52(5), Bw53, Bw57(17), Bw58(17), Bw59, Bw63(15), Bw77(15)
Bw6:	B7, B8, B14, B18, Bw22, B35, B39(16), B40, Bw41, Bw42, B45(12), Bw46, Bw48, Bw50(21), Bw54(w22), Bw55(w22), Bw56(w22), Bw60(40), Bw61(40), Bw62(15), Bw64(14), Bw65(14), Bw67, Bw70, Bw71(w70), Bw72(w70), Bw73, Bw75(15), Bw76(15)

The designations in parentheses in Table 1 indicate original broad specificities of each split antigen. A9 in parentheses next to A23 and A24 is the original broad specificity of these splits. In other words, HLA-A9 is subdivided into two split specificities, A23 and A24. The relationships between the original broad specificities and splits are listed in Table 2.

Bw4 and Bw6 are the supertypic antigens of the mutually exclusive diallelic genes. Every antigen of HLA-B locus shows the specific association with either Bw4 and Bw6. As shown in Table 3, individuals with HLA-B5, for example, are always HLA-Bw4 positive, and ones with HLA-B7 are always HLA-Bw6 positive.

In HLA-DR specificities, two supertypic antigens, DRw52 and DRw53, are generally accepted to be associated with the following specificities of HLA-DR.

DRw52: DR3, DR5, DRw6, DRw8, DRw11, DRw12, DRw13, DRw14, DRw17, DRw18
DRw53: DR4, DR7, DRw9

Typing Methods

Serological Typing for HLA Class I Antigens

The HLA class I antigens (HLA-A, B, C antigens) are typed by the lymphocytotoxicity test (LCT). Lymphocytes are isolated by centrifugation of heparinized blood over Ficoll-Hypaque solution. Density and viscosity of the solution are optimally adjusted for lymphocyte separation. The isolated lymphocytes are suspended in McCoy's 5a medium, and the cell count is adjusted to 2×10^6/ml. Typing trays are obtained commercially or prepared in-house using selected optimal antisera. One microliter of an antiserum is dotted into each well of the trays and the prepared typing trays are stored in a deep freezer. The trays are thawed several minutes before use. The lymphocyte suspension prepared as above is mixed thoroughly and 1 μl of the suspension is added to each well. After the incubation for 30 min at room temperature, 5 μl of rabbit complement is added to each well. The incubation of this step is 60 min at room temperature. At the end of the incubation, 2 μl aqueous 5% eosin Y solution is added. Five minutes later, the lymphocytes are fixed with 5 μl neutralized formalin. A coverslide is placed over the wells to flatten the top of the droplets. The typing results are read under inverted phase-contrast microscope by examining lymphocyte viability in each well in which a specific antiserum was placed. Dead lymphocytes are stained red while living cells are left unstained.

Serological Typing for HLA Class II Antigens

Among the HLA class II antigens, the HLA-DR and DQ antigens are typed by the modified cytotoxicity test with purified B lymphocytes. The Ficoll-Hypaque fractionated mononuclear cells are further separated into monocytes, B lymphocytes, and T lymphocytes. First, monocytes were removed by adhering them to the surfaces of the glass or plastic petri dishes. The remaining cells are incubated in a nylon wool column for 30 min at 37 °C. The nonadherent cells to nylon wool (T and null lymphocytes) are collected by allowing the McCoy's medium to pass through the column. After washing the column thoroughly, the nylon-adherent cells (B lymphocytes) are eluted by squeezing the column. The resulting B lymphocyte-rich suspension is then mixed with anti-DR and anti-DQ antisera.

The major source of these anti-DR and anti-DQ sera is multiparous women. Since most of the multiparous sera contain alloantibodies to HLA class I antigens and naturally occurring antibodies to human B lymphocytes, the alloantisera should be absorbed with equal volumes of pooled packed platelets prior to use. Mouse monoclonal antibodies are also extremely valuable reagents for B cell typing.

Antisera and B lymphocyte mixtures are incubated for 1 h at 37 °C. After adding rabbit complement, the mixture is further incubated for 2 h at 22 °C. Because rabbit serum sometimes contains naturally occurring antibodies to human B lymphocytes, the rabbit complement should be screened before use in terms of complement activity and the absence of nonspecific toxicity to human B lymphocytes.

Typing Methods for HLA-D Antigens: Mixed Lymphocyte Culture

Mixed lymphocyte culture (MLC) is a biological technique for detecting differences of cell surface antigens or antigen complexes encoded by a gene, or genes in the HLA-D region. When a population of immunogenetically competent cells (responders) from one individual is cultured with a population of irradiated mononuclear cells (stimulators) from a second individual whose HLA-D region antigens are not identical to those of the responder individual, the responder lymphocytes show blastogenic transformation and cellular proliferation. In the presence of tritiated thymidine at the end stage of the culture, the degree of blastogenic transformation can be measured by the uptake of this radioactive DNA precursor into the lymphocytes. If the culture is performed between two cell populations which are HLA-D identical, only marginal incorporation of thymidine is observed. HLA-D typing is based on this principle of MLC. If the homozygous cells of a certain HLA-D antigen are available and are used as stimulating cells in MLC after irradiation, responder cells are divided into two groups, namely blastogenic transformed and nontransformed. Individuals whose cells are not transformed are interpreted as having the same HLA-D antigen as the homozygous stimulating cells. These mononuclear cells from HLA-D homozygotes are called homozygous typing cells (HTCs). Now many HTCs have been collected and tested. Twenty-six HLA-D specificities were officially accepted by WHO after the 10th International Histocompatibility Workshop.

Typing Method for HLA-DP Antigens: Primed Lymphocyte Test

After Hayry and Anderson (1974) reported that memory T cells are generated in one-way MLC, the primed lymphocyte test (PLT) was introduced as a faster method for detection of HLA class II antigens by Sheehy et al. in 1975. If the responder lymphocytes in one-way MLC are maintained in culture for 10–14 days, they are still viable yet cease to proliferate. However, these "primed" responder lymphocytes have been "educated" to undergo vary rapid proliferation if exposed again to the same antigens present on the original stimulating cells. Shortly after the PLT system was first described, it was suggested that this technique can define new gene products in the HLA-D region in addition to HLA-D antigens. The studies of families with recombinant members demonstrated that the gene coding for the new antigen system are located between HLA-D and GLO loci (Mawas et al. 1978). Shaw et al. (1980) further defined five alleles in this segregant series using primed lymphocytes generated by MLC between unrelated individuals identical for HLA class I and II specificities. This secondary B-cell antigen system was called SB. In 1983, Watson et al. produced a murine monoclonal antibody, B7/21, specific for the SB antigen molecules. At the 9th International Histocompatibility Workshop, the SB antigens were given official designations from HLA-DPw1 through HLA-DPw6. Recently, Johnson et al. (1986) reported that it was possible to type HLA-DP gene products with alloantisera serologically.

Genetic Aspects of the HLA System

One of the important aspects in HLA genetics is haplotype. HLA antigens are inherited as simple Mendelian codominant traits. The combination of alleles at the segment of a single HLA chromosome is inherited from each parent. This is called haplotype. Each person has two haplotypes, one from the father and the other from the mother. In a typical two-generation family, two paternal and two maternal haplotypes can be identified from the phenotypes of the family members. In the HLA system, each parent transmits one of their haplotypes to each offspring. However, family studies indicate that exceptions, known as recombinations, occur less than 1% in transmission. These recombinations made it possible to map HLA loci in sequential order.

Another important aspect of HLA genetics is called linkage disequilibrium. It is sometimes observed that a certain allele in a locus associates nonrandomly with a specific allele in a different locus. For example, the frequency of A1-B8 haplotypes in the Caucasian population is much higher than the expected frequency from the gene frequencies of A1 and B8. The antigen combinations, which show strong linkage disequilibria, are often characteristic of a particular ethnic group. The linkage disequilibria in HLA antigens are of strong interest to anthropologists.

There have been so many reports on the associations between HLA and diseases. If the association is found between an HLA allele and a disease in a certain population, it may be due to a linkage disequilibrium between the HLA gene and a susceptibility or resistance gene to that disease in the ethnic group.

HLA Antigen Molecules

The gene products of the HLA system are glycoproteins and are believed to "float" or "swim" on the plasma membrane. HLA class I antigens are present on all the nucleated cells and platelets. As shown in Fig. 2, an HLA class I molecule is composed of noncovalently associated heavy (44 kd) and light (11 kd) chains. The light chain was found to be identical to $\beta 2$ microglobulin present in normal human serum. A $\beta 2$ microglobulin can reversibly associate and dissociate with the heavy chains of HLA class I molecules on cell surfaces. This is the case even be-

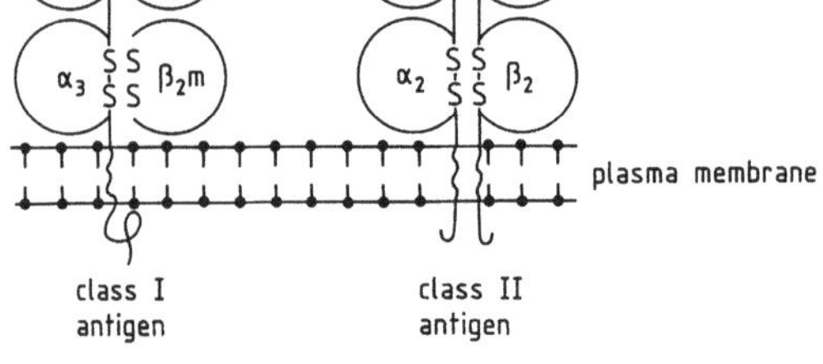

Fig. 2. Models of HLA antigen molecules. The class I and class II HLA antigens contain two immunoglobulin-like domains adjacent to the plasma membrane α_1: α_1 domain, α_2: α_2 domain, α_3: α_3 domain, β_1: β_1 domain, β_2: β_2 domain, β_2m: β_2 microglobulin

tween chains of different species. The heavy chain of the class I antigens consists of $\alpha 1$, $\alpha 2$, $\alpha 3$ domains, hydrophobic transmembrane segment, and a cytoplasmic tail. The $\alpha 2$, $\alpha 3$ domains, and $\beta 2$ microglobulin each contain an intradomain disulfide bond. The alloantigenic determinant is located on $\alpha 1$ and $\alpha 2$ domains.

The tissue distribution of class II antigens is limited to certain cell types, such as B lymphocytes, monocytes, macrophages, dendritic cells, and activated T lymphocytes. An HLA class II antigen is heterodimetric cell surface glycoproteins consisting of an α chain (33-34 kd) and a β chain (28-29 kd). These two chains are noncovalently associated and extend through the plasma membrane of the cells. The $\beta 1$, $\beta 2$, and $\alpha 2$ domains have an intradomain disulfide bond whereas the NH_2-terminal $\alpha 1$ domain has not. Comparison of the nucleotide sequences of the genes and of the deduced amino acid sequences revealed that three or four hypervariable regions spread across the NH_2-terminal domains ($\beta 1$ or $\alpha 1$). In addition to $\beta 2$ microglobulin, the membrane proximal domains of class II α and β chains and of class I heavy chain show strong homology in amino acid sequences to immunoglobulin constant region domains. This evidence suggests the existence of a common ancestor gene for genes responsible for the immune defense mechanisms.

The two-dimensional gel electrophoreses technique was introduced as an important tool for the analysis of the different HLA class II alloantigen molecules which reacted with monoclonal antibodies along with human alloantisera. The labeled molecules with radioisotopes were precipitated with a mouse monoclonal antibody or an alloantiserum, and then they were mapped by two-dimensional nonequilibrium pH/SDS-polyacrylamide gel electrophoresis. A group of laboratories performed a cooperative study as a part of the 9th Histocompatibility Workshop (1984) and compared the patterns of spots revealed by the different combinations of antibodies and class II molecules. It was confirmed that anti-DR antibodies precipitated one α and two β chains, while anti-DQ and anti-DP antibodies precipitated one α and one β chains. In total, three α chains and four β chains, namely DRα, DQα, DPα, DRβ1, DRβ2, DQβ, and DPβ, were identified. DRβ2 is generally believed to correspond with β chains of DRw52 and DRw53.

HLA Specificities and Isoelectric Points of Antigen Molecules

Yang et al. (1984) systematically analyzed the characteristic banding pattern for each HLA class I antigen by means of one-dimensional isoelectric focusing (1D-IEF). Radiolabeled membrane proteins were extracted, and HLA class I antigen molecules were specifically immunoprecipitated with three mouse monoclonal antibodies (MoAbs). MoAb4E recognized a common antigen determinant present on all the HLA-B locus antigens; MoAb4B identified a determinant shared by HLA-A2 and A28, and MoAbw6/32 recognized a common determinant on all HLA class I antigens. The isolated antigens were desialated by neuraminidase treatment. This treatment reduced the number of isoprotein bands. On a 1D-IEF gel, a single invariant $\beta 2$ microglobulin and variant heterogeneous heavy chain bands were revealed. The heavy chains of the HLA-A antigens had, in general, slightly

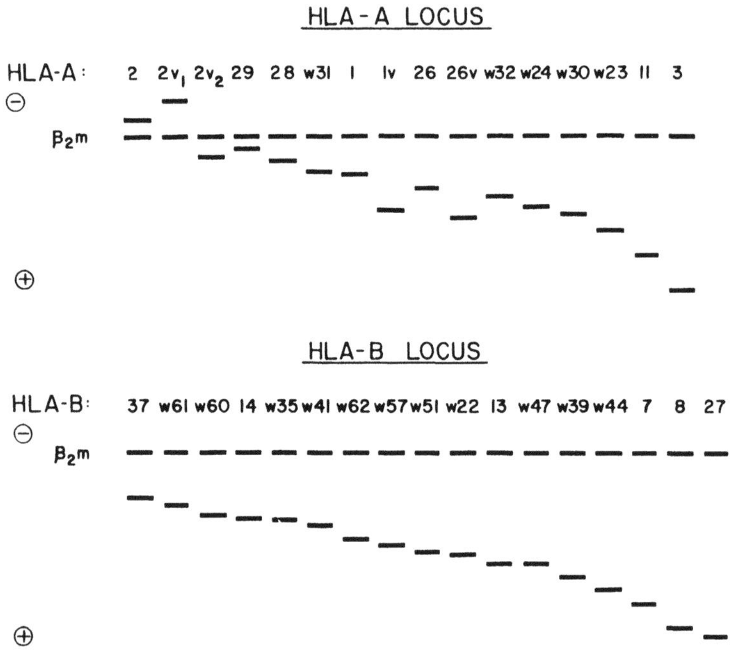

Fig. 3. Schematic representation of IEF banding patterns for desialated HLA-A and HLA-B antigens (Yang et al. 1984)

higher isoelectric points (pI) than those of the HLA-B antigens, while there were no locus specific banding patterns. Unfortunately HLA-C antigens could not be detected in their system. A schematic representation of the banding patterns for 12 HLA-A locus antigens and 17 HLA-B locus antigens is shown in Fig. 3. In addition to the identification of the characteristic pIs for each HLA class I allotype, IEF banding patterns have revealed structural differences between serologically indistinguishable subtypes of HLA-A2, A1, and A26. Similar analysis have been performed for HLA class II antigens.

Restriction Fragment Length Polymorphism (RFLP)

When cDNA clones of class I genes became available in 1980, (Ploegle et al. 1980) the Southern blot technique (Southern 1975) made it possible to analyze the HLA class I region at the DNA level (Sood et al. 1981). Genomic DNAs were extracted from established cell lines and peripheral blood leukocytes. The extracted DNAs were digested with various restriction endonucleases. These restriction fragments were separated in agarose gel by electrophoresis and transferred onto hybridization membranes. The transferred DNA fragments were hybridized with radioisotope-labeled cDNA probes specific for HLA genes. The characteristic patterns of restriction fragments were revealed according to the combination of leukocytes used and endonucleases. If there are differences in the distribution of sites recognized by an endonuclease between genes of two individuals, the patterns of fragments will be different. Each fragment has been analyzed for association with specific phenotypes of HLA antigens. Because whole DNA length of a class I gene is within 4 kb, two bands may represent one gene. However, a surprisingly large number of hybridized bands were identified by a class I probe. Dausset and Cohen (1984) analyzed the DNAs of the parents and children of 23 families using 5 different enzymes and class I and class II probes. They showed that by a class I probe 88 different fragments were polymorphic and always segregated with the HLA haplotypes. Of these polymorphisms, 63% correlated with the HLA-A locus alleles and only 13% and 5% with HLA-B and C alleles respectively. Also detected were 52 allogenotopes (fragments) using a DQβ probe and 6 different restriction enzymes. Most of these allogenotopes showed correlations with specificities of class II antigens. A large amount of RFLP data will be accumulated and will be discussed in the 10th International Histocompatibility Workshop.

Clinical Application of HLA

Transplantation

It has been recognized that the clinical outcome of a kidney transplantation from an HLA identical sibling is highly superior to that from a sibling with completely different HLA haplotypes. However, in cases of kidney transplantations from cadavers, the superiority of HLA compatibility diminishes. The postulation is as follows: there are so many other factors affecting the clinical outcome of a cadaveric transplantation such as the length of ischemic time, the level of pretransplant antibodies, the original disease of patient, the ages of patient and donor, the technical level of the transplantation center, and the number of pretransplant transfusions. The parallel increase in graft survival rates has been observed with the gradual widespread adoption of pretransplantation transfusions since 1975. In addition, a new immunosuppressive drug, ciclosporin-A, has proven to be a potent agent in improving graft survival rates.

Similar successful application of HLA has been reported in bone marrow transplantation. More than 70% of leukemic patients can be completely cured after bone marrow transplantation from an HLA identical sibling. Interestingly, while ABO incompatibility can be ignored unlike other organ transplantations, HLA identity appears to be extremely important, and no beneficial effect of pretransplant transfusions has been reported for bone marrow transplantations.

Platelet Transfusion

After repeated transfusions of random-donor platelets, many patients become refractory to further random-donor platelet transfusions. A lack of platelet increment with high fever after a platelet transfusion indicates refractoriness. In a refractory patient, transfused platelets are destroyed by alloantibodies, especially by those to HLA antigens on platelet surfaces, although antibodies to platelet-specific alloantigens may also be involved. Platelets obtained from an HLA compatible donor can be beneficial in about 90% of refractory patients. To ensure HLA compatible platelet donors, for such patients, a large number of HLA-typed donors who could donate their platelets by plateletapheresis willingly at any time on request must be registered in regional blood centers. Because of the extreme polymorphism of alleles in the HLA system, a pool of more than several thousand donors is necessary to provide sufficient HLA compatible donors to meet the needs of most patients.

HLA and Diseases

Before the introduction of HLA typing, many studies had been conducted to investigate possible associations between diseases and genetic markers other than HLA, such as blood groups, enzymes, and serum proteins. For example, Mourant et al. (1977) showed that a blood type A person is 1.22 times more likely to develop stomach cancer than those who are not type A by analysis of the data on 53155 patients with stomach cancer. In general, the relative risks in these studies were less than 2.

Since the HLA system has been introduced in the study of disease association, many diseases in which relative risk is greater than 2 have been reported. In 1973, an exciting discovery was made by two independent groups of investigators, Schlosstein et al. and Brewerton et al. They found an extremely strong association of HLA-B27 with ankylosing spondylitis. The relative risk was as great as 69. Their data suggested that HLA typing can be utilized as an important tool for the diagnosis of diseases.

Over the past 20 years, many diseases have been reported in more than 4000 papers with regard to HLA associations. Comprehensive reviews of the reported papers on HLA and diseases have been published by Dausset and Svejgaard (1977), Braun (1979), Ryder et al. (1977), and Tiwari and Terasaki (1985). These have served as important references in the field.

A statistically significant association between HLA and disease provides us with important information for the better understanding of the etiology and the pathogenetic pathway of the disease in question. It is not easy, however, to explain the underlying mechanisms in these empirically observed associations. A hypothesis, which enjoys a fair acceptance, proposes that HLA antigen itself is not directly involved in the development of a disease, but serves just as a genetic marker for a susceptibility gene of the disease which is in strong linkage disequilibrium with the HLA allele. According to an opposing hypothesis, an HLA antigen is directly involved in the pathogenesis and expresses itself as a receptor for pathogenic organisms, as a cross-reactive antigen with an organism, as a competitor to hormone receptors, and so on. The specific cross-reactivity between certain enteric bacteria and the cells of HLA-B27 positive patients with ankylosing spondylitis was first reported by Seager et al. (1979). Since then, these Australian investigators have continued their research by confirming that certain enteric bacteria were present in the bowel flora of patients with ankylosing spondylitis, but not in normal individuals. Geczy et al. (1980) demonstrated that rabbit antisera raised to the outer membrane component of these bacteria lyzed lymphocytes of HLA-B27 positive patients, but not lymphocytes of HLA-B27 positive normal individuals by a complement-dependent ^{51}Cr release assay. Upfold et al. (1986) revealed that lymphocytes of B27 positive normal individuals can be lyzed by antisera after incubation with the membrane component in question, namely the modifying factor, and confirmed it to be a polypeptide with a molecular weight of 30000 and an isoelectric point of 5.4–5.5. It has been suggested by van Rood (1986) that the class I antigens transfer, as their primary function, extracellular materials from the cell membrane to the cytoplasm where they can be degraded in the lysosomes. They explain that HLA-B27 molecules bind the modifying factor, but are ineffective in transporting it from the cell membrane to the cytoplasm. In failing to do so, the B27-modifying factor complex activates cytotoxic T cells. As a consequence the activated T cells attack the sacroiliac joints.

HLA for Paternity Testing

Because the HLA system is highly polymorphic and the seven loci link closely with each other, the parental haplotypes can be exactly specified in paternity testing. HLA typing alone can exclude about 90% of falsely accused males. With the addition of several red cell typings, the exclusion rate rises to more than 95%. Even if males share a haplotype with a child, the likelihood of their being the father can be calculated on frequencies of the HLA haplotypes in the population.

HLA System and Narcolepsy

It is generally accepted that the regulation of immune responses is mediated by the MHC. When macrophages present antigens to T lymphocytes, the T lymphocytes recognize the foreign antigen in the context of MHC class II antigens. In the effector phase of the immune responses, the cytotoxic T lymphocytes kill the target cells in the context of MHC class I antigens. Thus, the associations between diseases and HLA are usually explained by these regulatory functions of MHC for immune responses.

But strong associations with HLA were also demonstrated in some diseases in which the mechanisms of development are unrelated with immune responses. The adrenal 21-hydroxylase deficiency is associated with a deficient complement gene in the class III HLA system.

Narcolepsy is an important addition in this direction. There has been no actual evidence indicating the involvement of immunological mechanisms in narcolepsy. Our present research indicates that the HLA-DR2, Dw2, DQw1, 2.4-kb fragment of *Eco*R1-digested DQ beta DNA, and the 6.0-kb fragment of *Taq*-1-digested DQ alpha DNA are positive in 100% of narcoleptic patients. Since all of the markers in the HLA-DR and DQ alleles are positive in 100% of the patients, it is not possible to speculate an exact location of the susceptibility gene to narcolepsy.

Future discoveries of narcoleptic patients without any one of these markers will provide us a chance to map the susceptibility gene to narcolepsy.

This possibility opens a new horizon in the research of HLA in terms of additional clinical significance of the HLA system in the etiology of diseases that are unrelated to immune responses. On the other hand, HLA provides a very useful biological marker in the research of narcolepsy. Further cooperation and exchange of information between HLA specialists and investigators of sleep disorders are necessary for advances in both fields of medical science.

Acknowledgment. This paper was supported by Grant-In-Aid for Co-Operative Research from the Japanese Ministry of Education, Science, and Culture.

References

Braun WE (1979) HLA and disease: a comprehensive review. CRC, Boca Raton

Brewerton DA, Caffrey M, Hart FD, James DCO, Nicholls A, Sturrock RD (1973) Ankylosing spondylitis and HLA-A27. Lancet i: 904-907

Dausset J, Cohen D (1984) HLA at the gene level. In: Albert ED, Baur MP, Mayr WR (eds) Histocompatibility testing 1984. Springer, Berlin Heidelberg New York Tokyo, pp 22-28

Dausset J, Nenna A (1952) Présence d'une leuco-agglutinine dans le sérum d'un cas d'aggranulocytose chronique. C R Soc Biol 146: 1539-1541

Dausset J, Svejgaard A (eds) (1977) HLA and disease. Munksgaard, Copenhagen

Doan CA (1926) The recognition of biologic differentiation in the white blood cells, with especial reference to blood transfusion. JAMA 86: 1593-1597

Geczy AF, Alexander K, Bashir HV, Edmonds JP (1980) A factor(s) in *Klebsiella* culture filtrates specifically modifies an HLA-B27 associated cell-surface component. Nature 283: 782

Hayry P, Anderson L (1974) Generation of T memory cells in one-way mixed lymphocyte culture. II. Anamnestic responses of "secondary" lymphocytes. Scand J Immunol 3: 823-826

Johnson AH, Thorsby E, Nakatsuji T, Fang T, Moen T, Hartzyman RJ (1986) Recognition of an HLA-DPw1 specific alloantiserum raised by planned immunization. Hum Immunol 17: 21-29

Mawas C, Charmot D, Sivy M, Mercier P, North ML, Hauptmann G (1978) A weak human MLR locus mapping at the right of a crossing over between HLA-D, Bf and GLO. J Imunogenet 5: 583-588

Mourant AE, Kopec AC, Domaniewska-Sobczak K (1977) Blood groups and diseases. Oxford University Press, Oxford

Payne R, Rolfs MR (1958) Fetomaternal leukocyte in compatibility. J Clin Invest 37: 1756-1763

Ploegh HL, Orr HT, Strominger JL (1980) Molecular cloning of a human histocompatibility antigen cDNA fragment. Proc Natl Acad Sci USA 77: 6081-6085

Ryder L, Anderson E, Svejgaard A (eds) (1977) HLA and disease registry: third report. Munksgaard, Copenhagen

Schlosstein L, Terasaki PI, Bluestone R, Pearson G (1973) High association of an HL-A antigen, w27 with ankylosing spondylitis. New Engl J Med 288: 704-706

Seager K, Bashir HV, Geczy AF, Edmonds JP, de Vere-Tyndall A (1979) Evidence for a specific B27 associated cell surface marker on lymphocytes of patients with ankylosing spondylitis. Nature 277: 68

Shaw S, Johnson AH, Shearer GM (1980) Evidence for a new segregant series of B cell antigens that are encoded in the HLA-D region and that stimulate secondary allogeneic proliferative and cytotoxic responses. J Exp Med 152: 565-580

Sheehy MJ, Sondel PH, Bach ML, Bach FH (1975) HL-A LD (lymphocyte defined) typing: a rapid assay with primed lymphocytes. Science 188: 1308-1310

Sood AK, Pereira D, Weissman SM (1981) Isolation and partial nucleotide sequence of a cDNA clone for human histocompatibility antigen HLA-B by use of an oligo-deoxynucleotide primer. Proc Natl Acad Sci USA 78: 616-620

Southern EM (1975) Detection of specific sequences among DNA fragments separated by gel electrophoresis. J Mol Biol 98: 503-517

Terasaki PI, McClelland JD (1964) Micro-droplet assay of human serum cytotoxins. Nature 204: 998-1000

Tiwari JL, Terasaki PI (1985) HLA and disease associations. Springer, New York Berlin Heidelberg Tokyo

Upfold LI, Sullivan JS, Geczy AF (1986) Biochemical studies on a factor isolated from *Klebsiella* K43-B TS1 that cross-reacts with cells from HLA-B27 positive patients with ankylosing spondylitis. Hum Immunol 17: 224-238

Van Rood JJ (1986) HLA antigens as carrier molecules. Hum Immunol 17: 246-249

Van Rood JJ, Eernisse JG, Van Leeuwen A (1958) Leukocyte antibodies in sera from pregnant women. Nature 181: 1735-1736

Watson AJ, DeMars R, Trowbridge IS, Bach F (1983) Detection of a novel human class II HLA antigen. Nature 304: 358-361

Yang SY, Morishima Y, Colliens NH, Alton T, Pollack MS, Yunic EJ, Dupont B (1984) Comparison of one dimensional IEF patterns for serologically detectable HLA-A and B allotypes. Immunogenetics 19: 217-231

Chapter 2

Clinical Features of Narcolepsy: Japanese Experiences

Y. HONDA

In this chapter, narcolepsy is discussed from the clinical point of view. Several areas of recent concern in research are described based on my personal experiences with Japanese narcoleptic patients. There is a large Japanese literature on narcolepsy which has not been known to the researchers of other countries because of the language barrier. Some of these studies are cited and explained briefly. First, the symptomatology associated with narcolepsy is discussed. This leads to the definition of the term "narcolepsy" and issues in the diagnostic criteria for narcolepsy and in differential diagnosis. Next, the pathophysiology of narcolepsy, neuroendocrine, neuropharmacological, and epidemiological findings are described, followed by recommendations of practical treatment plans and an introduction of the activities of the Japan Narcolepsy Association.

Symptomatology of Narcolepsy

This section describes characteristic symptoms of narcolepsy. Data are taken from a series of narcoleptic patients who presented for treatment at the Sleep Disorders Clinic of the Tokyo University Hospital and at Seiwa Hospital during the years 1955-1986.

Recurrent Daytime Naps and/or Lapses into Sleep over Many Years

The most basic symptom of narcolepsy is recurrent daytime naps and/or lapses into sleep occurring almost daily over a period of many years. The daytime naps are characterized by repeated episodes of sleep of rather short duration due to overwhelming sleepiness. This sleepiness can be overcome by a patient if, with much effort and attention, he makes a strong effort to keep awake, or if he walks around or engages in physical exercise. Eventually, however, it is impossible to combat the recurrent somnolence which occurs daily (Fig. 1).

Often the patient grows so accustomed to such daytime sleepiness that he becomes unaware of it, and even denies that he feels sleepy. Frequently, taking naps in the daytime becomes a part of his daily life routine. The duration of daytime sleep episodes is usually less than 30 min and rarely exceeds 1 h (Fig. 2). The patient can be awakened easily by external stimuli. The patient typically sleeps for

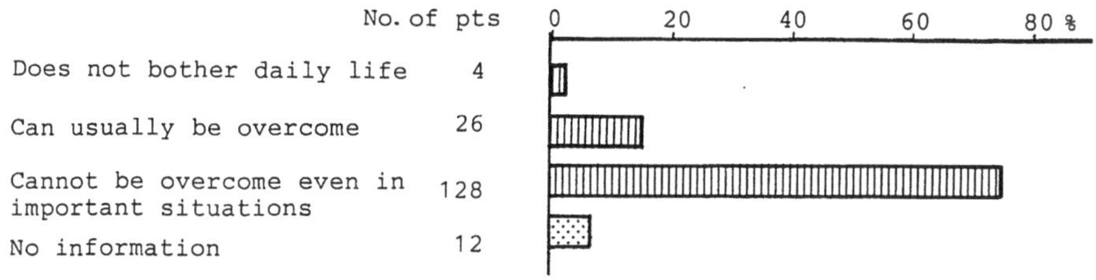

Fig. 1. Intensity of daytime somnolence ($n = 170$)

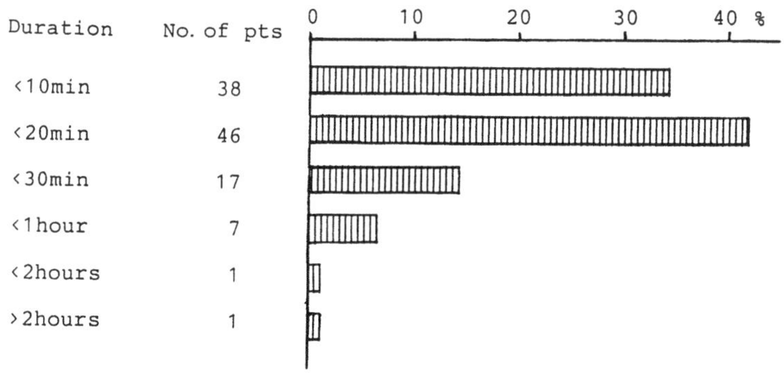

Fig. 2. Duration of usual daytime naps as reported by the patients ($n = 110$)

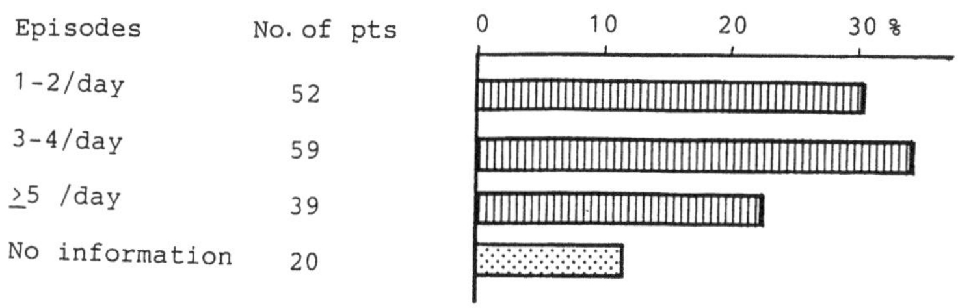

Fig. 3. Frequency of daytime sleep episodes ($n = 170$)

10–20 min and wakes up feeling refreshed, but within the next 2–3 h, he begins to feel sleepy again, and the pattern repeats itself. The frequency of sleep episodes in the daytime varies according to the severity of the disorder, from a few times in mild cases to several times in severe cases (Fig. 3). The narcoleptic patient falls asleep easily in circumstances in which ordinary people tend to feel sleepy, such as when seated on a bus, attending a monotonous meeting which requires no active participation, or listening to a boring lecture.

In addition, the narcoleptic patient has sleep attacks which are both sudden in onset and irresistible, and occur in circumstances where ordinary people would never sleep. For example, he may experience such attacks during an examination, at interactive business talks, while walking, while standing on guard, or at an important meeting attended by one's superiors or other very important people. The duration of a sleep attack is rather short, and usually only several minutes.

Sleep attacks have long been considered as the major symptom of narcolepsy. This is sometimes misleading, however, because it gives the impression that sleep episodes of narcolepsy are mainly composed of sudden, irresistible attacks of sleep resembling, in some respects, attacks of epilepsy. Although the sleep attack is an important and frequent symptom of narcolepsy, it is not the only manifestation of daytime sleep episodes. The sleep attacks may disappear after many years, but frequent naps and lapses into sleep, which the patient can resist with much effort, persist for a long period. Discrimination between sleep attacks and usual naps is often difficult. It has been suggested that, in contrast to naps, typical sleep attacks may be composed of daytime REM sleep (Suzuki 1966).

Cataplexy

Cataplexy is another fundamental symptom of narcolepsy, characterized by a sudden loss of bilateral skeletal muscle tone triggered by a strong wave of emotion. The duration of cataplexy is short, ranging from a few moments to several minutes, and recovery is immediate (Fig. 4; Roth 1962).

The grade of the loss of muscle tone at cataplexy also varies (Fig. 5). It is experienced vividly by the patient as a sensation of a sudden sinking of the body, or as buckling of the knees or difficulty of speech. Cataplexy may not be noticed by

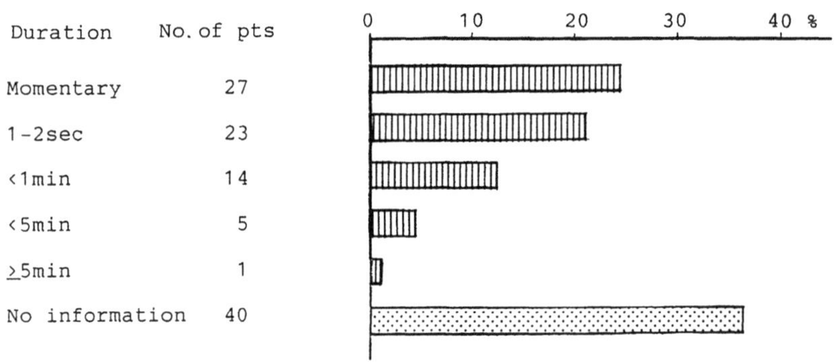

Fig. 4. Duration of cataplectic attacks as reported by the patients ($n=110$)

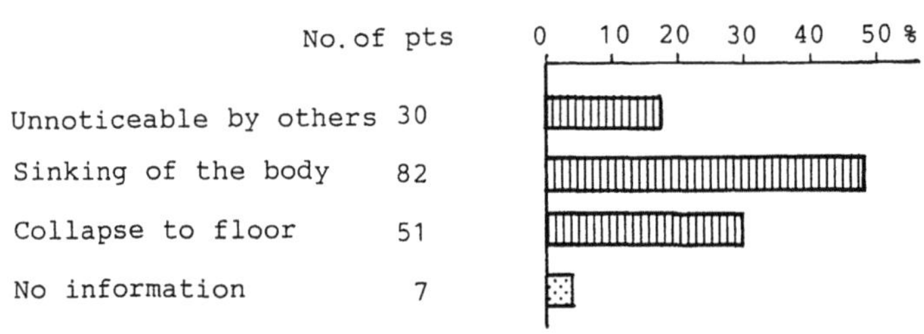

Fig. 5. Grade of loss of muscle tone at cataplexy ($n=170$)

others, or may be noticed as sudden sagging of the body or the face. Sometimes the patient may collapse to the floor. Although cataplexy itself is essentially not sleep, it is sometimes more easily provoked when a patient is sleepy, and is occasionally followed by a state of sleep, which is often composed of REM sleep.

Sometimes the emotional reactions of the patient in response to cataplexy provoke another episode of cataplexy in succession. This is called status cataplecticus; a repetition of numerous cataplectic attacks, which may last for several minutes or, rarely, even up to an hour. In such cases the patient cannot maintain an upright posture and may collapse to the floor. Consciousness remains clear during cataplexy; the patient remembers the surrounding situations well.

The presence of a wave of strong emotion as the triggering stimulus for cataplexy appears to be of special significance. The frequent triggering emotions are of exciting and pleasant nature, and touching to the heart of the patient. The most frequent emotional stimuli are laughter, feelings of elation, feelings of self-satisfaction, feelings of pride, attempts at repartee, anticipation just prior to showing off in front of others, tension, especially when meeting an important person unexpectedly, anger, and surprise (Fig. 6). Discouraging or frightful emotions seldom, if ever, precipitate cataplexy.

The sites of body affected at the time of cataplexy may include the whole body, knees, waist, lower half of the body, upper extremities, shoulders, neck, chin, muscles around the mouth, eyelids, or face (Fig. 7). Respiratory muscles are not affected. The average frequency of cataplexy tends to decrease over time, and is generally an indicator of the severity of illness (Fig. 8).

Case Study. Let me present a typical case of narcolepsy to describe cataplexy. A 64-year-old bookstore owner visited our clinic with the chief complaint of excessive daytime sleepiness. He developed the full tetrad of narcolepsy at the age of 12 years following a tonsillectomy. The severity of his symptoms was greatest between the ages of 15 and 20 years, when he had several sleep attacks daily and frequent cataplectic attacks whenever he laughed aloud or became angry. His symptoms gradually subsided, but at the time of consultation he still had three to four naps daily and about ten episodes of cataplexy per month. When he laughed

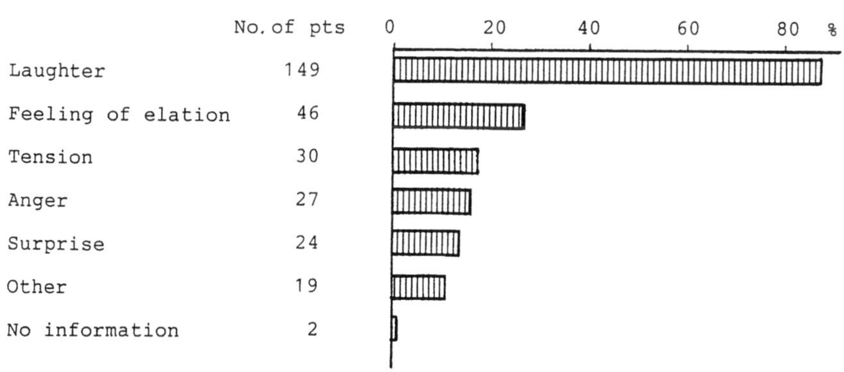

Fig. 6. Triggering emotion at cataplexy ($n = 170$, multiple responses)

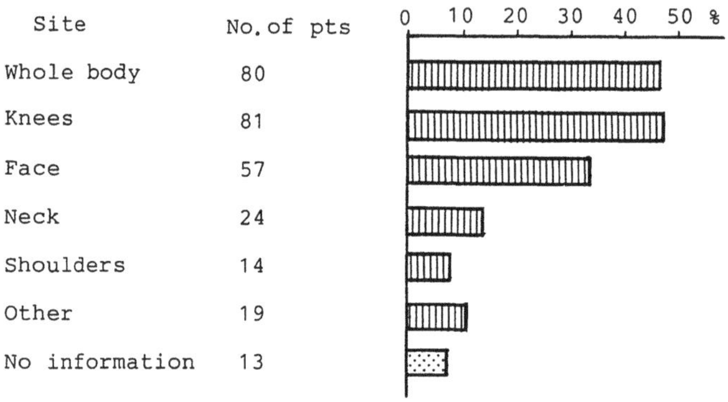

Fig. 7. Site of cataplexy ($n = 170$, multiple responses)

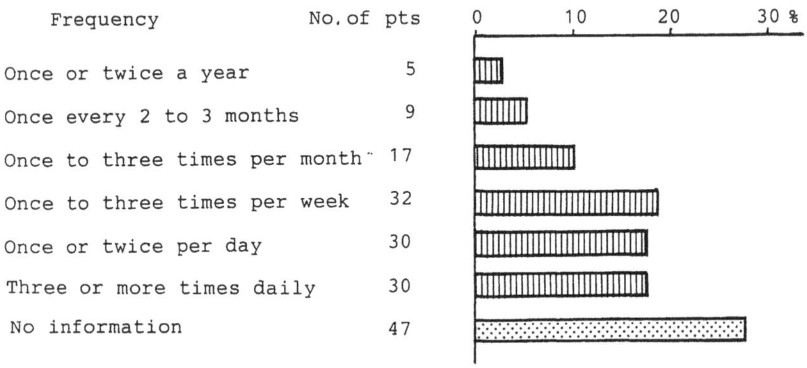

Fig. 8. Frequency of cataplexy at first consultation ($n = 170$)

aloud while watching exciting or humorous scenes on TV, his head drooped forward making him unable to watch the screen. Sometimes he fell to the floor. Similar cataplectic attacks developed when he scolded his grandchildren. His cataplectic attacks were often followed by episodes of short sleep. Polysomnography revealed marked sleep-onset REM activities. HLA typing results were Aw24, Aw31, Bw35, Bw39, Cw3, Cw7, DR2, DR4, DQw1.

As a further example, another narcoleptic patient experienced a sudden loss of power in his arms and hands and dropped a tile when he had a good hand while playing mahjongg. Still another narcoleptic patient was referred to our clinic because he did not run, but walked slowly and unsteadily when he made a clean hit during baseball games. His nickname was *"pyoko-tan"*, meaning "zigzag walk". It was found that he had repetitive mild cataplectic attacks of the lower extremities when he felt elation, preventing him from running. An unusual but dangerous situation has been reported in which a narcoleptic patient was subject to repetitive cataplectic attacks while he was taking a bath. He would involuntarily submerge under the hot water due to the loss of muscle tone of his whole body, with resultant inability to grasp onto anything for support.

Hypnagogic Hallucinations

Hypnagogic hallucinations are characterized by vivid dreaming with realistic sensations occurring during a drowsy state. They were first described by Maury (1848) in normal subjects and later by Lhermitte and Tournay (1927) as one of the frequent symptoms of narcolepsy. Soon after a narcoleptic patient gets into bed at night, and while he is half awake and aware of the environment of his bedroom, such as the location of the door or window, he starts to have unusual experiences. A typical example is having the sense that a burglar approaches his house, opens the door, climbs the stairs, enters his room, and assaults him. He may clearly hear the sound of the front door opening, and the sound of the burglar climbing the staircase. He may feel the presence of a frightening person standing at the foot of his bed. He may feel being slashed by a sword or shot by a gun by a burglar. Other patients have reported the sense that an amorphous black monster comes out of the closet and attacks. The patient often reports seeing dreadful reptiles, especially snakes, crawling around his body. He often feels the actual touch of snakes. He may feel as if he was brushing aside dead bodies as he walks through a blood-filled marsh. He may feel the biting of an animal such as a bear, or feels the fur of rabbits jumping around. The patient may feel as if being pressed down to the bed or being sexually harassed. Not a few patients report feeling as if they were flying through the air like Superman.

While this is happening the patient usually feels intense fear and tries to scream and escape. But his whole body is often paralyzed so he cannot move his arms or legs, and he cannot even shout for help. After fully awakening, the patient realizes that these dreadful experiences were only bad dreams. Some patients carry a wooden sword by the bed to defend themselves against the intruders at night. In some cases, after years of such experiences, the patient comes to realize while it is happening that this is not real but a bad dream, and he can ignore or mentally fight the intruders.

Sometimes the hypnagogic hallucinations appear during daytime napping and, on rare occasions, the dreamy experiences intrude into daytime consciousness resulting in the development of a hallucinatory-paranoid state which requires psy-

Frequency	No. of pts
None	30
Once or twice a year	1
Once every 2 to 3 months	6
Once to three times per month	9
Once to three times per week	29
Everyday	50
No information	45

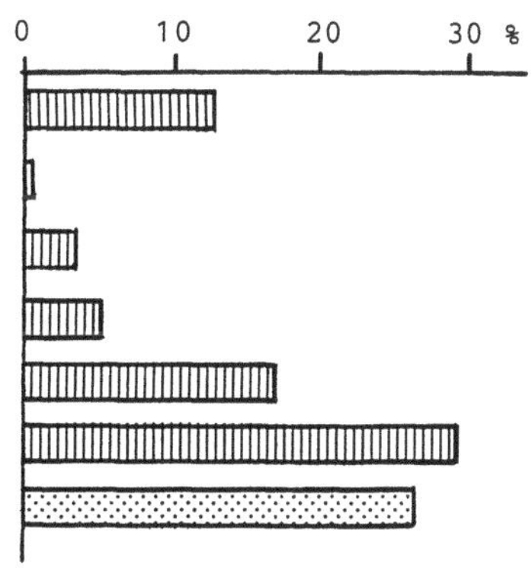

Fig. 9. Frequency of hypnagogic hallucinations at first consultation ($n = 170$)

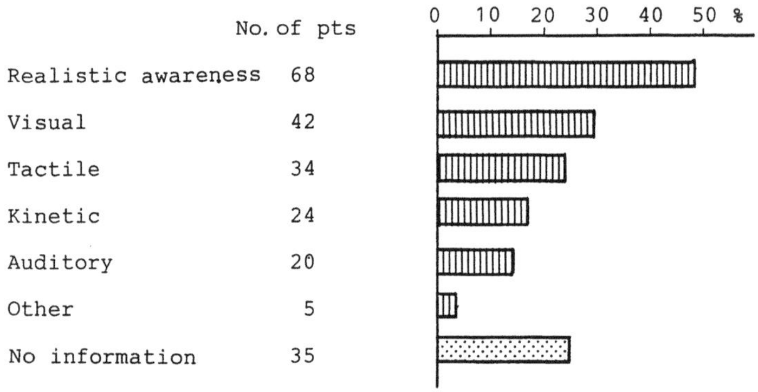

Fig. 10. Perceptual mode of hypnagogic hallucinations ($n = 140$, multiple responses)

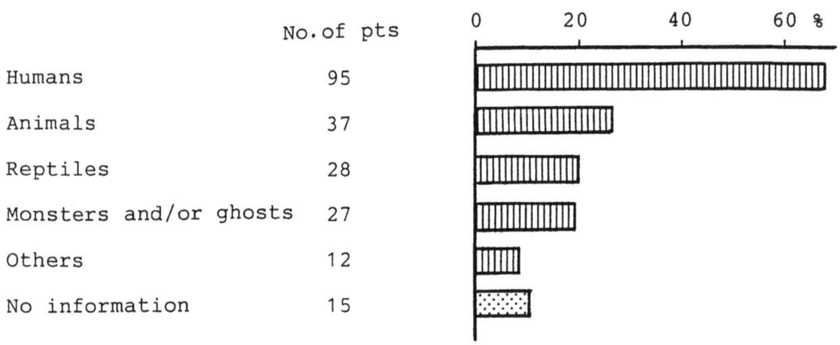

Fig. 11. Contents of hypnagogic hallucinations ($n = 140$, multiple responses)

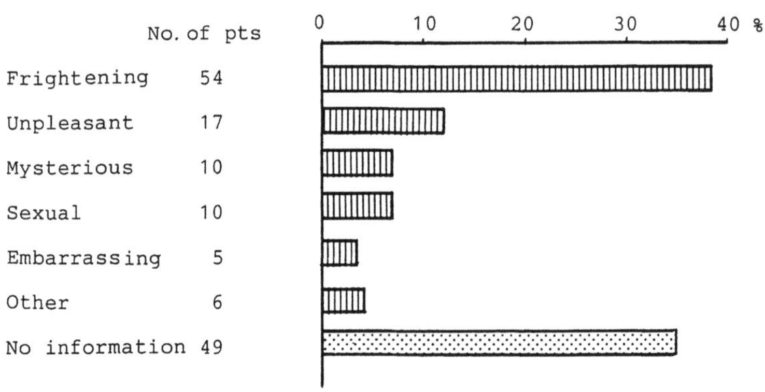

Fig. 12. Emotional responses to hypnagogic hallucinations ($n = 140$, multiple responses)

chiatric treatment (Honda and Takahashi 1971, Honda 1982a). The hypnagogic hallucinations almost always correspond with sleep-onset REM periods (Suzuki 1966).

The frequency of appearance, perceptual mode, and contents of hypnagogic hallucinations in narcoleptic patients are shown in Figs. 9–11. Frightful and unpleasant emotional responses are common, and pleasant experiences are rare during hypnagogic hallucinations (Fig. 12). Hypnagogic hallucinations were experienced by 82.3% of our narcoleptic patients.

Sleep Paralysis

The transient, generalized inability to move which develops at the stage between arousal and sleep is called sleep paralysis. Usually sleep paralysis occurs concomitantly with the experiences of frightening hypnagogic hallucinations. This experience was first described by Mitchell (1876) as night palsy and by Wilson (1928) as sleep paralysis. The association of sleep paralysis with narcolepsy was first described by Adie (1926).

The patient tries to get up to seek help, but his whole body is paralyzed as if a spell had been cast, rendering him helpless and unable to move or shout for help. He can only groan weakly, and the agonizing experiences are usually not noticeable enough to be recognized even by someone sleeping next to him.

Rosenthal (1928, 1939) described "hallucinatory-cataplectic anxiety syndrome" in narcoleptic patients and in schizophrenic patients. In Germany, the terms *"verzögertes psychomotorisches Erwachen"* (protracted psychomotor awakening) and *"Wachanfall"* (awaking attack) are used. Sleep paralysis was experienced by 80% of our narcoleptic patients.

Disturbed Nocturnal Sleep

The nocturnal sleep of a narcoleptic patient is usually shallow and is often disrupted by short awakenings and dreamings (Fig. 13). Evidence from all-night polysomnograms indicates that deep sleep is substantially reduced. The onset of nocturnal sleep is often disturbed by hypnagogic hallucinations.

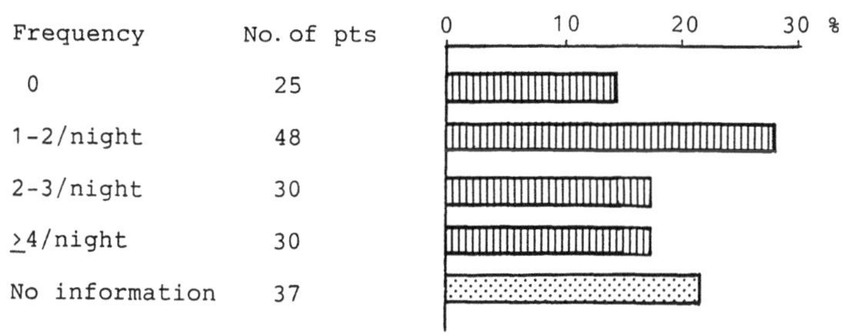

Fig. 13. Frequency of nocturnal awakenings at first consultation ($n = 170$)

Automatic Behaviors

Sometimes a narcoleptic patient has lapses of memory of routine daily behavior for a short period, from several seconds to several minutes. For example, he may not remember the entire situation of making a purchase, or he may find he has driven past a destination or brought unnecessary things out of the kitchen. Furthermore, he may find that he is no longer aware of feeling sleepy. These behaviors often occur when the patient tries to perform a task while unaware of his underlying sleepiness. They may thus be explained as conduct under altered consciousness with constriction of the field of consciousness. These behaviors are also explained as manifestations of recurrent microsleeps (Guilleminault et al. 1975). A loss of memory has been reported as one of the side effects of benzodiazepine medication. The possibility of this adverse effect of benzodiazepine may be worth consideration when the automatic behaviors occur at night while the patient is on benzodiazepines.

Decreased Psychic Tension and Narcoleptoid Personality

Due to the long-standing tendency to fall asleep in the daytime even during important situations where he is expected to be alert, the narcoleptic patient is often regarded by others as idle and unreliable, and he has to face frustrating situations almost everyday in his daily life at work and at home. The patient thus loses confidence and develops feelings of inferiority and self-depreciation. After years of such life, however, the patient grows accustomed to the somnolence, loses awareness of it, and even denies the feeling of frequent sleepiness. He instead develops decreased psychic tension, poor self-assertion, and good-naturedness. Punctuality decreases and the patient becomes easygoing and loses active concern about things around him. This characteristic personality observed frequently in chronic narcoleptic patients is termed "narcoleptoid personality" (Honda et al. 1965, Honda 1972). Table 1 shows a comparison between narcoleptic and epileptic personality changes. A narcoleptoid personality and an epileptoid personality can be considered to construct opposite ends of an axis which represents a physiological level of psychic tension and alertness. We could also place and evaluate normal subjects on this axis of psychic tension.

Other Complications

Obesity, headaches, lumbago, sweating, and diabetes mellitus are among complications of narcoleptic patients often observed in clinical situations. Many narcoleptic patients start to gain weight after the onset of illness. The average obesity index (Broca) of narcoleptic patients was reported to be 119.3 ± 17.3 (SD), and 42.1% of the 197 patients in our series had an obesity index above 120 (Honda et al. 1986b). Headaches are common complaints of narcoleptic patients (Roth 1962) and are often observed when the patients resist sleepiness and try to concentrate on their tasks. Lumbago sometimes is the result of irregular posture and collapsing due to cataplexy. Most narcoleptic patients are prone to parasympathicotonic con-

Table 1. Comparison of personality traits between chronic narcoleptic patients and chronic epileptic patients (grand mal type)

	Narcolepsy (narcoleptoid personality)	Epilepsy (epileptoid personality)
General feature	Decrease in psychic tension and alertness	Increase in psychic tension
Self-assertion	Low self-assertion, withdrawn, low spirited, unconfident, passive, feelings of inferiority, self-depreciation	Strong self-assertion, compulsive, thorough, confident, aggressive
Rapport	Natural, friendly, relaxed, unguarded, does not cause tension to others, does not resist changes in topics of conversation	Viscous, rigid, oppressive, causes tension to others, resists changes in topics of conversation
Affect	Good natured, sensitive, feels resigned, emotional tension and excitement do not persist, less explosive	Increased irritability, increased affective reactions, passionate, moodiness, persistence of emotional tension and excitement, explosive
Psychomotor activities	Slow, sluggish, less active, easygoing, not very punctual, inconsistent	Slow in tempo, punctual, circumstantial, compulsive about trifles, persevering
Intelligence	Absence of lowering of intelligence, preservation of personality integration	Lowering of intelligence, lowering of personality integration in untreated chronic patients
Social life	Decrease in punctuality, compromiser, less persistent in following social regulations, submissive, social introversion	Strict self-control, uncompromising, persistent about social regulations, excessive honesty, strong sense of righteousness sometimes inappropriately acted upon

stitution (Honda 1960, Roth 1962). Profuse sweating and obesity are often observed concomitantly. Increased frequency of non-insulin-dependent diabetes mellitus (12.5%) was also reported among narcoleptic patients (Honda et al. 1986b).

Concept of Narcolepsy

In this section, the concept of narcolepsy and the issue of whether narcolepsy is a symptom or a disease entity is discussed. Operational diagnostic criteria for narcolepsy based on clinical observation are proposed together with definitions of each symptom of narcolepsy. Differential diagnosis of narcolepsy is also discussed, especially that from epilepsy.

Definition of the Term "Narcolepsy"

The concept of narcolepsy has been subject to historical changes. Currently, the term is used in somewhat different ways according to the viewpoint of each investigator. Connotations of the term include:

(1) simply the symptom of excessive daytime sleepiness or sleep attacks;
(2) a clinical syndrome with one or more of the symptoms from the narcoleptic tetrad, which include sleep attacks, cataplexy, sleep paralysis, and hypnagogic hallucinations;
(3) a disease entity with excessive daytime sleepiness as a prototype, with or without the presence of one or more symptoms from the narcoleptic tetrad (Roth 1980); and
(4) a pathophysiological condition as defined by the results of the Multiple Sleep Latency Test (MSLT) as short sleep latency and more than two sleep-onset REM periods.

The expression of "narcolepsy-cataplexy" permits the presence of narcolepsy without cataplexy and indicates only the combination of the two symptoms.

When performing any biological research on narcolepsy, it is vital to employ clear and operational diagnostic criteria. Otherwise, other disorders of sleep may be diagnosed as narcolepsy according to the opinions of individual investigators. The diagnostic classification of sleep and arousal disorders adopted by the Association of Sleep Disorders Centers (ASDC) and the Association for the Psychophysiological Study of Sleep (APSS) in 1979 described essential features of narcolepsy as follows: Narcolepsy is a syndrome consisting of excessive daytime sleepiness and abnormal manifestations of REM sleep. The latter include frequent sleep-onset REM (SOREM) periods, which may be subjectively appreciated as hypnagogic hallucinations, and the dissociated REM sleep inhibitory processes, cataplexy and sleep paralysis. The appearance of REM sleep within 10 min of sleep onset is considered evidence for narcolepsy.

This description is quite ambiguous as diagnostic criteria; it permits conditions of both excessive daytime sleepiness (EDS) and dissociated REM sleep symptoms, such as hypnagogic hallucinations, sleep paralysis, or SOREM periods, regardless of the presence of cataplexy to be diagnosed as narcolepsy. Both hypnagogic hallucinations and sleep paralysis can be observed in a variety of pathological conditions as well as in normal subjects. If such unspecific symptoms are included in the diagnostic criteria, a rather strong possibility would emerge that various sleep disorders, with occasional complications of these unspecific symptoms, would be diagnosed as narcolepsy. Furthermore, the adoption of the highly specified item of a SOREM period is still problematic. The SOREM period is not narcolepsy specific and can be observed in cases of depression and even in normals (Nakagawa 1980). The SOREM period is sometimes absent in narcoleptic patients during a single polysomnography, especially when recorded without acclimation to the test environment or in the daytime after a nap (Takahashi 1977). To clarify this issue, electrophysiological test procedures sensitive to the detection of SOREM periods should be clearly and strictly defined. The adoption of SOREM periods for the diagnosis of narcolepsy should first be validated by demonstrating appearance of SOREM periods in all patients using large samples of narcoleptic patients already confirmed by clinical diagnosis of narcolepsy. It will also be necessary to prove that SOREM periods are a continuous finding throughout the long course of the disorder, especially when mild daytime naps become the only symptom after many years of clinical course. Should demonstration of SOREM periods always be required for the diagnosis of narcolepsy, the diagnosis of narcolepsy must be changed when SOREM periods are no longer demonstrated after many years during the course of the disorder.

Furthermore, another practical problem may arise with regard to the diagnostic importance of SOREM periods: If demonstration of SOREM periods by MSLT is adopted as a necessary diagnostic criterion for narcolepsy, the diagnosis cannot be made in clinical settings without sufficient equipment and facilities, and diagnosis will be deferred in patients without sufficient economic resources to afford the expense of polysomnographic test procedures.

Proposed Diagnostic Criteria for Narcolepsy

We view narcolepsy as an independent, specific disease entity on the basis of our observations that narcoleptic patients show consistent patterns in clinical symptomatology, distribution of ages at onset, clinical course and prognosis, familial loading, treatment responses, pathophysiological findings, and positive HLA-DR2 findings. We also believe that operational criteria for the diagnosis of narcolepsy based on a clinical syndrome and course are essential for more precise diagnostic reliability and clinical usefulness.

Our proposed diagnostic criteria for narcolepsy are as follows:

(A) Recurrent daytime naps and/or lapses into sleep occurring almost every day over a period of at least 6 months
(B) Clinical confirmation of cataplexy in a patient's history concurrent with (A)

We consider that the recurrent daytime naps or lapses into sleep in narcolepsy can be defined as follows:

(1) the duration of each episode of daytime sleep is usually less than an hour;
(2) the sleep can be terminated easily by external stimulation;
(3) the patient usually feels refreshed after the sleep;
(4) CNS stimulants such as methylphenidate, pemoline, and methamphetamine are effective against the somnolence; and
(5) the condition usually lasts over many years, but at the very least for 6 months.

Cataplexy can be defined as follows:

(1) cataplexy is a sudden bilateral loss of the tone of skeletal muscles;
(2) it is provoked by a sudden strong wave of emotion;
(3) consciousness and memory are not impaired during cataplexy;
(4) the duration of cataplexy is usually short, from moments to a few minutes; and
(5) clomipramine and imipramine are effective in markedly reducing cataplexy.

Since cataplexy may disappear in the course of the disease, diagnosis of narcolepsy can be made in patients without the presence of cataplexy at the time of examination if typical cataplexy is confirmed in the patient's history concurrent with the recurrent daytime naps.

Our clinical diagnostic criteria enabled us to select a homogeneous group of patients with common characteristics of clinical symptoms, a definite pattern of the distribution of ages of onset, a long-term clinical course, prognosis, polysomnographic findings, treatment responses, familial loading, and genetic predispositions including a positive HLA-DR2 antigen. Therefore we consider that our clinical diagnostic criteria have both validity and clinical usefulness. We also think that confirmation of SOREM periods on polysomnography and positive HLA-DR2 could be employed as valuable indicators for confirming narcolepsy when we perform research on narcolepsy.

Differential Diagnosis for Narcolepsy

The major conditions to consider in differential diagnosis are various excessive daytime somnolences (EDS) without cataplexy, respiratory-related sleep disorders, subwakefulness syndrome, neurotic disorders, and, most importantly, epilepsy.

Excessive daytime somnolence without cataplexy may be observed in subjects with other disorders of various origins. Poor sleep hygiene and disturbed nocturnal sleep may also produce daytime somnolence. In nocturnal sleep-apnea DOES (disorder of excessive daytime somnolence) syndrome or, in nocturnal myoclonus DOES syndrome, excessive daytime sleepiness is the major symptom. In these conditions, polysomnography shows frequent apneic or myoclonic episodes, and usually the daytime sleep is not refreshing, while CNS stimulants are effective.

Excessive daytime somnolence and subwakefulness syndrome may also be observed in states of altered or disturbed consciousness such as periodic somnolence and organic brain disorders. They are also observed in certain types of depression accompanied by decreased concentration and alertness, or even in schizophrenia with decreased initiative. In these conditions, the daytime sleep episodes are often lengthy and may persist for more than an hour without a refreshed feeling after awakening. CNS stimulants are generally ineffective in such cases. The patterns of daytime somnolence in these conditions are often unstable, and the duration of the condition does not usually exceed 6 months.

Certain types of conversion disorders and neurotic disorders also show daytime somnolence. The intensity of sleepiness in such cases usually fluctuates from day to day, and usually the continuation of sleepy days is much shorter than 6 months. CNS stimulants are usually ineffective in such cases, and may sometimes even aggravate neurotic anxiety.

Cataplexy must be differentiated from the muscle weakness of myasthenia gravis, multiple sclerosis, akinetic or astatic seizures of epilepsy, the drop attacks of the elderly, orthostatic hypotension, and vertigo.

Differential diagnosis of narcolepsy from epilepsy is not difficult when employing our diagnostic criteria for narcolepsy. However, narcolepsy is sometimes confused with epilepsy because both disorders have irresistible attacks of disturbed alertness and collapsing with origins in the central nervous system. Epileptic attacks are characterized by the loss or alteration of consciousness associated with convulsions, automatic behaviors, or sometimes akinetic or astatic seizures. Impairment of memory during the attacks is common, and termination of the attack is not possible by external stimulation.

Narcoleptic attacks consist of sleep and dissociated sleep, and lack the disturbance of consciousness. They can be terminated by external stimulation quite easily. While automatism in epilepsy shows a fixed pattern of purposeless movements along with disturbed consciousness, the automatic behaviors of narcolepsy replicate various daily habitual behaviors performed under incognizant somnolence. Postictal disturbance of consciousness is commonly observed after epileptic attacks, in contrast to a prompt restoration of alertness in narcolepsy. An emotional triggering is always required for cataplexy, while it is rare in epilepsy.

The EEGs show generalized or localized paroxysmal discharges in epilepsy, and the slowing of basic activities is usually observed in chronic epileptics indicating organic brain disturbances. EEGs of narcoleptic attacks generally show sleep patterns that are similar to those in normal subjects. Paroxysmal discharges and slowing of basic activities are usually absent even in the most chronic narcoleptic patients. The threshold of paroxysmal discharges on intravenous Metrazol (pentylenetetrazol) infusion is markedly lowered in epileptic patients, and sometimes clinical epileptic seizures are provoked during Metrazol infusion. Narcoleptic patients may show slightly lowered convulsive thresholds on Metrazol infusion, but provocation of sleep attacks or cataplexy never ensues. In addition, chronic epileptic patients often show lowered intelligence and lowered level of personality integration, and may show epileptoid personality changes with increased psychic tension. In contrast, chronic narcoleptic patients do not show a lowering of intelligence or lowering of the level of personality integration. They, instead, show narcoleptoid personality changes (Honda et al. 1965) which are characterized by a decrease in psychic tension and alertness (Table 1) (Honda et al. 1982c).

A familial loading for the disorder is sometimes observed in both narcolepsy and epilepsy, but they rarely mix with each other in the same family. The respective responses to drug treatments are also quite different. Anticonvulsants which are quite effective in epilepsy are not at all effective in narcolepsy, and CNS stimulants and tricyclic antidepressants effective in narcolepsy have little effect in epilepsy.

Thus, epilepsy and narcolepsy are essentially different and independent neuropsychiatric diseases and should not be confused with each other.

Pathophysiology

In this section, characteristic polysomnographic findings of narcolepsy, including sleep-onset appearance of REM sleep, especially at the Multiple Sleep Latency Test (MSLT), are described. The absence of sleep-onset secretion of growth hormone and specific effectiveness of CNS stimulants against daytime somnolence and specific anticataplectic effect of tricyclic antidepressants are described.

Polysomnographic Findings

The routine daytime EEGs of narcoleptic patients are characterized by persistent drowsiness patterns appearing soon after the onset of recording, which often turn out to be a sleep-onset REM (SOREM) period on polysomnography. The patient often lacks awareness of somnolence and often denies sleepiness even when his EEGs show drowsy or sometimes spindle sleep pattern. Upon the patient opening his eyes, the EEGs often show the appearance of diffuse alpha activities, which is called paradoxical alpha blocking. This phenomenon indicates a lowered level of wakefulness of the narcoleptic patient while his eyes are closed. Upon the opening of the eyes, the patient shows elevation of the wakefulness level similar to that of an ordinary resting condition of a normal subject with his eyes closed.

In addition to the increased tendency to fall asleep, a daytime polysomnogram often shows the appearance of a REM period within 10 min after the onset of sleep. This SOREM period is observed in narcoleptic patients frequently, but not in every instance (Wilson et al. 1972). The appearance of a SOREM period is subject to change by the recording conditions such as amount of sleep on the preceding night or napping on the same day prior to the recording, the use of drugs, time of day, anxiety, and psychological states. The frequency of appearance of SOREM periods in daytime polysomnography in 105 narcoleptic patients was reported to be 83.8% (Takahashi 1977).

The recent development of the Multiple Sleep Latency Test (MSLT) provides an objective measure to evaluate sleepiness (Carskadon and Dement 1977). A sleep latency of less than 5 min from "lights-out" to the first sleep epoch is considered a sign of increased sleepiness, or vulnerability to falling asleep (Carskadon et al. 1987). MSLT is also a valuable test to determine the presence of a SOREM period, with the appearance of more than two SOREM periods at an MSLT being considered indicative of narcolepsy (Richardson et al. 1978; Mitler et al. 1979).

On all-night polysomnography, sleep-onset REM is also a very frequent finding and is often associated with the experience of hypnagogic hallucinations and sleep paralysis (Vogel 1960; Rechtschaffen et al. 1963; Takahashi and Jimbo 1963). Nocturnal sleep cycles are usually irregular, and sleep is shallow and disrupted by frequent intermittent awakenings. The time spent for stages I and II is increased, while that for deep sleep stages III and IV is decreased.

Figure 14 shows an example of an all-night polysomnogram and MSLT performed on the following day in a 10-year-old girl 3 months after the onset of narcolepsy and before any drug treatment (Case 2 in Chap. 12). Marked tendency to fall asleep, frequent appearance of SOREM periods, increased amount (34.7%) of REM sleep, and decreased amount (15.1%) of stage IV sleep for the age of 10 years are demonstrated.

To summarize, the basic characteristic features of the electrophysiology of narcolepsy are the abnormality of sleep-wakefulness rhythm and frequent sleep-onset appearance of REM sleep. Cataplexy, hypnagogic hallucinations, and sleep paralysis have been considered to be related to REM sleep and are called "dissociated REM sleep manifestations".

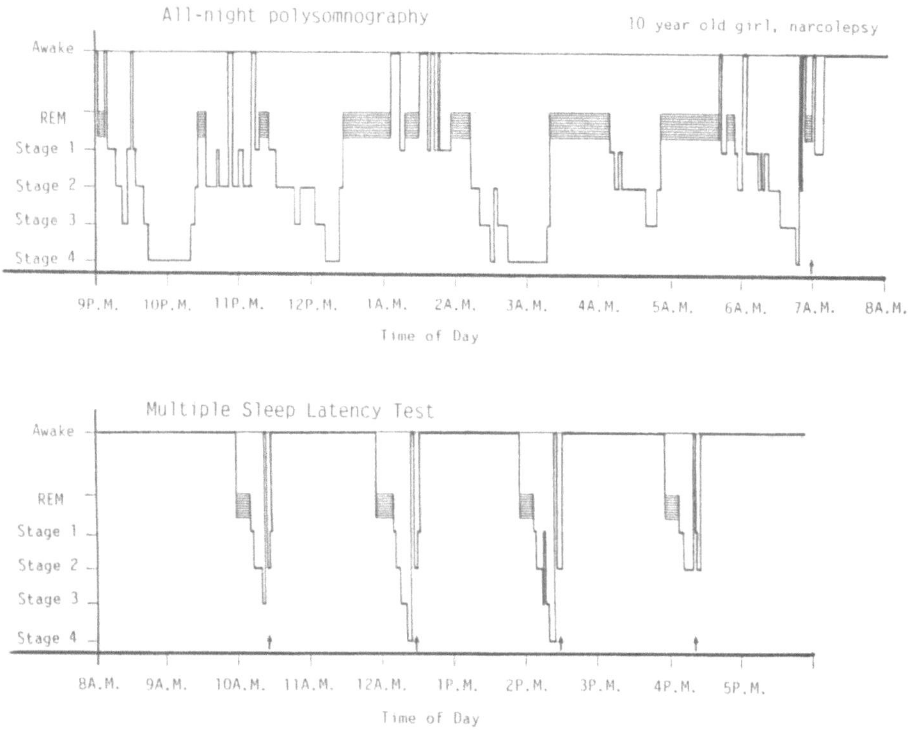

Fig. 14. An all-night polysomnogram and an MSLT performed on the following day, of a narcoleptic patient. The patient was a 10-year-old girl (Case 2 in Chap. 12), 3 months after the onset of illness and before any pharmacological treatment. Note appearance of sleep-onset REM periods and marked sleep tendency at each MSLT session. ↑ indicates a verbal call to awaken the patient at the end of each recording. After short arousal, however, the patient immediately fell asleep again until termination of the recording, showing increased sleepiness. Sleep parameters for the all-night polysomnography are as follows: total time in bed (TIB), 615 min; total sleep time (TST), 571 min; sleep latency, 3 min; REM latency, 0 min.

Sleep stage	Time spent for the stage	Percentage for TIB
Stage W	41 min	7.2%
Stage 1	91 min	15.9%
Stage 2	128 min	22.4%
Stage 3	68 min	11.9%
Stage 4	86 min	15.1%
Stage REM	198 min	34.7%

The software program for this diagrammatic illustration was kindly provided by Dr. Toshiyuki Kobayashi, at the Psychiatric Research Institute of Tokyo

Neuroendocrine Findings

The marked secretion of growth hormone at the onset of nocturnal sleep usually observed in normal subjects (Utena et al. 1968; Takahashi et al. 1968; Honda et al. 1969a) is often absent in narcoleptic patients (K. Takahashi et al. 1971) (Fig. 15).

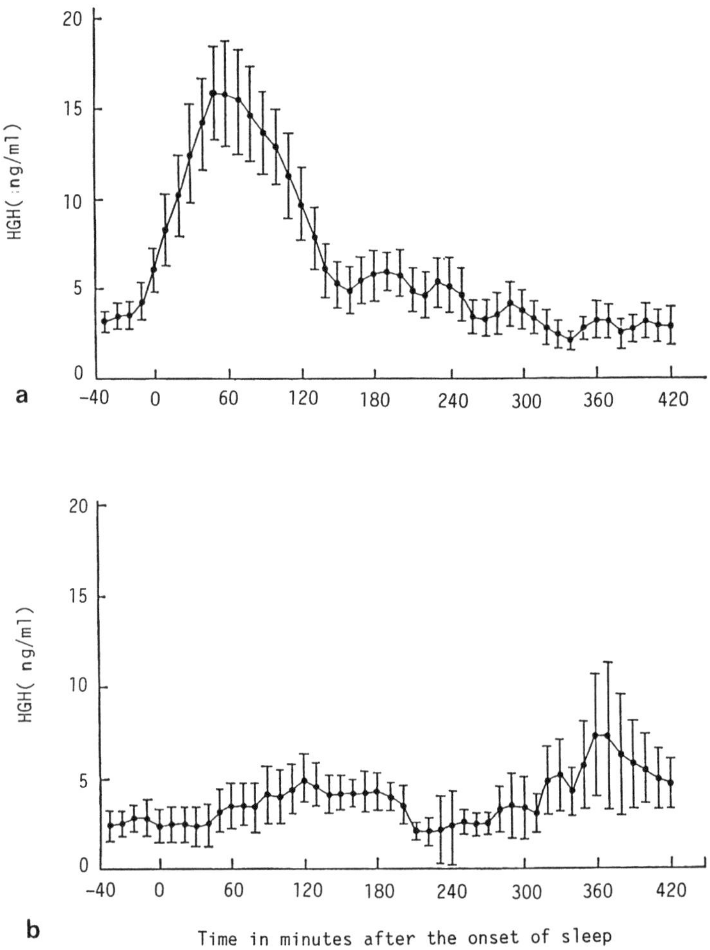

Fig. 15a, b. Growth hormone secretion during nocturnal sleep in normal subjects (**a**) and in narcoleptic patients (**b**). Note marked secretion of growth hormone at the onset of nocturnal sleep in normal subjects ($n = 10$) and absence of the secretion in narcoleptic patients ($n = 10$). (Takahashi et al. 1971)

Growth hormone secretion in response to insulin-induced hypoglycemia, however, is maintained in narcoleptic patients. The mechanisms of growth hormone secretion at sleep-onset in normal subjects and of its absence in most narcoleptic subjects are not clear.

Two hypotheses may be considered. One is that the neural pathways connecting the initiation of sleep and the mechanism of growth hormone secretion are inhibited in narcolepsy. The other hypothesis is that the accumulation of growth hormone during sustained wakefulness does not occur in narcoleptic patients due to frequent daytime nappings. The latter hypothesis is supported by animal experiments. Normal dogs show polyphasic, very frequent fluctuations of short sleeps and short arousals throughout a day, and a sleep-onset secretion of growth hormone is absent. The appearance of growth hormone secretion at the onset of sleep in the same dogs maintained in forced wakefulness for several hours (Takahashi 1979) seems to support that the onset of sleep acts as a priming mechanism for the release of the accumulated growth hormone during prolonged wakefulness.

Neuropharmacological Findings

Against the excessive daytime sleepiness in narcolepsy, CNS stimulants, such as methylphenidate, pemoline, pipradrol, and methamphetamine, are always effective (Yoss and Daly 1959; Akimoto et al. 1961; Takahashi and Honda 1964a; Honda et al. 1979, Honda and Hishikawa 1980). Anticonvulsants are ineffective against any of the narcoleptic symptoms including automatic behaviors. Tricyclic antidepressants, such as imipramine (Akimoto et al. 1960), desipramine and other tricyclic antidepressants (Takahashi and Honda 1964b), and clomipramine (Honda and Takahashi 1969), show marked and almost constant effectiveness against cataplexy, hypnagogic hallucinations, and sleep paralysis. So far, it is our experience that clomipramine is the most potent and reliable anticataplectic agent among many tricyclic antidepressants, and is still effective in narcoleptic patients for whom imipramine is no longer effective for cataplexy.

Since these agents are known to suppress REM sleep, the mechanism of action of the tricyclic antidepressants is considered to be related to their suppressing effect on REM sleep mechanisms.

Epidemiology

In this section, epidemiological aspects of narcolepsy in Japan are summarized. Five hundred and seventy-nine families of either narcoleptic or essential hypersomniac (EHS) probands were studied to deduce segregation ratios and the relative frequency (*K* value of Penrose), which are necessary for the analysis of genetic aspects of narcolepsy. A concentrated pattern during teens of the ages of onset for both somnolence and cataplexy in patients with a heavy familial loading, in contrast to a less concentrated pattern in patients without a remarkable familial loading, is shown. Sex differences in terms of younger ages of onset of both somnolence and cataplexy in female narcoleptic patients are pointed out.

Since 100% positive HLA-DR2 findings in narcoleptic patients are described fully in other chapters, and 100% presence of DNA findings is also described in Chap. 11, HLA and DNA findings in narcolepsy are omitted in this section. Findings on five genetic markers with significant associations with narcolepsy are briefly reviewed although they are discussed in Chap. 16, because these genetic markers appear to be important in understanding the genetic basis of liability to narcolepsy in addition to HLA. A new hypothetical model is proposed to explain both the two-threshold multifactorial mode, including various environmental factors, and the autosomal dominant inheritance mode of HLA-DR2, a prerequisite factor for the development of narcolepsy.

Genetic Markers Other than HLA in Narcolepsy

Several genetic markers are found to have associations with narcolepsy (Asaka 1981; Asaka et al. 1981; Honda et al. 1983 a). Haptoglobin (HP), a serum factor encoded by a gene on chromosome 16, showed a significant increase in the phenotype 1 ($P < 0.001$). Group-specific component (GC), a serum alpha-globulin (chromosome 4), showed a significant deviation from the expected phenotype distribution ($P < 0.01$). Soluble glutamate-oxalate transaminase (GOT), a serum enzyme (chromosome 10), showed a significant increase in its phenotypes of 2-1 and a rare variant 3-1 ($P < 0.025$). Esterase D (ESD), a serum enzyme (chromosome 13), showed a decrease in phenotype 1 and an increase in phenotype 2 ($P < 0.05$). Serum alpha-1-trypsin inhibitor (PI) (chromosome 14) showed a deviation from the expected phenotype distributions ($P < 0.05$). The result of a discriminant analysis using 16 genetic markers other than HLA showed 96% correct judgment of narcolepsy from a group including normal Japanese subjects. These findings will be further discussed in Chap. 16.

Family Study

Nevsimalova-Bruhova and Roth (1972) reported that 39.1% of 23 cases of idiopathic hypersomnia and 32.9% of 85 cases of narcolepsy showed a positive family history of hypersomnia or narcolepsy. They suggested a polyfactorial type of heredity with two or more genes to explain the transmission of narcolepsy. Kessler (1975) performed a family study on 130 families with an REM narcolepsy proband. Using Kessler's data, Thomson (1975) considered that a two-threshold multifactorial model, with narcolepsy as the more severe and EDS as the less severe form of the disorder, seemed to be the most appropriate. Baraitser and Parkes (1987) analyzed 50 families with a proband with the narcoleptic syndrome and found that 52% of the probands had an affected first-degree relative. They suggested a single dominant gene for the inheritance of the narcoleptic syndrome.

We performed a study including 232 families with a narcolepsy proband and 76 families with an EHS proband (Honda et al. 1983 b). We concluded that the development of narcolepsy and EDS fits well to the two-threshold multifactorial inheritance model with high heritability.

Extending our family study, we examined the frequencies of narcolepsy among parents and siblings of 579 somnolent patients. The total number of family members studied was 3557. As shown in Table 2, a total of 18 narcoleptic patients (4.3%) were found among parents and siblings of the 419 narcoleptic probands. The frequency of narcolepsy was 1.19% among 838 parents of these narcoleptic probands, and 0.58% among 1371 siblings except the probands. A total of 104 EDS subjects (24.8%) were found in the same families. The frequency of EDS was 8.00% among parents and 2.70% among siblings except the probands. It has been shown that the family members of a narcolepsy proband have a somewhat increased liability to narcolepsy, and an even more increased liability to EDS.

In addition to narcoleptic probands, we investigated families of 160 patients with EHS. Essential hypersomnia is defined by the following criteria:

Table 2. Frequency of narcolepsy and EDS among parents and siblings of 419 families with a narcolepsy proband

	Narcolepsy		EDS		Total	
Father (419)	6	>1.19%	28	>8.00%	34	>9.19%
Mother (419)	4		39		43	
Brother (720)	4	>0.58%	15	>2.70%	19	>3.28%
Sister (651)	4		22		26	
Total (2209)	18	0.81%	104	4.71%	122	5.52%
General population (12469)	20	0.16%	65	0.52%	85	0.68%

Table 3. Frequency of narcolepsy and EDS among parents and siblings of 160 families with an EHS proband

	Narcolepsy	EDS	
Father (160)	None	13	>8.13%
Mother (160)	None	13	
Brother (209)	None	2	>2.67%
Sister (240)	None	10	
Total (769)	None	38	4.94%
General population (12469)			0.52%

(a) EDS which occurs almost every day over a period of at least 6 months;
(b) absence of cataplexy; and
(c) not due to other known disorders associated with daytime somnolence, such as sleep-apnea syndrome (see Chap. 14).

The frequency of EDS among 160 families with an EHS proband showed a tendency similar to families with a narcolepsy proband (Table 3). There were no narcoleptic patients, and a total of 38 EDS subjects (23.8%) were found among these 160 families with an EHS proband.

In order to study the mode of inheritance, segregation ratios were calculated. Segregation ratio refers to the frequency of narcolepsy or EDS among siblings except the proband according to the condition of parents, and represents the susceptibility risk among the siblings. As shown in Table 4, there were 10 families with a total of 29 siblings in which 1 parent was affected with narcolepsy. There were 63 families with a total of 190 siblings in which one parent was affected with EDS. The remaining 346 families which included 1154 siblings had normal parents. The segregation ratios of narcolepsy were 0.0345 for the family group with a narcoleptic parent, 0.0105 for the family group with an EDS parent, and 0.0043 for the family group with normal parents. All of these values were much higher than the estimated frequency of narcolepsy (0.0016) among the general population (Honda 1979). The segregation ratios for EHS showed a similar tendency. The families with a narcoleptic parent showed the highest segregation ratio (0.1034) for EDS, followed by families with an EDS parent (0.0842), and lastly by families with nor-

Table 4. Segregation ratio of narcolepsy and EDS among 419 families with a narcolepsy proband

Parents	No. of families	Siblings with Narcolepsy	Siblings with EDS
Narcolepsy	10	0.0345 (1/29)	0.1034 (3/29)
EDS	63	0.0105 (2/190)	0.0842 (16/190)
Normal	346	0.0043 (5/1154)	0.0156 (18/1154)
Pooled	419	0.0058 (8/1373)	0.0269 (37/1373
General Population (12-16 yrs)		0.0016	0.0052

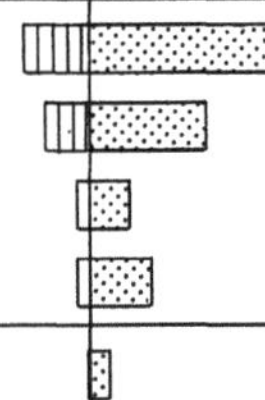

mal parents (0.0156). All of these findings were much higher than the estimated frequency of EDS (0.0052) among the general population. This similar tendency among the same group of subjects suggests the presence of a common genetic predisposition for both narcolepsy and EDS.

When we combine these data on both parents with narcolepsy and parents with EDS, the segregation ratio for somnolent subjects among siblings when one parent was affected was 0.1005 (22/219), which was much less than the expected value of 0.5 if the mode of inheritance was either autosomal dominant or recessive. The segregation ratio when both parents were normal was 0.0200 (23/1154), which was also much less than the value expected in the case of autosomal dominant (0.5) or autosomal recessive (0.25) inheritance. Thus, our data were not compatible with the classic Mendelian inheritance model.

In accordance with Penrose (1953), we divided the segregation ratio for all the siblings (s, 0.0328) of 419 narcolepsy probands by q (0.0068), the frequency among the general population, and the obtained value of K, a relative frequency, was 4.82 for both narcolepsy and EDS combined. It is expected that the value of K should be close to ½ q (73.5) in the case of dominant inheritance, and close to ¼ q (36.8) in the case of recessive inheritance. However, the observed value of K was closest to, and even less than, the expected value of $1/\sqrt{q}$ (12.3) for the multifactorial inheritance. Thus, the mode of inheritance of narcolepsy and EDS can be considered to be closest to the multifactorial inheritance model, where exogenous factors other than genetic factors also appear to play roles in the development of narcolepsy and EDS. When the sum of multiple genetic and environmental factors exceeds a certain threshold, EDS develops, and when the sum further exceeds the second threshold, narcolepsy develops. The heritability of liability to narcolepsy was calculated in three different ways, and similar values of 0.3364, 0.3587, and 0.3384 (Falconer 1965; Reich et al. 1972; Edwards 1967) were obtained. The heritabilities of liability to EDS including narcolepsy were also calculated. They were 0.6244, 0.6874, and 0.6267 respectively.

On the other hand, the inheritance of HLA DR2-Dw2 gene follows the Mendelian model. Thomson (1985) considered the mode of inheritance of the HLA-linked gene predisposing to narcolepsy as favoring an additive or dominant mode with possible incomplete penetrance. Thus it seems contradictory to which model, either multifactorial model with high heritability or autosomal dominant model with low penetrance, the true mode of inheritance of narcolepsy follows. In either case, various environmental stress factors must contribute to the development of narcolepsy. According to Krüger (1973), extreme cases of multifactorial inheritance with high heritability are theoretically not distinguishable from the extreme cases of dominant inheritance with low penetrance. It appears that the mode of inheritance of narcolepsy happens to fall into this particularly indistinguishable zone, and it is therefore futile to try to distinguish between the autosomal dominant mode and multifactorial mode of inheritance in the case of narcolepsy.

We consider that the HLA DR2-Dw2 is a prerequisite factor for the development of narcolepsy (Honda et al. 1984, 1986a). The presence of DR2-Dw2, however, is not sufficient in and of itself for the development of narcolepsy because the penetrance is low. Other genetic factors, such as HP, GC, GOT, ESD, and PI, also contribute to the development of narcolepsy. In cases of so-called symptomatic narcolepsy, various exogenous stress factors causing disturbances of consciousness, such as high fever, heavy bleeding, brain trauma, encephalitis, and general anesthesia, act as precipitating factors. Other somatic stress factors such as physical exhaustion and sleep deprivation may at times precipitate the onset of narcolepsy (somatogenic narcolepsy). Furthermore, profound psychological stress factors sometimes appear to contribute to the development of EDS and narcolepsy in some patients (psychogenic narcolepsy) (see Chap. 3). In all these cases, however, HLA DR2 is positive, indicating the presence of a common predisposition for the development of narcolepsy. We consider that these seemingly causative environmental stress factors eventually act only as precipitating factors, and that there is no independent symptomatic, somatogenic, or psychogenic narcolepsy in the true sense of the term.

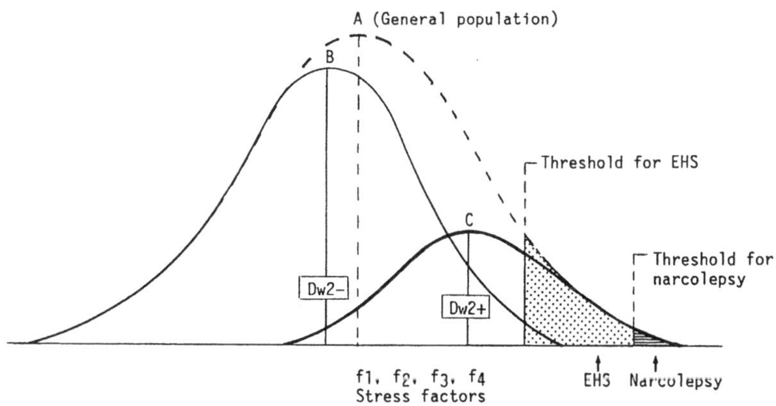

Fig. 16. A two-threshold multifactorial model with dominant HLA-Dw2 inheritance for the development of essential hypersomnia (EHS) and narcolepsy. *A*, distribution of liability to narcolepsy among the general population; *B*, distribution of liability to narcolepsy among HLA-Dw2-negative subjects; *C*, distribution of liability to narcolepsy among HLA-Dw2-positive subjects. *f1*, Fg(i): sum of genetic factors; *f2*, Fe(i): sum of exogenous factors; *f3*, Fs(i): sum of somatogenic factors; *f4*, Fp(i): sum of psychogenic factors

Our hypothetical model for the development of EHS and narcolepsy is shown in Fig. 16. This model can explain both aspects of autosomal dominant HLA-Dw2 inheritance as a prerequisite factor for the development of narcolepsy and of two-threshold multifactorial nature including the mechanism of development for so-called symptomatic narcolepsy.

The model is composed of three graphs. The graph at the center (A) shows a two-threshold multifactorial model for the development of EHS and narcolepsy among the general population. The abscissa shows the sum of multiple genetic factors as well as various exogenous, somatic, and psychological stress factors. The shaded area represents EHS, and the dark area shows narcolepsy. When the sum of various stress factors exceeds the first threshold, EHS develops, and when the sum further exceeds the second threshold, narcolepsy develops. The graph at the left (B) shows the model for the Dw2(−) population. Since the origin is placed to the left, the sum of multiple genetic and stress factors never reaches the second threshold for narcolepsy, and it only reaches the first threshold for EHS in rare occasions. The graph at the right (C) shows the model for the DR2(+)-Dw2(+) population, which comprises about one-tenth of the general population. The origin of the abscissa is located to the right, much closer to the threshold for EHS. Although this smaller population is predisposed to narcolepsy, multiple genetic and environmental stress factors are still needed to cross the first threshold for EHS, and additional factors to reach the second threshold for narcolepsy. The area for narcolepsy in graph C corresponds with the narcolepsy area in graph A.

Age of Onset

The ages of onset of recurrent daytime naps of 506 narcoleptic patients are illustrated in Fig. 17. A conspicuous peak in the middle of the teen years is noticed, followed by greatly lowered undulations after the age of 20 years. The peak age for all narcoleptic patients is 14 years, and 70.0% of these patients had the onset of somnolence between 10 and 19 years of age.

Figure 18 shows the distribution of the age of onset of cataplexy among 362 narcoleptic patients. An almost similar, but a slightly expanded, pattern and shift to the older ages is observed as compared with the pattern for daytime somnolence. The peak age of onset of cataplexy for all patients is 15 years, and 50.3% of them had the onset of cataplexy between 10 and 19 years. The patients with onset of cataplexy at or more than 30 years were 24.0%.

Figure 19 shows the distribution of the delay in years between the onset of daytime somnolence and the onset of cataplexy in 343 narcoleptic patients. Although a marked peak is present at year 0, indicating the dominance of simultaneous onset of both somnolence and cataplexy, there are some patients with delayed onset of cataplexy, sometimes even more than 30 years. The patients with a delay of less than 5 years comprised 65.6% of all patients.

Figure 20 shows the relationship between the age of onset of daytime somnolence and the age of onset of cataplexy in each narcoleptic patient. Patients who have parents and/or siblings affected with narcolepsy (NARCO+ group) are represented by solid circles. Patients with no relatives affected with either narcolepsy

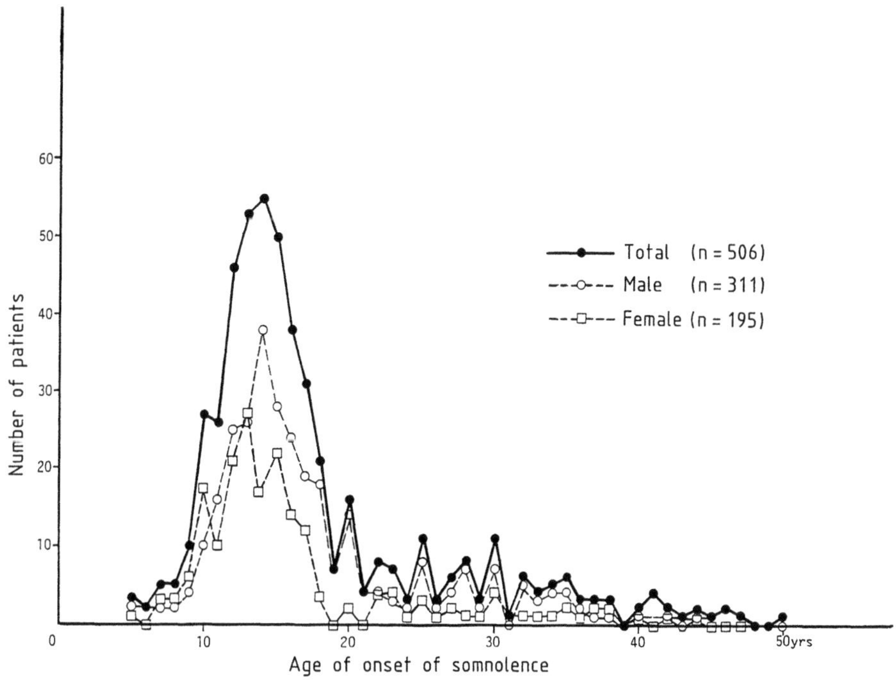

Fig. 17. Age of onset of daytime somnolence in 506 narcoleptic patients

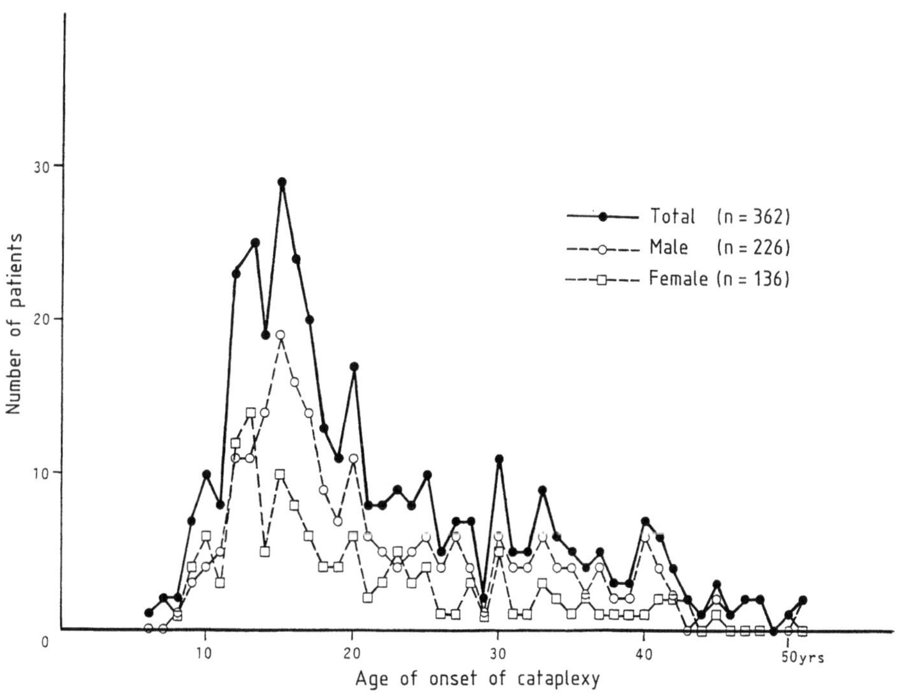

Fig. 18. Age of onset of cataplexy in 362 narcoleptic patients

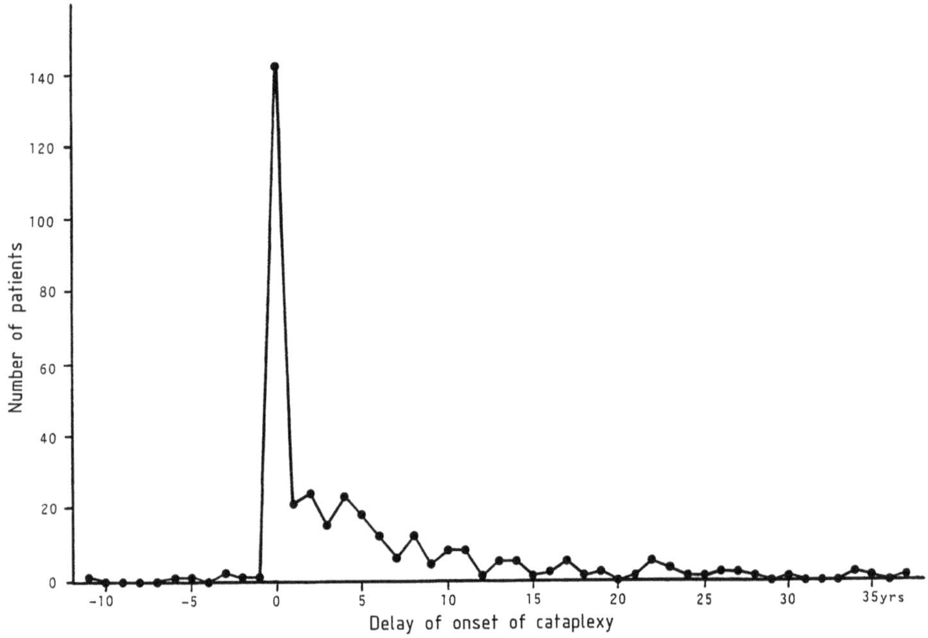

Fig. 19. Delay in years between onset of excessive daytime somnolence and onset of cataplexy in 343 narcoleptic patients (onset of cataplexy - onset of somnolence)

or EDS (NEG group) are shown with outlined circles. A concentrated pattern of ages of onset of both daytime somnolence and cataplexy is observed for the NARCO+ group, with 94.1% of them having ages of onset for both daytime somnolence and cataplexy between 10 and 20 years ($10 \leq age < 20$). On the other hand, the NEG group patients showed a much more widely distributed pattern of age of onset of both daytime somnolence and cataplexy. It is noteworthy that the onset of cataplexy showed varying periods of delays from the onset of daytime somnolence. Only 44.6% of NEG patients had ages of onset for both somnolence and cataplexy between 10 and 20 years. On the other hand, there are only a few patients with onset of cataplexy preceding the onset of daytime somnolence. The genetically loaded NARCO+ group showed a significantly younger mean age of onset of somnolence [12.7 years ± 3.1 (SD), $n = 17$] than the mean age for the genetically unremarkable NEG group [19.8 years ± 9.9 (SD), $n = 130$] (*t*-test, $P < 0.002$). It was also clear that the NARCO+ group had a significantly younger mean age of onset of cataplexy [15.4 years ± 4.5 (SD), $n = 17$] as compared with the one for the NEG group [24.7 years ± 11.5 (SD), $n = 130$] (*t*-test, $P < 0.001$).

Sex Difference

The number of narcoleptic patients who visited our hospital showed a male dominance, with a male: female ratio of 1:0.63. However, our family studies (Honda et al. 1983b and Table 2) showed no sex difference regarding the frequency of narco-

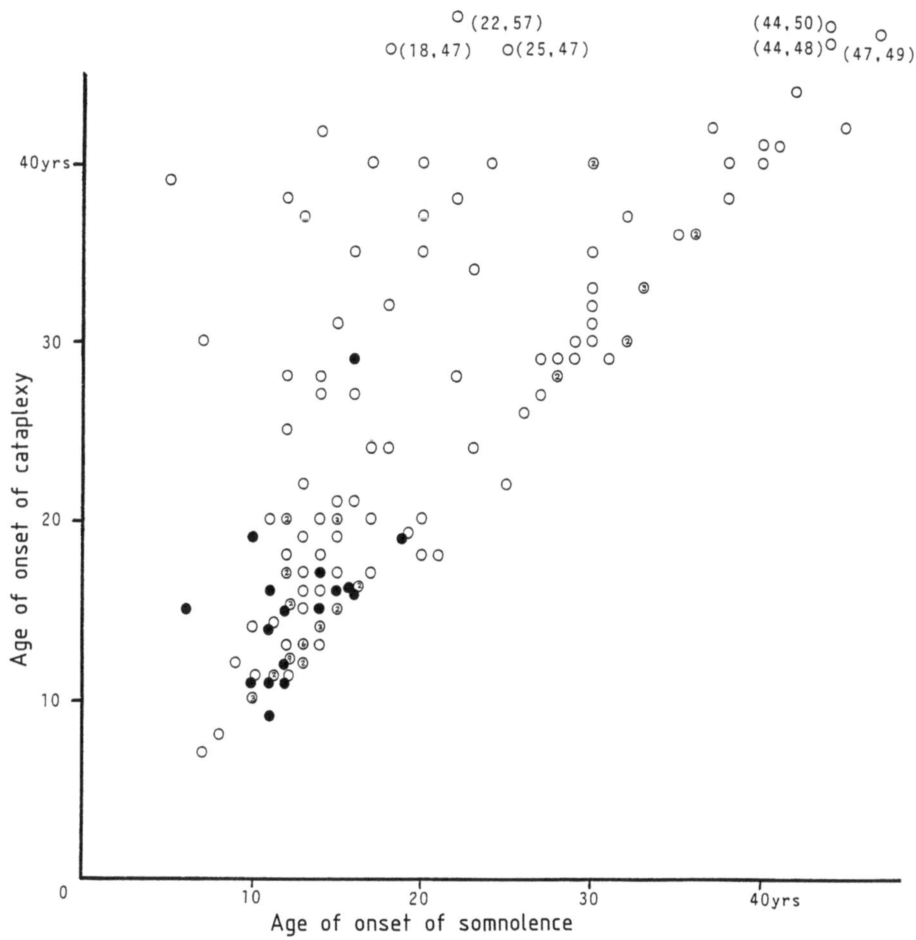

Fig. 20. Relationship between age of onset of daytime somnolence and age of onset of cataplexy. ○, narcoleptic patients without narcoleptic or EDS patients in their relatives (NEG group, $n = 130$). ●, narcoleptic patients with a narcoleptic patient in their first-degree relatives (NARCO+ group, $n = 17$)

lepsy among family members of narcolepsy probands. Therefore, the sex difference in the frequency of patients who visited our hospital is considered to be due to social factors.

The peak age of onset of daytime somnolence is 14 years in male patients and 13 years in female patients, showing a slightly younger age of onset in female patients (Fig. 17). The average age of onset of daytime somnolence is 18.22 years ± 8.16 (SD) in male patients, and 16.50 years ± 8.01 (SD) in female patients. This difference in the mean values of the age of onset of somnolence between male and female narcoleptic patients is statistically significant (t-test, $P < 0.011$), showing a slightly younger age of onset of somnolence for female narcoleptic patients.

The peak age of onset of cataplexy is 15 years for males and 13 years for female patients, showing a slightly younger age of onset in female patients (Fig. 18).

The average age of onset of cataplexy is 22.74 years ± 10.18 (SD) for males and 20.22 years ± 9.76 (SD) for females. The mean age of onset of cataplexy is slightly, yet significantly, younger in female than in male narcoleptic patients (*t*-test, $P <$ 0.011).

Prevalence of Narcolepsy

The prevalence of narcolepsy among the general population is not clear. Solomon (1945) reported 0.04%. Roth (1962) reported 0.02%-0.03% by comparing the frequency of his narcoleptic patients with that of epilepsy at his clinic in Prague. Dement et al. (1972) reported 0.06%-0.1% by using advertisements with monetary rewards to find narcoleptic patients in the San Francisco and Bay City areas. Honda (1979) reported 0.16% by a census survey on 12400 teenagers, which covered almost all of the teenagers between 12 and 16 years old in Fujisawa City, Japan, by using questionnaires filled out at school, and short, personal follow-up interviews with 500 high-scoring subjects. Prevalence of excessive daytime sleepiness without cataplexy was estimated to be 0.52%, three times higher than that of narcolepsy.

Prognosis

Reports on the long-term prognosis of narcolepsy are scarce. Ohta et al. (1980) made a 10- to 21-year follow-up study on 101 narcoleptic patients who visited the outpatient clinic, Department of Neuropsychiatry, Tokyo University Hospital, during the period 1955-1970. It was observed that each of the symptoms of the narcoleptic tetrad showed a general tendency toward gradual improvement during periods without medication. In cases without medication, disappearance of excessive daytime sleepiness was observed in 11 (10.9%) patients, cataplexy in 21 (20.8%) cases, hypnagogic hallucinations in 32 (34.8%) cases, and sleep paralysis in 39 (45.9%) cases (Table 5). There were four cases (4%) who were found free from all narcoleptic symptoms, and these were considered as cases with almost complete recovery. It was observed that so-called REM-related symptoms, such as cataplexy, hypnagogic hallucinations, and sleep paralysis improved rather early, but

Table 5. Disappearance of narcoleptic symptoms after 10-21 years (Ohta et al. 1980)

	Subject with the symptom in the past	Absence of symptom at the time of survey			Rate of disappearance
		No medication	On medication	Total	
S	101	11 (10.9%)	33	44	43.6%
C	101	21 (20.8%)	19	40	39.6%
HH	92	32 (34.8%)	17	49	53.3%
SP	85	39 (45.9%)	16	55	64.7%

S, daytime somnolence; C, cataplexy; HH, hypnagogic hallucinations; SP, sleep paralysis disorganized sleep-wake rhythm, such as recurrent daytime napping and disturbed nocturnal sleep, remained for longer periods, showing very slow improvement over many years. Aggravation and progressive worsening of the narcoleptic symptoms were rare.

Treatment

Pharmacotherapy

We usually start the treatment of narcolepsy by asking a patient to record a sleep log before administering medication (Fig. 21). This helps the patient to recognize his own disrupted patterns of nocturnal sleep. The initial effort of treatment is primarily directed to secure sound nocturnal sleep. Possible poor sleep habits and snoring at night should be treated first. Benzodiazepine derivatives or hypnotics may be administered to stabilize nocturnal sleep disruptions. We recommend a narcoleptic patient to sleep at least 7 h a night and to take a nap regularly after lunch or at a recess. Even when the patient does not feel sleepy, taking a rest on a

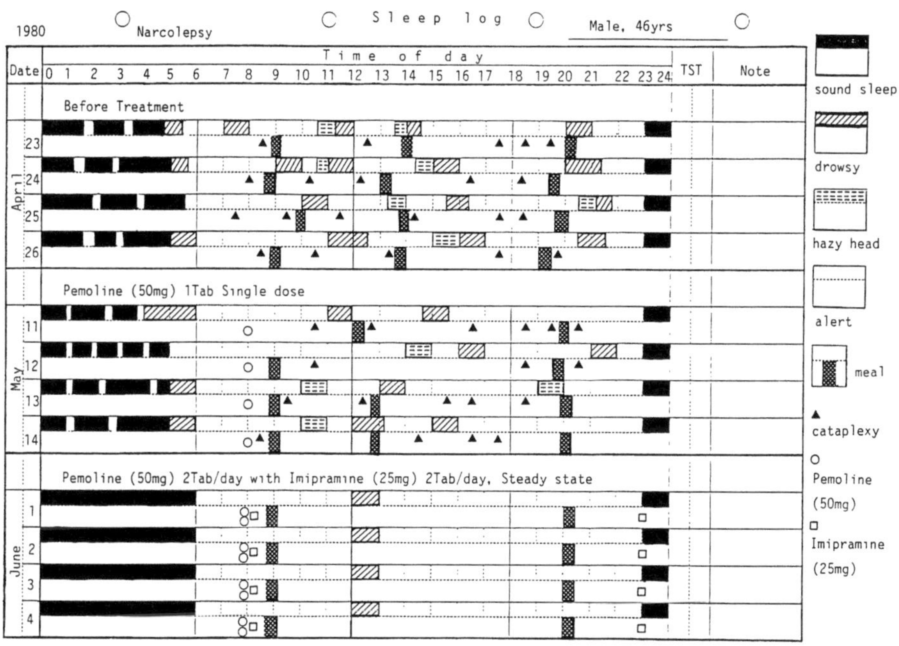

Fig. 21. A sleep log of a 46-year-old male narcoleptic patient at the beginning of pharmacotherapy. *Upper graph* shows a disrupted sleep pattern and frequent daytime napping and cataplexy recorded before medication. *Middle graph* shows slightly decreased napping in the daytime and persistence of cataplectic attacks while a single dose of 50 mg pemoline was administered in the morning. *Lower graph* shows a normalized sleep pattern and disappearance of cataplexy when a combination of 100 mg pemoline and 50 mg imipramine was administered

sofa with eyes closed for 15 min after lunch is recommended. This helps to establish the habit of taking a regularly scheduled nap, which is useful in alleviating afternoon somnolence.

After confirmation of progress in sleep habits as indicated by the sleep logs, we carefully start administration of CNS stimulants to suppress remaining daytime sleepiness. Pemoline and methylphenidate are often used in combination. Pemoline has a longer biological half-life of about 11 h, and has a rather weak potency of awakening action. Therefore, usually a single dose of 50-100 mg pemoline is given in the morning. When the awakening effect of pemoline is insufficient during the daytime, methylphenidate may be added. Methylphenidate has a much shorter half-life of about 2 h and has a sharp and strong awakening effect. Methylphenidate is given in doses of 10-40 mg both in the morning and in the early afternoon, but should not be given later than 5 p.m. The effectiveness of CNS stimulants is usually satisfactory unless the patient has complications of nocturnal sleep apnea or poor sleep habits, or is hampered by severe adverse effects such as tachycardia, a dry mouth sensation, and stomach ailments.

When adverse effects are intolerable, methamphetamine may be used to combat daytime sleepiness. The use of methamphetamine is a last resort because of the possible development of stimulant-induced hallucinatory paranoid states. Administration of CNS stimulants in the evening or at night is strictly avoided because of their possible stimulating effects on the dream mechanisms at night due to the remaining blood concentration of the stimulants. If available, determination of blood concentrations of pemoline (Nishihara et al. 1984) and methylphenidate (Nakagawa et al. 1986; Nakajima et al. 1986) is useful for adjusting doses and also for checking compliance with the prescribed medication. We recommend administering a small amount of phenothiazine derivatives before bedtime in order to block the possible remaining effect of CNS stimulants at night (Honda 1982b). Our experience shows that the development of a hallucinatory paranoid state as a result of the use of CNS stimulants in narcolepsy decreased markedly in the past 10 years since we have adopted these drug administration schedules.

To control cataplexy, 25-75 mg clomipramine or imipramine almost always show marked effectiveness. Administration of these tricyclic antidepressants more than 30 min before bedtime is also effective in suppressing hypnagogic hallucinations and sleep paralysis in addition to the removal of cataplexy on the following day. In severe cases of cataplexy, additional administration of clomipramine (10-25 mg) in the morning or before participation in exciting activities, such as making a speech, playing cards, fishing, etc., is recommended. Mild cataplexy can often be controlled by the administration of methylphenidate only.

Guidance for Living

It is necessary to secure both sufficient time and good quality of sleep at night. Routine recording of 24-h sleep-wake states by using a sleep log every day for a few months at the beginning of treatment is very helpful for motivating the patient to follow a regular schedule in his daily life. Development of oversensitive or psychotic states, such as ideas of reference and persecution or hallucinatory paranoid states, must always be carefully checked. If any sign of oversensitivity appears, the CNS stimulants should be discontinued immediately, and major tranquilizers without strong sedative effects, such as trifluoperazine, should be administered. The narcoleptic patient should be advised not to attempt to work for a longer period during the day than a normal person by increasing the amount of CNS stimulants in the daytime. This can be checked using the sleep log. Jobs involving long-distance driving, construction work in high places, heat treatment, or high-voltage cable works should be avoided. Narcoleptic patients can better adapt themselves to jobs where they can actively move around and can adjust the timing of work by their own judgment, and where there is no immediate danger involved should they fall asleep.

Activities of the Japan Narcolepsy Association (Narco-Kai)

The Japan Narcolepsy Association (JNA) is an autonomous organization composed of and managed by narcoleptic and excessively somnolent patients themselves. It was established in December 1967 at the Department of Neuropsychiatry of Tokyo University Hospital by a group of 71 narcoleptic patients (Japan Narcolepsy Association 1979; Honda 1983). The headquarters is now placed at Seiwa Hospital, Neuropsychiatric Research Institute, 91 Bentencho, Shinjuku-ku, Tokyo, 162, Japan. The aims of the JNA are cultivation of mutual friendship and support, and facilitation of self-help activities among the members. Further aims include enhancement of their social lives, a mass education campaign for a better public understanding of narcolepsy, and early detection and early treatment of narcoleptic patients. Cooperation with medical research for better medical treatment is another important objective.

The contributions of the JNA to the lives of narcoleptic patients are as follows:

(1) the patients have a place where they feel supported in talking about their embarrassing mistakes due to sleepiness, and find friends with similar needs for support and discussion;
(2) they can learn from the experiences of others in overcoming feelings of inferiority and frustrations in their daily lives; and
(3) they can have a chance to change their attitudes toward life in terms of social introvertedness, and acquire a motivation to engage in socially active and productive lives.

The activities of the JNA benefit physicians in the following ways:

(1) formation of an intimate and trustful therapeutic relationship between the physicians in charge and the patients;
(2) cultivation of patients' knowledge of narcolepsy, correct usage of medicines, and prompt detection of possible adverse effects and taking countermeasures;
(3) greater understanding of the social and home lives of the patients for better and more personalized guidance for living; and
(4) assurance of regular visits of the patients to the narcolepsy clinic and the opportunity for long-term observations about the clinical course of narcolepsy.

The social impact of the JNA includes:

(1) public education for a better understanding of narcolepsy and encouragement of narcoleptic patients to visit specialized clinics;
(2) offering information on narcolepsy to family members and to superiors and colleagues at the patient's place of employment;
(3) acquisition of necessary drugs available through the national health insurance system for the treatment of narcolepsy;
(4) appeals to increase the interest of physicians who have some interest in the treatment of narcolepsy;
(5) surveillance of misinformed descriptions of narcolepsy in the mass media, and providing correct advice; and
(6) communication and networking with other narcolepsy associations throughout the world.

Since its foundation, the Japan Narcolepsy Association has striven to achieve the above objectives and to reach out to narcoleptic patients and their families. Of special significance will be its contribution in facilitating early detection and early treatment of narcoleptic patients in their mid-teens. It is at this time when narcoleptic patients are most liable to develop personal difficulties in self-perception and are likely to confront strong and stressful challenges such as entrance into college and seeking good jobs. The handling of sleepy students at school will be an important yet hopefully manageable educational as well as social problem in the future.

Acknowledgments. Our appreciation is extended to the members of the Japan Narcolepsy Association who willingly cooperated with our research. Thanks are also due to Mrs. Mitsuko Matsuyama and Miss Kimiko Sugiyama for their secretarial and technical assistance. We are also grateful to Patricia McDonald-Scott, Ph. D. and Ms. Nancy Baxer for their critical comments and help in preparing the manuscript. This paper was supported in part by Grant-In-Aid for Co-Operative Research from the Japanese Ministry of Education, Science, and Culture.

References

Adie WJ (1926) Idiopathic narcolepsy: a disease sui generis, with remarks on the mechanism of sleep. Brain 49: 257-306

Akimoto H, Honda Y, Takahashi Y (1960) Pharmacotherapy in narcolepsy. Dis Nerv Syst 21: 704-706

Akimoto H, Nakakuki M, Honda Y, Takahashi Y, Toyoda J, Sasaki K, Machiyama T (1961) Clinical evaluation of the effect of central stimulants, MAO inhibitors, and imipramine in the treatment of affective disorders. Proceedings of the third world congress of psychiatry, Montreal, pp 958-963

Asaka A (1981) Genetic markers and neuropsychiatric disorders (in Japanese). Jpn J Clin Psychiat [Rinsho Seishin Igaku] 10: 401-414

Asaka A, Park K, Honda Y, Kuroiwa Y, Tsuji S, Hamaguchi H, Akizuki M, Matsumoto H, Omoto K (1981) Studies on genetic markers in intractable diseases. In: Watanabe I (ed) Annual report of Research Committee on Host Factors of Intractable Diseases, for the year 1980 (in Japanese). Ministry of Health and Welfare, Tokyo, pp 123-131

Association of Sleep Disorders Centers and Association for the Psychophysiological Study of Sleep (1979) Diagnostic classification of sleep and arousal disorders. Sleep 2: 1-137
Baraitser M, Parkes JD (1987) Genetic study of narcoleptic syndrome. J Med Genet 15: 254-259
Carskadon MA, Dement WC (1977) Sleep tendency: an objective measure of sleep loss. Sleep Res 6: 200
Carskadon MA, Dement WC, Mitler MM, Roth T, Westbrook PR, Keenan S (1987) Guidelines for the multiple sleep latency test (MSLT): a standard measure of sleepiness. Sleep 9: 519-524
Dement W, Zarcone V, Varner V, Hoddes E, Nassau S, Jacobs B, Brown J, McDonald A, Horan K, Glass R, Gonzales P, Friedman E, Phillips R (1972) The prevalence of narcolepsy. In: Chase MH, Stern WC, Walter PL (eds) Sleep research, vol. 1. Brain Information Service/Brain Research Institute, UCLA, Los Angeles, p 148
Edwards JH (1967) Familial predisposition in man. Br Med Bull 25: 58-64
Falconer D (1965) The inheritance of liability to certain diseases estimated from the incidence among relatives. Ann Hum Genet 29: 51-76
Guilleminault C, Phillips R, Dement W (1975) A syndrome of hypersomnia with automatic behavior. Electroencephalogr Clin Neurophysiol 38: 403-413
Honda Y (1960) Clinical studies on the diencephalon-related psychic symptoms (in Japanese). Psychiatr Neurol Jpn 62: 297-325
Honda Y (1972) Treatment of narcolepsy (in Japanese). In: Hirai T, Hara T, Hozaki H (eds) Treatments in psychiatry [Seishinka Chiryo-gaku]. Kanahara, Tokyo, pp 327-333
Honda Y (1979) Census of narcolepsy, cataplexy and sleep life among teenagers in Fujisawa city. Sleep Res 8: 191
Honda Y (1982a) A trial of application of DSM-III diagnosis to narcoleptic patients with hallucinatory paranoid states (in Japanese). Jpn J Clin Psychiatry [Rinsho Seishin Igaku] 11: 239-246
Honda Y (1982b) Narcolepsy and related hypersomnias. In: Ueda H, Shimazono Y, Takeuchi J, Toyokura Y (eds) Sleep disorders (in Japanese). Nankodo, Toyko, pp 199-224
Honda Y (1982c) Narcolepsy and its differential diagnosis from epilepsy (in Japanese). Neurol Med 16: 34-40
Honda Y (1983) Activities of the Japan Narcolepsy Association (in Japanese). Jpn J Clin Psychiatry [Rinsho Seishin Igaku] 12: 1525-1530
Honda Y, Hishikawa Y (1980) A long-term treatment of narcolepsy and excessive daytime sleepiness with pemoline (Betanamin). Curr Ther Res 27: 429-441
Honda Y, Takahashi Y (1969) Clinical evaluation of some psychotropic drugs (lithium carbonate, pyrithioxine, chlomipramine) in narcolepsy (in Japanese). Annu Rep Pharmacopsychiatry Res Foundation 1: 56-60
Honda Y, Takahashi Y (1971) Psychotic states observed during long-term administration of psychostimulants in narcolepsy (in Japanese). Annu Rep Pharmacopsychiatry Res Foundation 3: 164-169
Honda Y, Takahashi Y, Suzuki J, Nishiyama A, Hosoki A, Ohno H, Furusawa Y, Nagatsuka K (1965) Psychic symptoms of narcoleptics, with special reference to their personality characteristics (in Japanese). Psychiatr Neurol Jpn [Seishin Shinkeigaku Zasshi] 67: 195
Honda Y, Takahashi K, Takahashi S, Azumi K, Irie M et al. (1969) Growth hormone secretion during nocturnal sleep in normal subjects. J Clin Endocrinol Metab 29: 20-29
Honda Y, Hishikawa Y, Takahashi Y (1979) Long-term treatment of narcolepsy with methylphenidate (Ritalin). Curr Ther Res 25: 288-298
Honda Y, Asaka A, Tanaka Y, Juji T (1983a) Discrimination of narcoleptic patients by using genetic markers and HLA. Sleep Res 12: 254
Honda Y, Asaka A, Tanimura M, Furusho T (1983b) A genetic study of narcolepsy and excessive daytime sleepiness in 308 families with a narcolepsy or hypersomnia proband. In: Guilleminault C, Lugaresi E (eds) Sleep/wake disorders; natural history, epidemiology and long-term evolution. Raven, New York, pp 187-199
Honda Y, Doi Y, Juji T, Satake M (1984) Narcolepsy and HLA: postive DR2 as a prerequisite for the development of narcolepsy. Folia Psychiatr Neurol Jpn 38: 360
Honda Y, Juji T, Matsuki K, Naohara T, Satake M, Inoko H, Someya T, Harada S, Doi Y (1986a) HLA-DR2 and Dw2 in narcolepsy and in other disorders of excessive somnolence without cataplexy. Sleep 9: 133-142

Honda Y, Doi Y, Ninomiya R, Ninomiya C (1986b) Increased frequency of non-insulin-dependent diabetes mellitus among narcoleptic patients. Sleep 9: 254-259

Japan Narcolepsy Association (1979) Toward the better understanding of narcolepsy - invitation to the Japan Narcolepsy Association (Narco-Kai). Japan Narcolepsy Association, Tokyo

Kessler S (1975) Genetic factors in narcolepsy. In: Guilleminault WC, Dement C, Passouant P (eds) Narcolepsy. Spectrum, New York, pp 285-302

Krüger J (1973) Zur Unterscheidung zwischen multifaktoriellem Erbgang mit Schwellenwerteffekt und einfachem diallelem Erbgang. Humangenetik 17: 181-252

Lhermitte J, Tournay A (1927) Le sommeil normal et pathologique. Rev Neurol (Paris) 1: 751-822; 885-887

Maury A (1848) Des hallucinations hypnagogiques (ou des erreurs de sens). Ann Med Psychol II: 26-40

Mitchell SW (1876) On some of the disorders of sleep. Virginia Med Monthly 2: 769-781

Mitler MM, van den Hoed J, Carskadon MA et al. (1979) REM sleep episodes during the multiple sleep test in narcoleptic patients. EEG Clin Neurophysiol 46: 479-481

Nakagawa F, Saitoh Y, Kotaki H, Nakajima K, Honda Y (1986) Dosage adjustment of methylphenidate for patients with narcolepsy: determination of methylphenidate and its main metabolite in plasma by gas chromatography-chemical ionization mass spectrometry (in Japanese). Annu Rep Pharmacopsychiatry Res Foundation 17: 15-20

Nakagawa Y (1980) Continuous observation of EEG patterns at night and in daytime of normal subjects under restrained conditions. I. Quiescent state when lying down. Electroencephalogr Clin Neurophysiol 49: 524-537

Nakajima K, Kotaki H, Saitoh Y, Nakagawa F (1986) Determination of methylphenidate and its main metabolite in plasma by gas chromatography-chemical ionization mass spectrometry. Chem Pharm Bull (Tokyo) 34: 1701-1708

Nevsimalova-Bruhova S, Roth B (1972) Heredofamilial aspects of narcolepsy and hypersomnia. Arch Suisses Neurol Neurochir Psychiatr 110: 45-54

Nishihara K, Kohda Y, Saitoh Y, Nakagawa F, Honda Y (1984) Determination of pemoline in plasma, plasma water, mixed salive, and urine by high-performance liquid chromatography. Ther Drug Monit 6: 232-237

Ohta T, Honda Y, Kameyama T, Kurita H, Takahashi Y (1980) A long-term prognosis of narcolepsy: 10-20 year follow-up study of patients diagnosed as narcolepsy during 1958-1969 (in Japanese). Jpn J Clin Psychiatr [Rinsho Seishin Igaku] 9: 485-493

Penrose LS (1953) The genetical background of common diseases. Acta Genet 4: 257-265

Rechtschaffen A, Wolpert W, Dement W, Mitchell S, Fischer C (1963) Nocturnal sleep of narcoleptics. Electroencephalogr Clin Neurophysiol 15: 599-609

Reich T, James J, Morris C (1972) The use of multiple thresholds in determining the mode of transmission of semi-continuous traits. Ann Hum Genet 36: 163-184

Richardson GS, Carskadon MA, Flagg W, van den Hoed J, Dement WC, Mitler MM (1978) Excessive daytime sleepiness in man: multiple sleep latency measurement in narcoleptic and control subjects. Electroencephalogr Clin Neurophysiol 45: 621-627

Rosenthal C (1928) Über die krankhaften Dissoziationszustände bei der echten Narkolepsie und dem verzögerten psychomotorischen Erwachen (Wachanfälle). Arch Psychiatr 84: 120-180

Rosenthal C (1939) Über das Auftreten von halluzinatorisch-kataplektischem Angstsyndrom, Wachanfällen und ähnlichen Störungen bei Schizophrenen. Monatsschr Psychiatr Neurol (Basel) 102: 11-38

Roth B (1962) Narkolepsie und Hypersomnie vom Standpunkt der Physiologie des Schlafes. VEB Verlag Volk und Gesundheit, Berlin

Roth B (1980) Narcolepsy and hypersomnia. Karger, Basel

Solomon P (1945) Narcolepsy in negroes. Dis Nerv Syst 6: 179-183

Suzuki J (1966) Narcolepsy syndrome and paradoxical sleep. Folia Psychiatr Neurol Jpn 20: 123-149

Takahashi K, Takahashi S, Azumi K, Honda Y, Utena H (1971) Changes of plasma growth hormone during nocturnal sleep in normals and in hypersomniac patients (in Japanese). Adv Neurol Sci [Shinkei Kenkyu-no Shimpo] 14: 743-754

Takahashi Y (1977) Pathophysiology of narcolepsy (in Japanese). Clin Physiol [Rinsho-seiri] 7: 5-15

Takahashi Y (1979) Growth hormone secretion related to the sleep and waking rhythm. In: Drucker-Colin R, Shkurovich M, Sterman MB (eds) The functions of sleep. Academic, New York, pp 113-145
Takahashi Y, Honda Y (1964a) Pharmacotherapy in narcolepsy; part I: effects of central nervous system stimulants (in Japanese). Clin Psychiatry [Seishin Igaku] 6: 673-682
Takahashi Y, Honda Y (1964b) Pharmacotherapy in narcolepsy; part II: effects of thymoleptics and other psychotropic drugs (in Japanese). Clin Psychiatry [Seishin Igaku] 6: 775-784
Takahashi Y, Jimbo M (1963) Polygraphic study of narcoleptic syndrome with special reference to hypnagogic halucinations and cataplexy. Folia Psychiatr Neurol Jpn [Suppl] 7: 343-347
Takahashi Y, Kipnis DM, Daughaday WH (1968) Growth hormone secretion during sleep. J Clin Invest 47: 2079-2090
Thomson G (1975) Narcolepsy: theoretical aspects of a genetic study. In: Guilleminault C, Dement WC, Passouant P (eds) Narcolepsy. Spectrum, New York, pp 303-310
Thomson G (1985) The mode of inheritance of the HLA-linked gene predisposing to narcolepsy. Tissue Antigens 26: 201-203
Utena H, Honda Y, Takahashi S, Takahashi K (1968) Correlation between brain activities during sleep and humoral changes - time course of changes of plasma growth hormone and cortisol levels during nocturnal sleep. In: Shimazono Y (ed) Annual Report of Research Committee on the Mechanism of Development of Disturbance of Consciousness, for the year 1967 (in Japanese). Ministry of Education, Science and Culture, Tokyo
Vogel G (1960) Studies in psychophysiology of dreams. III. The dream of narcolepsy. Arch Gen Psychiatry 3: 421-428
Wilson R, Raynal D, Guilleminault C, Zarcon V, Dement W (1972) REM latencies in daytime sleep recordings of narcoleptics. Sleep Res 2: 166
Wilson SAK (1928) The narcolepsies. Brain 51: 63-109
Yoss RE, Daly DD (1959) Treatment of narcolepsy with Ritalin. Neurology 9: 171-173

Chapter 3

HLA in Narcolepsy in Japan

K. MATSUKI, Y. HONDA, M. SATAKE, and T. JUJI

In April 1973, two independent groups in the United States (Schlosstein et al. 1973) and in England (Brewerton et al. 1973) reported a strong association between ankylosing spondylitis and HLA-B27. This was the strongest association between a disease and an HLA antigen for more than 10 years. The association between ankylosing spondylitis and B27 had a relative risk of 70 (Brewerton et al. 1973): a person with B27 was 70 times more likely to develop ankylosing spondylitis than a person without B27. No other diseases had shown a higher relative risk until 1984.

In 1984, a disease with a higher relative risk than that of ankylosing spondylitis was first described: narcolepsy. All the patients with narcolepsy had DR2. The relative risk was theoretically infinite: a person without DR2 had virtually no chance of developing narcolepsy. This strong association was first observed in Japanese (Honda et al. 1984a, b, 1985, 1986; Juji et al. 1984, 1985; Matsuki et al. 1985a) and later in Caucasians in England (Langdon et al. 1984), France (Billiard and Seignalet 1985), Canada (Poirier et al. 1986), the Federal Republic of Germany (Mueller-Eckhardt et al. 1986; Andreas-Zietz et al. 1986), Czechoslovakia (Andreas-Zietz et al. 1986), and Australia (Juji et al. 1986).

In this chapter, we will summarize current findings on HLA and narcolepsy in the Japanese population.

Definition of Narcolepsy

The first step in biological research on any disease is to define the disease clearly using strict operational diagnostic criteria. This vital process appears to have been previously absent in research on narcolepsy. Because the ideas conveyed by the word "narcolepsy" are different among investigators, the first issue to be addressed must be the definition of narcolepsy.

Narcolepsy. Narcolepsy is a very homogeneous disease entity defined by the following criteria: (a) recurrent daytime naps and/or lapses into sleep which occur almost every day over a period of at least 6 months and (b) clinical confirmation of cataplexy in the patient's history. Daytime napping and cataplexy must be present concurrently in the patient's history.

In the above-mentioned criteria, cataplexy also needs clarification. It is defined as attacks of sudden bilateral loss of the tone of skeletal muscles, triggered by sudden wave(s) of strong emotion, such as laughter, feelings of elation, anger, or surprise. Cataplectic attacks should not be accompanied by loss of consciousness. Muscle weakness occurring at sleepy moments or occurring when emotional excitement is absent cannot be considered a pathognomonic symptom.

One of the characteristics of narcoleptic cataplexy is its responsiveness to clomipramine treatment. Drop attacks of the elderly, collapse of the whole body from orthostatic hypotension, akinetic or astatic seizures of epilepsy, and muscle weakness of such neuromuscular disorders as multiple sclerosis may mimic narcoleptic cataplexy, but they are generally unresponsive to clomipramine.

Essential Hypersomnia. This category is defined by the following criteria:

(a) recurrent daytime sleepiness which occurs almost every day over a period of at least 6 months;
(b) absence of cataplexy, and
(c) not due to other known disorders associated with daytime somnolence, such as sleep-apnea syndrome.

Unlike narcolepsy, which is a single homogeneous disease entity, essential hypersomnia is a heterogeneous mixture of various etiologies.

Excessive Daytime Somnolence. This term is used to denote morbid daytime somnolence without confirmation of cataplexy based on the information obtained from family members.

HLA Antigen Frequencies in Japanese Narcoleptic Patients

Up to now, we have typed HLA antigens for 190 patients with narcolepsy, with all the previously reported cases included. All met the aforementioned criteria. The diagnosis of each patient was made clinically before the HLA typing.

HLA antigen frequencies in the patients are listed in Tables 1 and 2. There were no patients who did not express DR2 or DQw1. Complete association between DR2, DQw1, and narcolepsy still holds true in our series. The frequencies of DQw3 and DR antigens other than DR2 were generally lower than those of controls. Relative risks were 753 and 174 for DR2 and DQw1, respectively.

As for class I antigens, A2, B35, Bw67, Cw3, and Cw7 increased in frequency. B7, which increased in Caucasian narcoleptics (Seignalet and Billiard 1984; Langdon et al. 1984; Mueller-Eckhardt et al. 1986), decreased in the Japanese patients. Aw33 and B44, which are in linkage disequilibrium with DRw13 in normal Japanese (Fujii et al. 1983), also decreased. Bw52 and Bw59 decreased significantly, too.

Splits of the DQw1 Antigen

Only three DQ antigen specificities are known at present, namely DQw1, DQw2, and DQw3. However, evidence has accumulated to indicate that the DQ antigens can be split into more than three specificities (Park and Terasaki 1984; Ferrara et

Table 1. HLA class I frequencies in Japanese narcolepsy

Ag	Patient (n=190)	Control[a] (n=310)	χ^2	Relative risk	$\log_{10} P$
A1	1 (0.5%)	3 (1.0%)			
A2	104 (54.7%)	127 (41.0%)	8.99	1.74	−2.57
A3	0 (0.0%)	5 (1.6%)			
A11	41 (21.6%)	56 (18.1%)			
A24	95 (50.0%)	185 (59.7%)	− 4.48	0.68	−1.46
A26	52 (27.4%)	65 (21.0%)			
A31	30 (15.8%)	50 (16.1%)			
Aw33	18 (9.5%)	50 (16.1%)	− 4.44	0.54	−1.46
B7	5 (2.6%)	35 (11.3%)	−12.00	0.21	−3.27
B13	1 (0.5%)	11 (3.5%)			
B27	2 (1.1%)	1 (0.3%)			
B35	64 (33.7%)	55 (17.7%)	16.51	2.35	−4.32
B37	2 (1.1%)	3 (1.0%)			
B39	24 (12.6%)	23 (7.4%)			
B44	12 (6.3%)	39 (12.6%)	− 5.05	0.47	−1.61
Bw46	8 (4.2%)	26 (8.4%)			
Bw48	9 (4.7%)	14 (4.5%)			
B51	41 (21.6%)	53 (17.1%)			
Bw52	13 (6.8%)	72 (23.2%)	−22.41	0.24	−5.66
Bw54	27 (14.2%)	45 (14.5%)			
Bw55	6 (3.2%)	21 (6.8%)			
Bw56	5 (2.6%)	3 (1.0%)			
Bw59	1 (0.5%)	13 (4.2%)	− 4.55	0.12	−1.48
Bw60	20 (10.5%)	41 (13.2%)			
Bw61	34 (17.9%)	56 (18.1%)			
Bw62	46 (24.2%)	65 (21.0%)			
Bw67	17 (8.9%)	5 (1.6%)	15.07	5.99	−3.98
Bw4	66 (34.7%)	170 (54.8%)	−19.10	0.44	−4.91
Bw6	173 (91.1%)	274 (88.4%)			
Cw1	42 (22.1%)	85 (27.4%)			
Cw3	118 (62.1%)	142 (45.8%)	12.54	1.94	−3.40
Cw4	12 (6.3%)	33 (10.6%)			
Cw5	0 (0.0%)	3 (1.0%)			
Cw7	53 (27.9%)	60 (19.4%)	4.91	1.61	−1.57

[a] Controls were randomly selected healthy Japanese

al. 1984; Duquesnoy and Marrari 1984; Satake et al. 1986; Matsuki 1986; Matsuki et al. 1985b, 1986). At the DNA level, DQw1 can be divided further into several clusters. Cohen et al. (1984) first described clusters of restriction fragments within DQw1 using a DQ beta gene probe. They designated one such cluster as "DQR1." This cluster is included in DQw1 and associated with most of DR1, a part of DRw6, and a short split of DR2. Another cluster, named "DQR2,6", is also included in DQw1 and associated with most of DR2 and a part of DRw6.

It is unclear at this time if there are phenotypical counterparts to these gene clusters. We have presented a possible split of DQw1, TB23 (Satake et al. 1986; Matsuki 1986; Matsuki et al. 1985b, 1986). This split is associated with most of DR1, a part of DRw6, and DR2 short, and is considered to be a serological coun-

Table 2. HLA class II frequencies in Japanese narcolepsy

Ag	Patient ($n=190$)	Control[a] ($n=310$)	χ^2	Relative risk	$\log_{10} P$
DR1	4 (2.1%)	45 (14.5%)	−19.15	0.13	− 4.92
DR2	190 (100.0%)	104 (33.5%)	211.99	752.89	−35.0
DR4	63 (33.2%)	125 (40.3%)			
DRw8	17 (8.9%)	84 (27.1%)	−24.07	0.26	− 6.03
DRw9	20 (10.5%)	85 (27.4%)	−20.26	0.31	− 5.17
DRw10	1 (0.5%)	2 (0.6%)			
DRw11	8 (4.2%)	20 (6.5%)			
DRw12	17 (8.9%)	41 (13.2%)			
DRw13	10 (5.3%)	51 (16.5%)	−13.77	0.28	− 3.68
DRw14	5 (2.6%)	8 (2.6%)			
DRw52	57 (30.0%)	178 (57.4%)	−35.55	0.32	− 8.61
DRw53	83 (43.7%)	189 (61.0%)	−14.19	0.50	− 3.78
DQw1	190 (100.0%)	213 (68.7%)	71.77	173.99	−16.6
DQw3	70 (36.8%)	157 (50.6%)	− 9.05	0.57	− 2.58

[a] Controls were randomly selected healthy Japanese

Table 3. Frequencies of possible DQw1 split antigens

Ag	Patients	Controls[a]	χ^2	Relative risk	Pc[b]
TB22	($n=140$) 15 (10.7%)	($n=102$) 30 (29.4%)	− 5.18	0.48	0.046
TB23	($n=139$) 17 (12.2%)	($n=142$) 32 (22.5%)	−13.63	0.29	0.00045

[a] Controls were DQw1-positive normal Japanese
[b] *P* values corrected by multiplying the number of examined antigens

terpart of "DQR1" (Matsuki 1986). The presence of a serological counterpart of the "DQR2,6" cluster has been postulated but is yet to be confirmed (Ferrara et al. 1984).

Another possible serological split of DQw1 in Japanese is called TB22. This antigen is associated with most of the Bw52-DR2-Dw12 haplotypes (Maeda et al. 1983).

The frequencies of TB22 and TB23 in narcoleptics are shown in Table 3. These possible splits of the DQw1 antigen decreased significantly. This indicates that TB22 and TB23 are not associated with narcolepsy. Analysis with restriction fragment length polymorphism (RFLP) revealed that it is the "DQR2,6" cluster that is associated with narcolepsy (Inoko et al. 1986; Juji et al. 1986; Marcadet et al. 1985).

Table 4. Estimated haplotype frequencies

Haplotypes	Narcolepsy[a] (*n*=190)		Controls[b] (*n*=414)		*P*
	Mean	SD	Mean	SD	
B35-DR2	186	55	11	2	<0.001
Bw62-DR2	129	54	16	3	<0.025
B51-DR2	114	54	9	2	<0.05
Bw61-DR2	94	53	6	2	<0.05
Bw54-DR2	74	53	3	2	
Bw52-DR2	35	52	110	7	

[a] Haplotype frequencies and standard deviations (SD) in narcoleptics (per 1000) were calculated with the formulae given by Mittal et al. (1972)

[b] Control haplotype frequencies and standard deviations (SD) in the general Japanese population (per 1000) were obtained from the family study data at the Eighth Japan HLA Workshop (Fujii et al. 1983)

Haplotype Frequencies

One of the intriguing findings in the HLA class I antigens in Japanese narcoleptics is the significant decrease of the Bw52 frequency. In normal Japanese, the association between DR2 and Bw52 is strong: about 60% of the DR2-positive Japanese have Bw52 (Fujii et al. 1983). When we first found this decrease of Bw52 (Honda et al. 1983a), our initial assumption was that DR2 would be decreased. Actually, DR2 was present in all the patients.

The large number of the narcoleptic patients enabled us to analyze haplotype frequencies statistically. A haplotype is a group of closely linked genes on a chromosome inherited from one parent. Table 4 shows the estimation of haplotype frequencies computed using the formulae of Mittal et al. (1972). The frequency of Bw52-DR2 decreased to about one-third of that in the normal controls ($0.05 < P < 0.10$). On the other hand, the frequencies of the less common haplotypes in normal Japanese, such as B35-DR2, Bw62-DR2, and B51-DR2, increased significantly.

HLA-D specificities appear to differ between these haplotypes. The haplotye Bw52-DR2 usually carries Dw12 (Reinsmoen et al. 1978), while other haplotypes which increased in narcolepsy, such as B35-DR2, Bw62-DR2, and B51-DR2, carry Dw2 (Matsuki et al. 1985a; Honda et al. 1986). The differences between these haplotypes are summarized in Table 5. It is the Dw2 haplotype and not the Dw12 haplotype that is associated with Japanese narcoleptics.

Family Study

Seventeen families were examined to deduce disease-susceptibility HLA haplotypes (Fig. 1). Table 6 shows the DR2-positive haplotypes which were associated with narcolepsy.

Table 5. A schematic representation of the differences between the two DR2 haplotypes in Japanese

Allele	Dw2 haplotype	Dw12 haplotype
HLA-B[a]	35, 51, w62	w52
C4	A3 B2	A2 BQ0
BF	F	S
C2	C	C
HLA-DR	2	2
HLA-D	w2	w12
HLA-DQ	w1	w1
TB22	Negative	Positive
DQ RFLP EcoRI	2.4 kb	18 kb
PstI	12 kb	12 kb
BamHI	2.9 kb	
Frequencies[b]		
in DR2 positive normals	40%	60%
in narcoleptics	100%	3.5%

[a] Only the most common HLA-B, C4, BF, and C2 antigens were listed

[b] About 40% and 60% of the DR2-positive normal subjects have the Dw2 and Dw12 haplotypes, respectively. The Dw12 haplotypes were found in 3.5% of the narcoleptics (see Table 4), probably only in DR2/DR2 homozygotes. Our hypothesis is that Dw2 is present in all the patients (Juji et al. 1984)

Table 6. DR2 haplotypes in families studied

Family	Narcolepsy-associated DR2-positive haplotype				
1	a:A2	Cw1	Bw54	DR2	DQw1
2	a:A24	C-	Bw52	DR2	DQw1
3	a:A24	Cw3	B51	DR2	DQw1
4	a:A26	Cw3	B35	DR2	DQw1
5	a:A24	C-	B51	DR2	DQw1
6	a:A31	Cw3	B35	DR2	DQw1
7	a:A2	Cw3	B35	DR2	DQw1
8	a:A24	Cw3	BW62	DR2	DQw1
9	a:A2	Cw1	Bw54	DR2	DQw1
	c:A11	Cw7	Bw67	DR2	DQw1
	d:Aw33	C-	B44	DR2	DQw1
10	a:A30	C-	B13	DR2	DQw1
11	a:A24	C-	Bw61	DR2	DQw1
12	a:A11	Cw7	Bw67	DR2	DQw1
13	a:A24	C-	Bw61	DR2	DQw1
14	a:A26	Cw3	Bw61	DR2	DQw1
15	a:A2	Cw3	B35	DR2	DQw1
16	a:A2	Cw3	B35	DR2	DQw1
17	a:A26	C-	Bw60	DR2	DQw1

Haplotype *a* was considered to be disease associated in all the families, except for the family 9 where three haplotypes were DR2 positive; C-, C blank

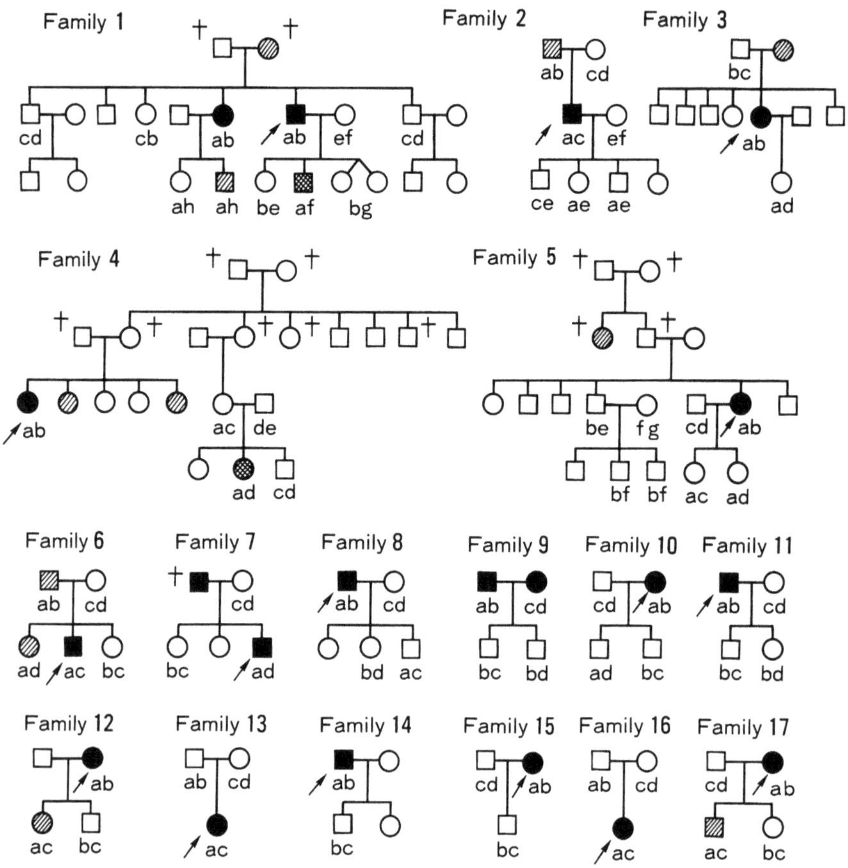

Fig. 1. Family pedigrees. *Arrows* indicate probands; *closed symbols*, narcolepsy; *cross-hatched*, essential hypersomnia; hatched, excessive daytime sleepiness; *open*, normal. *a, b, c, etc.* indicate deduced haplotypes

The most frequent haplotype was Cw3-B35-DR2-DQw1, but various other haplotypes were also deduced from the families. This is in contrast with the data on German narcoleptic patients (Mueller-Eckhardt et al. 1986). In the German study, the haplotypes in association with narcolepsy were fairly constant: 10 DR2 haplotypes deduced from 14 families carried B7. This is mainly due to the ethnic difference in the haplotype association. In Caucasians, the association between B7 and DR2/Dw2 is fairly strong, while in Japanese, various B-locus antigens are associated with DR2/Dw2, and the associations are generally weak.

The common haplotype in normal Japanese, A24-C blank-Bw52-DR2, was less frequent in narcoleptic patients. Only one haplotype (family 2 in Fig. 1 and Table 6) carried Bw52. It should be noted that this haplotype was different from the usual Bw52-DR2-Dw12 haplotype: this haplotye carried a complement allele, C4A13J (Matsuki et al. 1985a), whereas the usual Bw52-DR2-Dw12 haplotype carries C4A2 (Tokunaga et al. 1985).

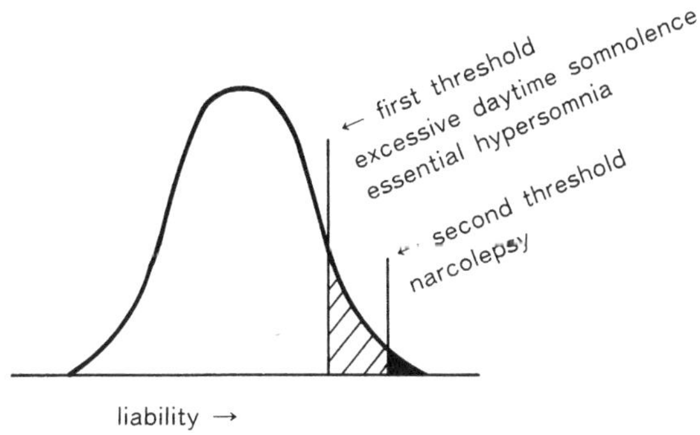

Fig. 2. Multifactorial inheritance with two thresholds. The disease liability shows a normal distribution. Individuals to the right of the first threshold and to the left of the second threshold *(in the hatched area)* develop excessive daytime somnolence or essential hypersomnia. Only those to the right of the second threshold *(in the black area)* develop narcolepsy

Genetic Model

Two-Threshold Multifactorial Model

Our study also showed that familial occurrence of narcolepsy is not a very frequent phenomenon. Many family members shared the same disease-susceptibility HLA haplotype as the proband and never developed narcolepsy. Actually, in the 17 families, 22 subjects shared the same disease-susceptibility haplotype as the proband. Among them, 1 subject suffered from narcolepsy, 2 from essential hypersomnia, 6 from excessive daytime somnolence, and the remaining 13 subjects did not show any symptoms of narcolepsy. This finding indicates that some factor(s) other than DR2 is required for the full manifestation of narcolepsy.

The two-threshold multifactorial model (Kessler et al. 1974; Honda et al. 1983b) provides one possible explanation for these results. According to this model, multiple factors contribute to the liability for narcolepsy (Fig. 2). When the sum of the liability exceeds the first threshold, excessive daytime somnolence or essential hypersomnia will develop. Narcolepsy becomes manifest when the total liability crosses the second threshold.

When a subject has DR2, the manifestation of the disease will be dependent on other liability factors. If the total liability is below the first threshold, then narcolepsy will never develop even if the subject is DR2 positive. It is only after the total liability exceeds the second threshold that the subject develops narcolepsy.

When a subject is DR2 negative, the subject is most likely never to develop narcolepsy even if all other liability factors are present. The DR2-linked susceptibility gene has a special significance in this model as a prerequisite factor.

The heritability of this liability was previously computed from the frequencies of narcolepsy in the general population and in relatives of the patients. The calculated heritabilites were generally high: 0.82 by Leckman and Gershon (1976), 0.741 by Kessler (1976), and 0.63 by Honda et al. (1983b)

Dominant Mode of Inheritance with Incomplete Penetrance

Another possible model for narcolepsy is a single-allele dominant model with incomplete penetrance. Previous analyses on the HLA antigen genotype frequencies among patients favored the additive and dominant mode of inheritance for the DR2-linked disease susceptibility gene (Langdon et al. 1984; Matsuki et al. 1985a; Thomson 1985; Mueller-Eckhardt et al. 1986). We can calculate expected antigen genotype frequencies according to the strict dominant, additive, and recessive models (Thomson 1980). In the present series, for the dominant and additive model, the expected values of the DR2 homozygotes (including DR2/DR blank heterozygotes) and DR2 heterozygotes are 36.78 and 153.22, respectively. For the recessive model, the expected values are 190 and 0. The observed numbers of 45 and 145 are well in agreement with the expected numbers under the dominant and additive model ($P=0.30$).

We can calculate the penetrance under the strict dominant model on the assumption that DR2/Dw2 itself is the disease susceptibility gene. The frequency of narcolepsy in the general Japanese population is 0.16% (Honda et al. 1983b). The gene frequency of DR2/Dw2 is 4.0% (Sasazuki et al. 1980). The penetrance is calculated as 0.02 from these two values (Vogel and Motulsky 1986).

The next question is why certain subjects with a disease susceptibility HLA haplotype develop only incomplete forms of narcolepsy. This is explained by "variable expressivity" (Vogel and Motulsky 1986): the degree of manifestation of a dominant gene can vary in each individual. When the "expressivity" is low, a subject may develop only an incomplete form of the disease.

Thus, this model gives a good explanation for the mode of inheritance of the DR2-linked disease-susceptibility gene. However, this model does not provide explanation as to why the penetrance is incomplete and why the expressivity is variable. It is likely that the penetrance and expressivity are determined by multiple factors, possibly including other predisposing genes and environmental factors.

Which Model is Appropriate?

The distinction between a single-locus dominant model with low penetrance and a multifactorial model with high heritability is often impossible (Kruger 1973). There is a considerable overlapping area where neither model can be excluded theoretically. Narcolepsy falls into this equivocal area (see Chap. 2, 16).

An integration of both models might be more appropriate. In this model, multiple genes and environmental factors are postulated to determine disease manifestation. The DR2-linked disease-susceptibility gene is one of such genes that contribute to the disease development. This gene itself is an additive gene, i.e., heterozygous expression of this gene is sufficient and required for the development of narcolepsy. For the full manifestation of narcolepsy, however, other genes are also required; environmental factors may also contribute to the development of narcolepsy.

At present we do not know the exact number of these susceptibility genes. The minimum is two: one is the DR2-linked susceptibility gene, the other is a gene that modifies the manifestation of the former gene. However, since at least five genetic markers other than DR2 on different chromosomes show significant associations with narcolepsy (see Chap. 16), the total number is more likely over two.

Under this integrated model, the penetrance and expressivity in the single-locus dominant model are considered as variables determined by these multiple factors other than the DR2-linked gene. The liability in the multifactorial model is the total effect of the DR2-linked gene and other genetic and environmental factors.

DR2 in Healthy Subjects

We found different haplotype frequencies between Japanese narcoleptics and normals. However, this is mainly because about two-thirds of DR2-positive normal Japanese have Bw52-DR2/Dw12 haplotypes (Table 5). When we compare normal DR2/Dw2 haplotypes with narcoleptic DR2 haplotypes, we may not find any difference. In Caucasians, most of the DR2 haplotypes carry Dw2, and frequent haplotypes in narcoleptics are apparently the same as the most common DR2 haplotype in Caucasians (Mueller-Eckhardt et al. 1986).

Moreover, we have not yet found any difference between DR2/Dw2 in narcoleptics and DR2/Dw2 in normal subjects either in the restriction fragment length polymorphism (Inoko et al. 1986; Marcadet et al. 1985) or in isoelectric points of the HLA proteins (Maeda et al. 1987). Furthermore, the HLA-D specificity is identical between the narcoleptics and normal HLA-Dw2 subjects (see Chap. 9). There is no evidence at present to indicate that DR2/Dw2 in normals and DR2/Dw2 in narcoleptics are different.

One of the possible predictions from this observation is that all of the DR2/Dw2-positive individuals might have the DR2/Dw2-linked narcolepsy-susceptibility gene. Most of them do not develop narcolepsy, but this is explained by lack of other liability factors (according to the multifactorial model) or by very low penetrance of the disease gene (according to the single-allele dominant model). Schulz et al. (1986) reported that rapid-eye-movement (REM) latencies are shorter in apparently healthy DR2 subjects than in those with other DR antigens. If this is confirmed,[1] this would imply that at least some of the apparently healthy DR2 subjects have a certain REM-related aberration.

Clinical Value of HLA Typing in Narcolepsy

The strong association between HLA-DR2 and narcolepsy caused DR2 to become a most useful cytological marker in the diagnosis of narcolepsy. We may use the HLA typing to detect family members at high risk. It provides us with the hope that the HLA typing will lead to prevention of narcolepsy under certain circumstances.

---

[1] Later, the same authors reported that they could not reproduce their finding (Schulz et al. 1987).

In family 1 in Fig 1, for example, the HLA typing was useful for detecting a family member at risk for narcolepsy (Matsuki et al. 1985a; Honda 1986). The second child of the proband shared a DR2 haplotype with his father. He had not been seriously aware of his somnolence before being interviewed during this study. He often fell asleep in the classroom throughout the previous year and could not concentrate on studying, which resulted in low grades. He attributed all of these problems to his baseball practice. Although cataplexy, sleep paralysis, or hypnagogic hallucinations were not observed, a polysomnogram examination revealed a marked tendency to fall asleep and a rapid eye movement period at the onset of sleep. He was diagnosed as having essential hypersomnia and is now doing well in college under medication with pemoline.

In family 10, the HLA typing was helpful in differentiating other sleepy conditions from narcolepsy. The mother, who was a narcoleptic, worried about her second child because he seemed to fall asleep often during the daytime. His HLA typing revealed that he was DR2 negative. His sleepiness was due to poor sleep habits; no signs of narcolepsy were detected.

Bayes' Theorem

According to Bayes' theorem, the probability that a patient has a certain disease can be calculated from four parameters: the HLA frequencies in normal and diseased populations, the HLA typing result, and the "prior probability" that the subject has the disease before the HLA typing is performed. The formulae are given as below:

$$P[D+/A+] = \frac{P \times PP}{(P \times PP) + C \times (1 - PP)}$$

$$P[D+/A-] = \frac{(1-P) \times PP}{(1-P) \times PP + (1-C) \times (1-PP)}$$

where $P[D+/A+]$ = The probability that a patient has the disease when the antigen is present

$P[D+/A-]$ = the probability that a patient has the disease when the antigen is absent

P = frequency of the antigen in the patients

C = frequency of the antigen in the controls

PP = prior probability

The prior probability that the patient has the disease in question is dependent on the physician's clinical evaluation. When the physician is 50% certain that the patient has the disease, the prior probability is 0.5.

The results when this theorem is applied to narcolepsy are shown in Table 7. Consider a case in which the prior probability is 0.5. After the HLA typing, suppose the patient is found DR2 positive, then the probability will be raised to 74.9%, but not 100%. The negative result of DR2 will lower the probability to 0%.

This calculation shows two important things. First, the HLA typing will never lead to the definite diagnosis: the diagnosis can only be made clinically. Second, the subject without DR2 has little, if any, possibility of having narcolepsy.

Table 7. The diagnostic value of DR2 in narcolepsy

Prior probability of narcolepsy	Probability of narcolepsy when the patient is: DR2 +	DR2 −
0.20	0.427	0.000
0.40	0.666	0.000
0.50	0.749	0.000
0.60	0.817	0.000
0.80	0.923	0.000

Frequency of DR2 in the patients = 1.000
Frequency of DR2 in the controls = 0.335

Table 8. "Symptomatic" and "idiopathic" narcolepsy

	Relationship with exogenous stressors	Male *n*	Female *n*	Total *n*
Symptomatic	Clear	5	7	12
	Vague	3	2	5
	Ambiguous	48	27	75
Idiopathic	Absence of causes	68	30	98
Total		124	66	190

"Symptomatic" and Other Types of Narcolepsy

Narcolepsy has been subclassified as either idiopathic or symptomatic. "Symptomatic" narcoleptic patients are those who develop the disease immediately after an exposure to exogenous stress factors such as head trauma, encephalitis, or heavy bleeding. Those without any apparent preceding histories are classified as "idiopathic."

Among the 190 patients reported here, 17 experienced clear preceding episodes of disturbed consciousness within 3 months prior to the onset of narcolepsy (Table 8). Table 9 shows these episodes. Among them, 11 patients (cases 1-9 and cases 14, 15) felt that these episodes definitely triggered the development of narcolepsy.

One of the cases with a clear preceding episode is presented here (case 9 in Table 9). The patient had been well until 30 years old, when she was diagnosed as having cholecystolithiasis and appendicitis and underwent two consecutive operations under general anesthesia. Ten days after the second operation, she developed attacks of sudden loss of body muscle tone. She often collapsed when she laughed or was surprised, although she did not lose consciousness. Two years later, sleep attacks and daytime somnolence developed, along with sleep paralysis and hypnagogic hallucinations. Her body weight had been 60 kg; after the operations, she began to gain weight and weighed 83 kg when she first came to our hospital.

Table 9. "Symptomatic" narcolepsy

Case	Sex	Age at onset	Stressors	Interval to onset	HLA typing DR	HLA typing DQ
1	F	29	Four consecutive days of high fever and disturbed consciousness	Immediate	2,w9	w1,w3
2	M	17	Loss of consciousness for 3 h after a judo match	Immediate	2,4	w1,w3
3	F	28	Five days of disturbed consciousness after an operation for empyema	1 day	2,-	w1,-
4	M	12	Two days of high fever and disturbed consciousness after tonsillectomy	1 day	2,4	w1,-
5	F	36	Spontaneous abortion resulting in heavy bleeding and curettage under general anesthesia	1 day	2,4	w1,-
6	F	22	Heavy bleeding due to a motorcycle accident	1 day	2,w9	w1,w3
7	F	30	Cesarean section	1 day	2,w11	w1,w3
8	M	11	Brain contusion	4 or 5 days	2,w9	w1,w3
9	F	30	Cholecystectomy and appendectomy under general anesthesia	10 days	2,w12	w1,w3
10	M	12	Seven days of hospitalization for enteritis and disturbed consciousness	20 days	2,w8	w1,w3
11	F	15	Carbon monoxide intoxication	1 month	2,w8	w1,-
12	M	14	Operation for hernia	1 month	2,-	w1,-
13	M	11	High fever following hiking on a hot day	1 month	2,w12	w1,w3
14	M	11	Two days of disturbed consciousness after an operation for hernia	2 months	2,-	w1,-
15	M	15	Encephalitis and 4 days of high fever	<3 months	2,4	w1,w3
16	F	6	High fever with disturbed consciousness	<3 months	2,4	w1,-
17	F	11	High fever with disturbed consciousness	<3 months	2,4	w1,-

Clomipramine was effective against her cataplexy. Her clinical features were indistinguishable from those of "idiopathic" narcolepsy. Her HLA typing results were A26, B51, B35, C blank, DR2, DRw12, DQw1, and DQw3.

Ninety-eight patients, on the other hand, did not recall any episode of disturbed consciousness in their histories (Table 8). The remaining 75 patients recalled preceding episodes that might have been accompanied by disturbed consciousness, but the intervals between the episodes and the onset of the illness were longer than 3 months. All the patients with or without direct triggers had DR2.

Among the 173 cases without immediate histories of disturbed consciousness, 7 cases stated that their disease developed on days of extreme physiological fatigue, overtime work, night shift work, sleep deprivation, etc. (Table 10). These cases may be classified as "fatigue-induced", "insufficient-sleep-induced", or "somatogenic" narcolepsy. They were all DR2 positive.

In addition to these cases, four patients claimed that their disease developed following psychological stresses. Their purported causes are listed in Table 11.

Table 10. "Somatogenic" narcolepsy

Case	Sex	Age at onset	Stressors	Interval to onset	HLA typing	
					DR	DQ
1	F	27	Overtime work for 6 months	Concurrent	2,4	w1,-
2	M	25	All-night driving and trucking work for 6 months	Concurrent	2,w9	w1,w3
3	M	40	Hard work and short sleep hours for 3 months	Concurrent	2,4	w1,w3
4	F	13	1 month of hard training for dancing and long distant travel	Concurrent	2,w12	w1,w3
5	M	15	Going to school, 12 km distant from home by bicycle, every day for 3 years	Concurrent	2,4	w1,w3
6	F	11	1 week of hard training for an athletic cvcnt	Concurrent	2,4	w1,w3
7	F	36	Short sleep hours for taking care of her mother	Concurrent	2,w8	w1,-

Table 11. "Psychogenic" narcolepsy

Case	Sex	Age at onset	Stressors	Interval	HLA typing	
					DR	DQ
1	M	11	Change of schools	Concurrent	2,w12	w1,w3
2	M	20	Listening to a shocking wartime story	Concurrent	2,w14	w1,-
3	F	9	Sexual harassment	Several days	2,4	w1,-
4	F	43	Informed of having syphilis	Several days	2,-	w1,-

These cases were tentatively classified as "psychogenic." This is only for the sake of convenience. We do not believe in a "psychogenic" etiology of narcolepsy in a literal sense. They were all DR2 positive (Table 11).

All of these cases with apparent exogenous stressors expressed DR2. This fact demonstrates that narcolepsy with or without any kind of exogenous trigger has the same DR2-related genetic predisposition. Various triggers, such as disturbed consciousness, physical fatigue, or poor sleep habits, might precipitate the onset of narcolepsy. In the cases in Table 9-11, the preceding episodes appeared as if they had been the direct causes. However, in all of the cases, the DR2-related genetic predisposition was prerequisite for the development of narcolepsy.

This observation also suggests that dualistic classifications like "symptomatic" and "idiopathic" or "psychogenic" and "somatogenic" should be used only as a convenient way to describe the relationships between exogenous triggers and the development of narcolepsy. There is no essential difference in etiopathology and symptomatology of various "subtypes" of narcolepsy.

Exogenous Factors and Narcolepsy. As described above, exogenous factors per se cannot produce narcolepsy. However, they do increase the total liability and can precipitate the onset of narcolepsy. They might even act as "the final straw" in the development of narcolepsy. Such cases might have been previously classified as "symptomatic."

Up to now, no reliable way to avert contracting narcolepsy has been known. However, in order to reduce exogenous liability factors, it may be wise for a subject at risk to keep a regular sleep/wake schedule and practice good sleep hygiene.

Are There Any DR2-Negative Narcoleptic Patients?

We have examined 190 patients so far and have not found a single patient without HLA-DR2. Other investigators reported the presence of DR2-negative narcoleptics, though they HLA-typed only a small number of the patients (Andreas-Ziets et al. 1986; Langdon et al. 1986; Guilleminault and Grumet 1986; Mueller-Eckhardt et al. 1986). What causes this difference?

The typing of DR2 is not very difficult nowadays. Most HLA laboratories can type DR2 quite accurately. It is not likely that this difference resulted from poor HLA typing.

The difference may be attributed to the ethnic difference of the patient groups. In Japanese, DR2 may be tightly linked to narcolepsy; in Caucasians, it may not.

The other likely reason is the difference in the individual investigator's concept of narcolepsy and the application of the diagnostic criteria. A number of conditions can mimic narcolepsy. Sleepiness may be due to various causes: shift work, medical illness, psychological disturbance, keeping late hours, etc. Sudden muscle weakness can be seen in many circumstances. A patient may feel weak when the patient is drowsy. Sudden loss of muscle tone may be found in senile drop attacks. Some children may experience physiological cataplexy.

If vague and unspecified diagnostic criteria for narcolepsy are adopted, the chances are high that DR2-negative patients with essential hypersomnia or other narcolepsy-like conditions will be labeled as narcoleptics. The most critical step in the study of HLA and narcolepsy does not lie in the HLA typing but in the diagnosis and definition of narcolepsy.

It is practically impossible to prove that *all* narcoleptic patients are DR2 positive. However, since we have studied the largest number of patients reported anywhere to date and yet have not found any DR2-negative narcoleptics, we remain skeptical about the presence of DR2-negative narcolepsy.

Underlying Mechanism for the Strong Association

As is always the case with the HLA and disease association, no definite explanation is available for the mechanisms behind the strong narcolepsy-DR2 association. The following discussion thus has a speculative nature.

Because most of the HLA-associated diseases have underlying immunological mechanisms, one of the possibilities is that narcolepsy is an immunological disorder. Routine laboratory tests generally have failed to demonstrate abnormal immune parameters in narcolepsy, but this does not preclude the possibility that narcolepsy is an immunological disorder. Discussions on this possibility are presented in Chap. 12.

The second possibility is that HLA-DR2 itself has a certain function in the sleep mechanism. Since one of the major roles of the HLA proteins in immune reaction is cell-cell recognition, the HLA proteins may participate in intercellular recognition in the nervous system.

The third possibility is that some gene(s), different from but closely linked to the HLA genes, play(s) a role in sleep and arousal mechanisms. This gene may encode an enzyme, a receptor, a structural protein, or a sleep substance that is essential for normal sleep. The single mutation hypothesis (Terasaki and Mickey 1976) provides a possible explanation. According to this hypothesis, the normal function of this putative gene was lost by mutation in a single prehistoric individual who happened to be DR2/Dw2 positive. The mutated gene was spread in the population and transmitted from generation to generation, but the tight linkage with DR2 remained because of the very close localization in the chromosome.

Acknowledgments. We are grateful to all the members of "Narco-Kai," the Japan Narcolepsy Association, who were willing to cooperate with our studies. We also thank Ms. Honoka Yoshida, Mr. Sumio Takahashi, Ms. Machiko Okuyama, Ms. Angela Yu, and Ms. Mariko Aoyagi for their excellent technical assistance, Dr. Tohru Naohara and Dr. Patricia McDonald-Scott for their critical comments, and Ms. Nancy Baxer for her help in preparing the manuscript. This paper was supported in part by Grant-In-Aid for Co-Operative Research from the Japanese Ministry of Education, Science and Culture.

References

Andreas-Zietz A, Keller E, Scholz S, Albert ED, Roth B, Nevsimalova S, Sonka K, Docekal P, Ivaskova E, Schulz H, Geisler P (1986) DR2 negative narcolepsy. Lancet ii: 684-685

Billiard M, Seignalet J (1985) Extraordinary association between HLA-DR2 and narcolepsy. Lancet i: 226-227

Brewerton DA, Caffrey M, Hart FD, James DCO, Nicholls A, Sturrock RD (1973) Ankylosing spondylitis and HL-A27. Lancet i: 904-907

Cohen D, Le Gall I, Marcadet A, Font M, Lalouel J, Dausset J (1984) Clusters of HLA class II restriction fragments describe allelic series. Proc Natl Acad Sci USA 81: 7870-7874

Duquesnoy RJ, Marrari M (1984) Antigen report: HLA-DQw3. In: Albert ED, Baur MP, Mayr W (ed) Histocompatibility testing 1984. Springer, Berlin Heidelberg New York, pp 209-211

Ferrara GB, Park MS, Tanigaki N, Terasaki PI (1984) Antigen report: HLA-DQw1. In: Albert ED, Baur MP, Mayr W (ed) Histocompatibility testing 1984. Springer, Berlin Heidelberg New York, pp 205-207

Fujii T, Juji T, Kaihara N (1983) Family study of HLA-A, B, C, and DR in Japanese. Ishoku 18: 189-203

Guilleminault C, Grumet C (1986) HLA-DR2 and narcolepsy: not all narcoleptic-cataplectic patients are DR2. Hum Immunol 17: 1-2

Honda Y, Asaka A, Tanaka Y, Juji T (1983 a) Discrimination of narcoleptic patients by using genetic markers and HLA. Sleep Res 12: 254

Honda Y, Asaka A, Tanimura M, Furusho T (1983b) A genetic study of narcolepsy and excessive daytime sleepiness in 308 families with a narcolepsy or hypersomnia proband. In: Guilleminault C, Lugaresi E (eds) Sleep/wake disorders. Raven, New York, pp 198-229
Honda Y, Doi Y, Juji T, Satake M (1984a) Positive HLA-DR2 finding as a prerequisite for the development of narcolepsy. In: Proceedings of the 9th meeting of Japanese Society of Sleep Research, May 11, 1984, p 8
Honda Y, Doi Y, Juji T, Satake M (1984b) Narcolepsy and HLA: positive DR2 as a prerequisite for the development of narcolepsy. Folia Psychiatr Neurol Jpn 38: 360
Honda Y, Harada S, Someya T, Juji T, Matsuki K, Naohara T, Satake M (1985) HLA-DR2 and Dw2 in narcolepsy and other DOES without cataplexy. In: Proceedings of the Second International Symposium on Narcolepsy, 6-7 July 1985, Stanford
Honda Y, Juji T, Matsuki K, Naohara T, Satake M, Inoko H, Someya T, Harada S, Doi Y (1986) HLA-DR2 and Dw2 in narcolepsy and in other disorders of excessive somnolence without cataplexy. Sleep 9: 133-142
Inoko H, Ando A, Tsuji K, Matsuki K, Juji T, Honda Y (1986) HLA-DQ beta chain DNA restriction fragments can differentiate between healthy and narcoleptic individuals with positive HLA-DR2. Immunogenetics 23: 126:128
Juji T, Satake M, Honda Y, Doi Y (1984) HLA antigens in Japanese patients with narcolepsy. All the patients were DR2 positive. Tissue Antigens 24: 316-319
Juji T, Matsuki K, Naohara T, Satake M, Honda Y (1985) Extraordinary association between HLA-DR2 and narcolepsy. Lancet i: 227
Juji T, Honda Y, Matsuki K, Bashir H (1986) Narcolepsy: joint report. In: Aizawa M (ed) HLA in Asia-Oceania 1986. Hokkaido University Press, Sapporo, pp 346-348
Kessler S (1976) Genetic factors in narcolepsy. In: Guilleminault C, Dement WC, Passouant P (eds) Narcolepsy. Spectrum, New York, pp 285-302
Kessler S, Guilleminault C, Dement WC (1974) A family study of 50 REM narcoleptics. Acta Neurol Scand 50: 503-512
Kruger J (1973) Zur Unterscheidung zwischen multifaktoriellem Erbgang mit Schwellenwerteffekt und einfachem diallelem Erbgang. Hum Genet 17: 181-252
Langdon N, Welsh KI, Dam MV, Vaughan RW, Parkes D (1984) Genetic markers in narcolepsy. Lancet ii: 1178-1180
Langdon N, Lock C, Welsh K, Vergani D, Dorow R, Wachtel H, Palenschat D, Parkes JD (1986) Immune factors in narcolepsy. Sleep 9: 143-148
Leckman JF, Gershon S (1976) A genetic model of narcolepsy. Br J Psychiatry 128: 276-279
Maeda H, Hirata R, Okuyama M (1983) TB22. Ishoku 18: 165
Maeda H, Hirata R, Matsuki K, Juji T, Honda Y (1987) Analysis of HLA-DR2 and DQw1 molecules in narcolepsy. J Jpn Soc Blood Transfusion 33: 149
Marcadet A, Gebuhrer L, Betuel H, Seignalet J, Freidel AC, Confavreux C, Billiard M, Dausset J, Cohen D (1985) DNA polymorphism related to HLA-DR2 Dw2 in patients with narcolepsy. Immunogenetics 22: 679-683
Matsuki K (1986) TB22, TB23, and TB24. In: Aizawa M (ed) HLA in Asia-Oceania 1986. Hokkaido University Press, Sapporo, pp 191-193
Matsuki K, Juji T, Tokunaga K, Naohara T, Satake M, Honda Y (1985a) HLA haplotype frequencies estimated from the data on HLA class I, II, and III antigens in 111 Japanese narcoleptics. J Clin Invest 76: 2078-2083
Matsuki K, Takahashi S, Juji T (1985b) Analysis of TB22, TB23, TB24 antigens. In: Naito S (ed) Joint report of the 9th Japan HLA Workshop, pp 155-158
Matsuki K, Watanabe S, Nanzai Y, Nakatate M, Juji T (1986) DR2 short antigen in Japanese. A strong association with Bw67 and TB23. Tissue Antigens 27: 239-243
Mittal KK, Hasegawa T, Ting A, Mickey MR, Terasaki PI (1972) Genetic variation in HL-A system between Ainus, Japanese, and Caucasians. In: Terasaki PI (ed) Histocompatibility testing 1972. Munksgaard, Copenhagen, pp 187-195
Mueller-Eckhardt G, Meier-Ewert K, Schendel DJ, Reinecker FB, Mueller-Eckhardt C (1986) HLA and narcolepsy in a German population. Tissue Antigens 28: 163-169
Park MS, Terasaki PI (1984) Second DR locus. In: Terasaki PI (ed) Histocompatibility testing 1980. UCLA Tissue Typing Laboratory, Los Angeles, pp 578-582
Poirier G, Montplaisir J, Decary F, Momege D, Lebrun A (1986) HLA antigens in narcolepsy and idiopathic central nervous system hypersomnolence. Sleep 9: 153-158

Reinsmoen NL, Sasazuki T, Kaneoka N, Ohta H, Noreen HJ, Greenberg LJ, Kersey JH (1978) Two distinct HLA-D specificities (DHO and Dw2) in linkage with HLA-DRw2 as defined in white and Japanese populations. Transplant Proc 10: 789-791
Sasazuki T, Kaneoka H, Tsuji K, Nose Y, Kashiwagi N, Kaneoka T (1980) HLA-D in Japan. In: Terasaki PI (ed) Histocompatibility testing 1980. UCLA Tissue Typing Laboratory, Los Angeles, pp 274-276
Satake M, Matsuki K, Yabe T, Suzuki M, Juji T (1986) A possible split of antigen DQw1 identified by antiserum T3516. Tissue Antigens 27: 155-162
Seignalet J, Billiard M (1984) Possible association between HLA-B7 and narcolepsy. Tissue Antigens 23: 188-189
Schlosstein L, Terasaki PI, Bluestone R, Pearson GM (1973) High association of an HL-A antigen, W27, with ankylosing spondylitis, N Engl J Med 288: 704-706
Schulz H, Geisler P, Pollmaecher T, Andreas-Zietz A, Keller E, Scholz S, Albert ED (1986) HLA-DR2 correlates with rapid-eye-movement sleep latency in normal human subjects. Lancet ii: 803
Schulz H, Geisler P, Pollmaecher T, Andreas-Zietz A, Keller E, Scholz S, Albert ED (1987) HLA-DR2 and rapid-eye-movement sleep latency: failure to replicate. Lancet i: 627
Terasaki PI, Mickey MR (1976) A single mutation hypothesis for multiple sclerosis based on the HL-A system. Neurology (NY) 26: 56-58
Tokunaga K, Omoto K, Akaza T, Akiyama N, Amemiya H, Naito S, Sasazuki T, Satoh H, Juji T (1985) Haplotype study on C4 polymorphism in Japanese. Associations with MHC alleles, complotypes, and HLA-complement haplotypes. Immunogenetics 22: 359-365
Thomson G (1980) A review of theoretical aspects of HLA and disease associations. Theor Popul Biol 20: 168-208
Thomson G (1985) The mode of inheritance of the HLA-linked gene predisposing to narcolepsy. Tissue Antigens 26: 201-203
Vogel F, Motulsky FV (1986) Human genetics. Problems and approaches. Springer, Berlin Heidelberg New York Tokyo

Chapter 4

HLA in Narcolepsy/Cataplexy in the United Kingdom

C. B. Lock, K. I. Welsh, J. D. Parkes, A. So, D. C. Briggs, R. W. Vaughan, and M. Van Dam

Introduction

Familial cases of narcolepsy in the United Kingdom have been known for a considerable time (Barraitser and Parkes 1978), but the genetic factors involved have in the past, been uncertain. In 1984 however, Langdon et al. showed that the HLA system provided a strong genetic marker for the disease in UK Caucasoids.

This discovery, as well as being diagnostically useful, raised several important questions. These are outlined below:

HLA in Other Sleep Disorders

Since no other sleep disorders had previously been investigated for HLA associations, the specificity of the finding for narcolepsy was not proven initially. The HLA system might have provided a marker for sleep disorders in general rather than narcolepsy/cataplexy in particular.

Significance of Cataplexy

As described in detail in the previous chapter, the subjects in our original UK study all had unequivocal narcolepsy-cataplexy. The question of whether or not the actual genetic link was with cataplexy specifically rather than the complete syndrome remained open.

Table 1. Narcolepsy and HLA DR2/DQw1 association

Stud	No. of subjects	DR2	DQw1
Langdon et al. 1984	$n=42$	100% (21.5%)	100%
Billiard and Seignalet 1985	$n=8$	100% (33.6%)	100%
Juji et al. 1985	$n=92$	100% (21.8%)	100% (70.9%)
Gaetan et al. 1985	$n=20$	100% (35.4%)	100%

NB, control frequencies are in parentheses

Is DR2 the Best Disease Marker?

High degrees of linkage disequilibrium are a characteristic of the HLA genetic region. Although DR2 appears to be the antigen which is the most closely associated with narcolepsy, it is only one of a family of tightly linked genes, any one of which might be the actual "disease marker."

Does Narcolepsy Have an Immune Basis?

The main biological role of HLA antigens is in the induction and control of the immune response. Why therefore does a disease, not thought to be an immune disorder, have the strongest HLA association known?

Is There a Common Genetic Link Between Narcolepsy and Other DR2-Associated Diseases?

Are there any other diseases, neurological or otherwise, which have a similar genetic basis? Would comparison with other and better-defined DR2-associated diseases yield clues to the pathogenesis of narcolepsy?

The purpose of this chapter is to describe the progress made in answering each of these questions and to update our original finding (Langdon et al. 1984) for narcolepsy per se.

To the latter end we have now class II typed (serology and Southern blotting) 71 patients with narcolepsy/cataplexy. In addition class III MHC typing (i.e., allotypes of the complement components C2, C4, Bf) have been determined on a limited number of patients (37) (see Table 5).

Further Results

In Table 2 we show the HLA class I and II antigen frequencies of the UK Caucasoid patients compared with UK Caucasoid controls, and in Table 5 show a similar analysis for class III.

Several conclusions can be drawn from Table 2. The frequencies of the class I antigens A3, B7, and Cw7 are all raised, B7 and Cw7 significantly so. The results

Table 2. Relevant HLA class I and II antigens (%) in UK patients with narcolepsy

Antigen	Control	Caucasoid patients	Non-Caucasoid patients
HLA A3	27.5	48.7	
HLA B7	28.5	73.4	
HLA Cw7			
HLA DR2	30.0	98.6	60.0

Table 3. Comparison of class I antigens in Caucasoid and Japanese subjects

Japanese	A2, Bw6, B35, B51, Bw67, and Cw3 increased B52 and B7 decreased
Caucasoid	A3, B7, Bw6, and Cw7 increased A2, A23, B35, B51, and Cw3 decreased or unchanged

are as expected when the population differences in linkage disequilibrium between class I antigens and DR2 are taken into account. There is no evidence of a single class I antigen in both populations being a second marker for the disease.

Table 3 compares the UK and other Caucasoid results with the Japanese population results (Honda et al. 1982, 1984a, b; Juji et al. 1985).

All UK Caucasoids, bar one, carry the marker DR2. The single subject who is DR2 negative has two sisters, one of whom has monosymptomatic narcolepsy; the other is normal. Neither sister has HLA-DR2.

Is there any evidence for a second class II antigen being important in narcolepsy/cataplexy? In HLA-linked diseases (for review see Batchelor and Welsh 1982) such as rheumatoid arthritis (DR4 and DR1 raised, DR2 lowered), juvenile onset diabetes (DR3 and DR4 raised, DR2 lowered), and celiac disease (DR3 and DR7 raised) there is evidence that more than one class II gene product can exert influence over susceptibility or progression of the disease.

We have therefore removed one DR2 from each class II tissue type and looked at the remaining antigens. As a control we have carried out the same exercise on 60 DR2-positive controls. Where DR2 was the only DR antigen determined, the person has been assumed to be a DR2 homozygote. In cases where a second antigen was thought to be present (e.g., reactions with some sera but not others) a blank has been assumed.

As can be seen in table 4 both DR2 and DR5 are higher than expected in the patient group but these differences are not significant. In the first study (Langdon et al. 1894) 11 out of 37 patients were homozygous for DR2, although only 5 would be expected from control data. Homozygosity for DR2 might be associated

Table 4. Second class II antigens in 60 narcolepsy/cataplexy patients and 60 DR2-positive controls

Second antigen	Narcolepsy/ cataplexy	Controls
DR1	3	5
DR2	13	8
DR3	11	9
DR4	8	10
DR5	13	6
DR6	5	7
DR7	4	9
DR8	1	2

All patients and all but three controls were DQw1 positive

with a slightly increased risk. A larger number of UK patients and a similar analysis on non-Caucasoid patients might prove more informative but, on present evidence, there is only a weak suggestion of a second class II antigen being additive and no evidence at all of a second class II antigen being protective for narcolepsy.

MHC-Encoded Complement Components in Narcolepsy

The class III data, especially the association with Bf, is significant, but the findings can be explained by the known linkage disequilibrium within the HLA region. BfS is in positive and BfF in negative linkage disequilibrium with DR2. This finding is similar to that noted in multiple sclerosis (Stewart et al. 1979). In spite of the significant associations between class III alleles and narcolepsy, it is not, therefore, likely that complement is involved in the pathogenesis of the disease. The absence of an independent complement association supports the class II association as being primary.

Narcolepsy in Non-Caucasoids in the United Kingdom

We have also HLA typed several patients of West Indian or African extraction. Although the numbers are small (7) the results are of extreme interest since two of the five subjects of West Indian origin did not type as DR2. One

Table 5. C4 and factor B (Bf) allotypes in narcolepsy

Allotype	Narcolepsy		Controls (307) (%)
	(n=36)	(%)	
C4A 3	34	94.4	84.7
C4A Q0	13	36.1	26.4
C4A 2	2	5.5	17.9
C4A 6	1	2.1	8.5
C4A 4	0	--	8.5
C4A 21	1	2.1	1.3
C4A 12	1	2.1	0.3
C4B 1	35	97.2	92.2
C4B Q0	10	27.2	27.0
C4B 2	4	11.1	17.3
C4B 5	1	2.7	1.0
Bf S	36	100.0	86.5[a]
Bf F	5	13.9	41.4[b]
Bf SO.7	1	2.7	3.0

[a] Frequency of Bf S is significantly raised [P(Fisher's) =0.0073]
[b] Frequency of Bf F is significantly reduced [P(Fisher's) =0.0065]

DR2-negative subject was from a family with a clear history of the disease (see Table 2).

So far single cases from African countries have proven to be DR2 positive but clearly it is too early to draw any firm conclusions. Such studies in non-Caucasoids need extensive follow-up, and are discussed more fully under "Is DR2 the Best Disease Marker?" below.

HLA in Other Sleep Disorders

In the initial studies (Honda et al. 1984a, b, Billiard and Seignalet 1985, Langdon et al. 1984) only well-defined narcolepsy/cataplexy patients were studied. We have tissue typed a further 49 individuals with monosymptomatic narcolepsy and other sleep disorders in order to examine this question. A study of similar design has been carried out in Japan (Honda et al. 1985).

The results of both studies are shown in Table 6. The footnotes to the table highlight differences in disease defintion, i.e., there may be a margin of error in a direct comparison of the results presented in the table. In summary, in narcolepsy, all 122 Japanese patients and 70 of 71 UK Caucasoid subjects were DR2 positive. Of seven non-Caucasoids two were non-DR2 and these were both of West Indian extraction. It is apparent from the table that other sleep disorders do not have the same strong DR2 association. In results not shown there was no significant HLA region link with any other sleep disorder although there were some interesting trends. For example, half the monosymptomatic narcolepsy patients were DR2 whereas of seven definite sleep apnea patients none were DR2 (although two others with asymptomatic sleep apnea were DR2).

In conclusion, narcolepsy is unique among sleep disorders investigated in its almost 100% association with DR2. Indeed the absence of DR2 in Caucasian subjects can almost but not entirely exclude the diagnosis.

Table 6. Class II MHC antigen frequencies in Japanese and UK Caucasoid patients with sleep disorders

Disease	Incidence of DR2	
	Japan	UK
Narcolepsy without cataplexy	14/27	6/12
Narcolepsy/cataplexy	122/122	70/71
Sleep apnea	1/5	2/9
Postencephalitic Parkinson's disease		3/7
periodic somnolence	2/5	7/16
Sleep/wake rhythm disorders	0/4	
Other sleep problems	1/5	0/3

"Idiopathic hypersomnolence" in the UK study = "periodic somnolence" in the Japanese study

Significance of Cataplexy

Could it be that cataplexy is actually the component of the narcoleptic syndrome which is DR2 associated? Would it fit the data if susceptibility to monosymptomatic narcolepsy was totally HLA independent but if DR2 was present in a sufferer then the full syndrome including cataplexy would eventually result? Longitudinal studies on monosymptomatic patients would show if all those that are DR2 will indeed eventually develop the full syndrome. The question of whether it is narcolepsy per see or cataplexy that is HLA linked is still open.

Is DR2 the Best Disease Marker?

Our study of the telomeric class I and class III MHC alleles indicate that the DR2 is the best protein marker for narcolepsy. However, in recent years, molecular analysis of the class II region has shown a high degree of complexity. Further analysis of the DR2 association in narcolepsy by Southern blotting and RFLP analysis is therefore necessary.

Southern Blotting

Southern blot hybridization has been used to try to identify the exact nature of the base sequence associated with susceptibility to narcolepsy. Class II molecules are heterodimers of one alpha and one beta chain unit. The MHC class II region con-

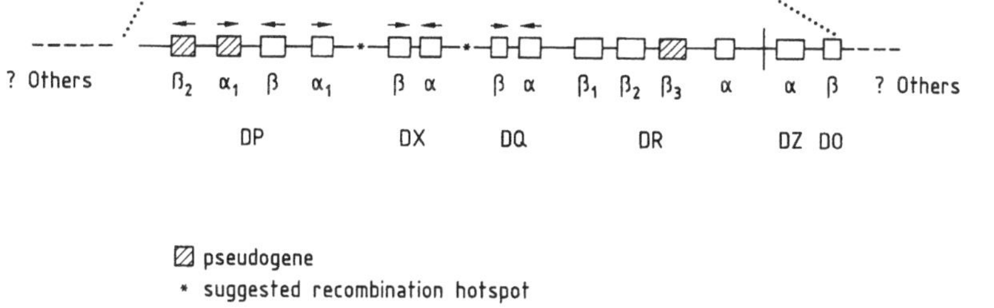

Fig. 1. Schematic map of the HLA-D region

sists of at least six alpha and seven beta chain genes, organized into three subregions, DR, DQ, and DP (see Trowsdale et al. 1985).

The complexity of this region and high degree of polymorphism makes serological analysis inadequate, for example, only three DQ alleles are detected by serology. Southern blotting (Southern 1975) detects differences between individuals in genes probed with a specific DNA sequence.

Restriction fragment length polymorphisms (RFLPs) can be defined by Southern blotting, which correlates with the DR2 serological type. DR2 can be further "split" by cellular typing in an MLR into five subtypes, termed Dw2, Dw12, MN2, FJO and DB9 (Albert et al. 1984). RFLPs which correlate with these DR2 subtypes can also be identified (Segall et al. 1986).

Results

DNA from 25 unrelated narcoleptic subjects was analyzed by Southern blotting for an RFLP in linkage with the disease. Twenty-two subjects were Caucasian; one of these was non-DR2. Three subjects were West Indian; of these, two were non-DR2, and the third had monosymptomatic narcolepsy.

DNA was digested with the restriction enzyme *Taq*I. Blots were probed with DQ alpha (Trowsdale et al. 1983) and DQ beta probes (Larhammar et al. 1983).

With DQ alpha, a 6.5-kb fragment was identified which was strongly associated with the disease, and was present in 24 out of 25 subjects. This fragment correlated with the DR2 serological type in normal controls. The band was also present, however, in two West Indian non-DR2 narcoleptics. There did not appear to be any correlation of narcolepsy with the DX alpha polymorphism.

With the DQ beta probe, a 2.8-kb fragment was identified, which was also associated with the disease, although less strongly. The fragment was present in 22 out of 25 narcoleptics. From DNA analysis of homozygous cell lines this RFLP correlated with the Dw2 subtype of DR2 (A. So, unpublished data).

Narcoleptics who did not have the expected bands were as follows. With DQ alpha the single narcoleptic who lacked the 6.5-kb band is one of three sisters; all three sisters are non-DR2. One sister has monosymptomatic narcolepsy (without cataplexy) and the other is unaffected. The index case (and her sisters; data not shown) did not have the normal DR2Dw2 2.8 DQ beta band. Instead a 2.4-kb band was present, not so far seen in any other narcoleptics or controls. In addition, two West Indian subjects had different DQ beta bands; these were consistent with their DR serotypes.

These results agree with other published RFLP studies in narcolepsy. It is important to note that, to date, RFLP studies do not distinguish narcoleptics from healthy DR2Dw2 controls. It is of interest, however, that some non-DR2 subjects in the present study share a fragment, defined with the DQ alpha probe, with DR2 +ve subjects.

Marcadet et al. (1985a) analyzed DNA from 22 French Caucasian narcoleptics, and found bands with *Eco*RI and *Eco*RV using the DQ beta probe. All the narcoleptics had the DR2Dw2 pattern, which the authors term the DQR 2,6 fragment cluster (some DR6 haplotypes have this same RFLP).

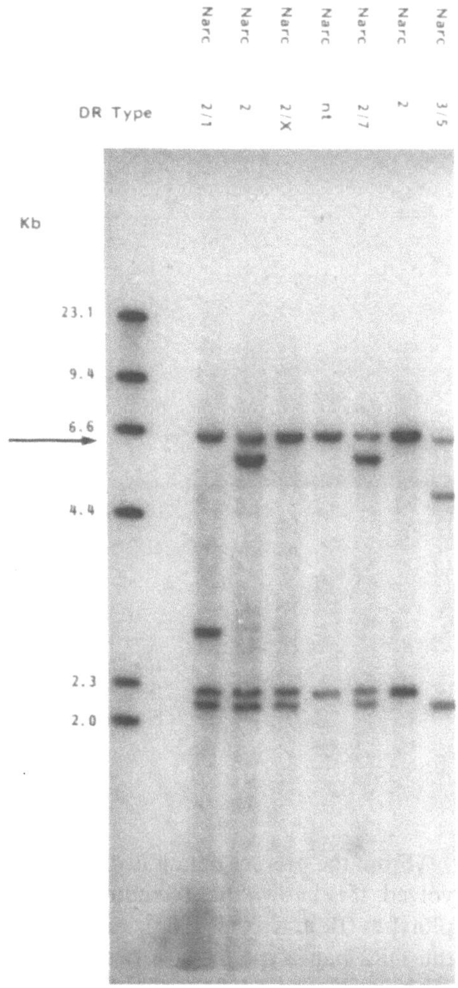

Fig. 2. Restriction fragment patterns detected in narcoleptics using a DQ alpha probe. The 6.5-kb band is *arrowed*; this band correlates with DR2, but is also seen in some non-DR2 narcoleptics. The *two lower bands* are the DX alpha polymorphism. *Additional bands* correlate with the second DR allele. A molecular weight marker appears *in the left-hand track* (lambda-*Hind* III digest). (*nt*, not DR typed)

Holloman et al. (1985) report the study of DNA from 12 narcoleptics using DR beta and DQ beta probes with several enzymes. RFLPs showed the DR2Dw2 allele to be present in 9 out of 12 subjects. Three patients lacked the RFLP pattern, and serological typing showed them to be non-DR2.

Inoko et al. (1986) also identified the same subtype of DR2 in all 33 Japanese narcoleptics studied, using *Eco*RI, *Pst*I, and *Bam*HI with the DQ beta probe. The Dw2 subtype is relatively uncommon among normal DR2 Japanese. An additional 18-kb fragment with *Eco*RI was noted in 100% of controls, but was only present in 42.4% of narcoleptics.

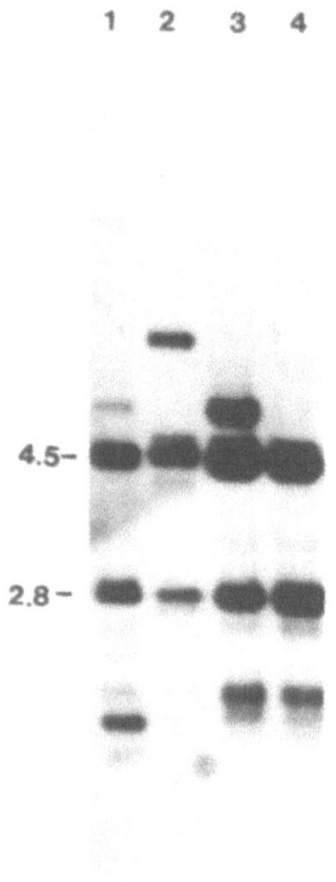

Fig. 3. Restriction fragment patterns in four narcoleptics identified using a DQ beta probe. The 2.8-kb band is *arrowed;* this band correlates with the DR2Dw2 subtype

From the present data it is not clear which gene within the class II region is involved. It is known that the number of DR beta genes varies between different haplotypes (Bohme et al. 1985). Analysis of DNA from homozygous cell lines shows the DR2 haplotype to have two DR beta chain genes (A. So, unpublished data). Nishimura et al. (1984), using two-dimensional SDS-IEF protein analysis, have shown that Dw2 and Dw12 vary in the structure of one of their two DR beta chains. Both subtypes share an invariant chain, termed beta 1, but vary in the structure of the second chain, termed beta 2.

In our study there is no RFLP which is common to all subjects when DQ alpha and DQ beta genes are probed. DQ alpha has the closer linkage with DR beta and appears to have the tighter disease association. We have speculated that the gene coding for the DR beta 2 chain, or a very closely linked gene, is implicated in narcolepsy. The non-DR2 narcoleptics in our study may share a similar beta chain gene or linked gene, or there may be a different genetic mechanism in these subjects.

DNA sequencing should resolve some of these questions.

Of further note is the finding that the DQ beta RFLP associated with narcolepsy is also associated with DR2-positive multiple sclerosis in 97% of subjects (Marcadet et al. 1985b), but negatively associated with insulin-dependent diabetes (Cohen et al. 1986).

Table 7. Restriction fragment lengths (DQ probes) in narcolepsy/cataplexy patient DNA

DR	DQαRFLP (kb)	DXαRFLP (kb)	DQ β RFLP (kb)
2	6.5	2.2	4.6, 2.8
2/4 or 7	6.5	2.2	2.8
2/6	7.8 6.5	2.2	9 4.6, 2.8
2/4	6.5, 5.9	2.1	5.2, 4.6, 2.8
2/5	6.5, 4.8	2.2, 2.1	4.6, 2.8
2	6.5	2.2, 2.1	4.6, 2.8
2	6.5	2.2	4.6, 2.8
NT	6.5, 5.9	2.2, 2.1	4.6, 2.8
2/X	6.5	2.2, 2.1	4.6, 2.8
2	6.5	2.2	2.8
2/3	6.5 4.8	2.2	4.6, 2.8
2/7	6.5, 5.9	2.2, 2.1	7.5 2.8
2/X	6.5	2.2, 2.1	5.2 2.8
2/4	6.5	2.2	2.8
2/1	6.5 2.7	2.2, 2.1	5.2 2.8
2	6.5, 5.9	2.2, 2.1	4.6, 2.8
2/3	6.5	2.2	5.2, 4.6, 2.8
2/7	6.5, 5.9	2.2, 2.1	7.5 4.6, 2.8
5	4.8	2.1	12 4.6, 2.4
3/6[a]	6.5 4.8	2.2, 2.1	5.2, 4.6 2.5
2/6	6.5	2.2	5.2, 4.6, 2.8
2/4	6.5, 5.9	2.2	5.2, 4.6, 2.8 1.9
3/5[a]	6.5 4.8	2.1	4.6
2[a]	6.5	2.2	5.2 2.8
2/7	6.5, 5.9	2.2	7.5, 4.6, 2.8

[a] West Indian

Table 8. Marker frequencies in narcoleptics and controls

	Frequency %		Chi square	Relative risk
	Patients	Controls		
DR 2	92	31	27	24
DQ 6.5 kb	96	40	23	34
DQ 2.8 kb	87.5	33	22	14

Note. The group chosen for the RFLP analysis was selected to contain the non-DR2-positive patients. It should be stressed also that more RFLP data are needed on non-Caucasoid controls

Chromosomal Morphology

High-resolution chromosomal banding studies with particular reference to chromosome 6 have been normal in two of our subjects (C. Berry, personal communication).

Does Narcolepsy Have an Immune Basis?

In the preceding chapter we outlined clinical and other evidence for immune factors in narcolepsy and will, therefore, restrict ourselves here specifically to the HLA system.

Narcolepsy is linked to HLA-DR2; and that link may be with the DR beta chain genetic locus. It is known that the major function of this and closely associated loci is an immunological one. Further there are no detected non-class II genes in the immediate vicinity and we have shown that the association lessens outside this vincinity. Narcolepsy must therefore be an immune disorder associated with a class II gene, or, alternatively, DR beta chain genes must be capable of fulfilling a nonimmune function. The differences between DR2 beta chain sequences and those of other class II DR beta chain sequences are known to be small and to exist in restricted molecular sites. A nonimmune function must involve the same fine discrimination as the immune function, at least in certain instances.

Is There a Common Genetic Link Between Narcolepsy and Other DR2-Associated Diseases?

Multiple sclerosis (MS) (Welsh 1984, review), older-onset (over 40) myasthenia gravis (MG) (Compston et al. 1980), antiglomerular basement membrane disease (aGBMD) (Rees et al. 1978), dermatitis herpetiformus (DH), certain forms of Guillain-Barré syndrome (GBS), and specific allergies, for example, to ragweed pollen antigen (RPA) (Marsh et al. 1982), have been reported to have a positive HLA-DR2 association. Rheumatoid arthritis (RA) and juvenile onset diabetes (JOD), especially the latter, have a lowered incidence of HLA-DR2.

Co-occurrence of narcolepsy and multiple sclerosis has been described, but there is no evidence that such co-occurrence occurs more often than would be expected if, for example, different environmental agents are acting on a common genetic background.

There is by no means general agreement on whether or not a particular answer in Table 9 is "Yes" or "No"; it is apparent that except for narcolepsy, in all diseases which are linked in a positive or negative way to DR2, there has been at least some evidence of antibody or T-cell involvement and in most there has also been evidence of infection, other environmental agents, or other genes. It must be remembered, however, that to date few immunological studies have been carried out in narcolepsy.

Unfortunately, although several Nobel prize groups and a host of other laboratories have published on HLA and disease associations, the contribution of this research to the elucidation of specific disease mechanisms has been limited. It is not known how DR2 operates in Goodpasture's disease, multiple sclerosis, juvenile onset diabetes, etc. Despite this, can any clues be obtained for narcolepsy by comparison with other diseases which are DR2 linked? Certain allergies (to ragweed,

Table 9. DR2-linked diseases: comparison with narcolepsy

	Neuro-logical	Cooccur-rence with narcolepsy	Antibody present	T-cell involve-ment	Viral agent	Environ-mental-agent	Poly genic
Old-MG	Yes	No	Yes	No	No	Yes	Yes
aGBMD	No	No	Yes	No	No	Yes	Yes
Wegeners	No	No	Yes	No	No	No	No
DH	No	No	Yes	No	No	No	No
GBS	Yes	No	Yes	No	Yes	No	Yes
RPA	No	No	Yes	Yes	No	Yes	No
RA	No	No	Yes	Yes	No	No	Yes
JOD	No	No	Yes	Yes	Yes	No	No
MS	Yes	Yes	Yes	Yes	Yes	No	Yes
N	Yes		No	No	No	No	No

The factor need not be pathogenic to warrant a "yes," however; thus antibody is well documented in RA but the evidence for its damaging effect is slight

for example), certain neurological disorders (see above), Wegener's vasculitis, Goodpasture's disease, SLE in certain studies, as well as dermatitis herpetiformis are DR2 linked. With MS, IDD, and narcolepsy, all appear to be linked with the same subset of DR2, implying that there may be a common link even though such a link is not immediately obvious.

References

Albert ED, Baur MP, Bayr WR (ed) (1984) Histocompatibility testing 1984. Springer, Berlin Heidelberg New York, pp 186-187

Barraitser M, Parkes JD (1978) Genetic study of narcoleptic syndrome. J Med Genet 15: 254-259

Batchelor JR, Welsh KI (1982) Association of HLA antigens with disease. In: Lachmann PJ, Peters DK (eds) Clinical aspects of immunology. Blackwell, Oxford pp 283-309

Billiard M, Seignalet J (1985) Extraordinary association between HLA-DR2 and narcolepsy. Lancet i: 226-227

Bohme J, Andersson M, Andersson G, Moller E, Peterson P, Rask L (1985) HLA DR-beta genes vary in number between different DR specificities, whereas the number of DQ-beta genes is constant. J Immunol 135 (3): 2149-2155

Cohen N. Brautbar C, Font M-P, Dausset J. Cohen D (1986) HLA-DR2 associated Dw subtypes correlate with RFLP clusters: most DR2 IDDM patients belong to one of these clusters. Immunogenetics 23 (2): 84-89

Compston DA, Vincent A, Newsom-Davis J. Batchelor JR (1980) Clinical, pathological, HLA antigen and immunological evidence for disease heterogeneity in myasthenia gravis. Brain 103 (3): 579-601

Gaetan P, Montplaisir J, Andre L et al. (1985) HLA antigens in narcolepsy (abstract). Second international symposium on narcolepsy, Stanford, 6-7 July 1985

Holloman JD, Bell JI, Lee T et al. (1985) Major histocompatibility complex restriction fragment length polymorphism in narcolepsy (abstract). Second international symposium on narcolepsy, Stanford 6-7 July 1985

Honda Y, Asaka A, Tanaka Y, Juji T (1982) Discrimination of narcoleptic patients by using genetic markers and HLA. Fourth international congress of sleep research, Bologna, 19-22 July 1982

Honda Y, Doi Y, Juji T, Satake M (1984a) Narcolepsy and HLA-positive DR2 as a prerequisite for the development of narcolepsy. Folia Psychiatr Neurol Jpn 38: 360

Honda Y, Doi Y, Juji T, Satake M (1984b) Positive HLA-DR2 finding as a prerequisite for the development of narcolepsy. Proceedings of the 9th meeting of the Japanese Society of sleep Research, May 11th, 1984, p 28
Honda Y, Harada S, Someya T (1985) HLA-DR2 and Dw2 in narcolepsy and other DOES without cataplexy (abstract). Second international symposium on narcolepsy, Stanford, 6-7 July 1985
Inoko H. Ando A, Tsuji K et al. (1986) HLA-DQ beta chain DNA restriction fragments can differentiate between healthy and narcoleptic individuals with HLA-DR2. Immunogenetics 23: 126-128
Juji T, Matsuki K, Naohara T et al. (1985) HLA antigens in Japanese patients with narcolepsy. Lancet i: 227
Langdon N. Welsh KI, van Dam M et al. (1984) Genetic markers in narcolepsy. Lancet ii: 1178-1180
Larhammer D, Hylding-Nielson JJ, Servenious B, et al. (1983). Exon-intron organisation and complete nucleotide sequence of a major histocompatibility antigen DC beta gene. Proc Natl Acad Sci USA 80: 7313
Marcadet A, Gebuhrer L, Betuel H et al. (1985a) DNA polymorphism related to HLA-DR2 Dw2 in patients with narcolepsy. Immunogenetics 22: 679-683
Marcadet A, Massart C, Semana G et al. (1985b) Association of class II HLA-DQ beta chain restriction fragments with multiple sclerosis. Immunogenetics 22: 93-96
Marsh DG, Hsu SH, Roebber M et al. (1982) HLA-Dw2: a genetic marker for human immune response to short ragweed pollen allergen Ra5. I. Response resulting primarily from natural antigenic exposure. J Exp Med 155: 1439-1451
Nishimura Y, Tsukamoto K, Sone T et al. (1984) In: Albert ED, Baur MP, Mayr WR (eds) Histocompatibility testing 1984. Springer, Berlin Heidelberg New York Tokyo, pp 504-508
Ress AJ, Peters DK, Compston DAS, Batchelor JR (1978) Strong association between HLA-DR2 and antibody-mediated Goodpasture's syndrome. Lancet i: 966-969
Segall M. Noreen H, Schluender L, Bach FH (1986) DNA restriction fragment length polymorphisms characteristic for Dw subtypes of DR2. Hum Immunol 15: 336-343
Southern EM (1975) Detection of specific sequences among DNA fragments separated by gel electrophoresis. J Mol Biol 98: 503-517
Stewart GJ et al. (1979) Strong linkage disequilibrium between HLA-Dw2 and BfS in multiple sclerosis and in the normal population. Tissue Antigens 14: 86-97
Trowsdale J, Lee J, Carey J et al. (1983) Sequences related to HLA-DR alpha chain on human chromosome 6: restriction enzyme polymorphism detected with DC alpha chain probes. Proc. Natl Acad Sci USA 80: 1972
Trowsdale J et al. (1985) Structure, sequence and polymorphism in the HLA-D region. Immunol Rev 85: 5-43
Welsh KI (1984) Genetic markers in neurological diseases. In: Behan P, Spreafico F (eds) Neuroimmunology. Raven, New York, pp 469-473

Chapter 5

HLA in Narcolepsy in France

M. BILLIARD, J. SEIGNALET, H. BETUEL, A. MARCADET, L. GEBUHREL, A. C. FREIDEL, C. CONFAVREUX, A. BESSET, and J. CADILHAC

The genetic aspect of narcolepsy in man has long been considered, with the first report of a positive family history of narcolepsy made by Westphal (1877) even before the term "narcolepsy" was coined by Gelineau (1880). Since then a number of series have been published showing variable rates of probands with a positive family history of narcolepsy and suggesting either an autosomal dominant mode of inheritance with incomplete penetrance (Krabbe and Magnussen 1942; Daly and Yoss 1959; Baraitser and Parkes 1978) or a two-threshold multifactorial system (Nevsimalova-Bruhova and Roth 1972; Kessler 1976; Honda et al. 1983a).

The first report of a significant increased frequency of HLA-B35 and Cw3 and of a significant decreased frequency of HLA-Bw52 and B7 in 56 Japanese narcoleptic subjects was published by Honda et al. (1983b). These results prompted us to investigate HLA antigens in French narcoleptic subjects. We found a significantly incresed frequency of B7 and a nonsignificantly increased frequency of A3, an antigen in linkage disequilibrium with B7, in 38 subjects (Seignalet and Billiard 1984). The discrepancy between Honda's results and ours was not surprising since several associations between HLA and diseases have been found to be different in Mongoloids and Caucasoids. For instance, myasthenia gravis is associated with B12 in Mongoloids and with B8 in Caucasoids, Grave's disease with B35 in Mongoloids and with B8 in Caucasoids. Later, two reports simultanenously appeared, one in London (Langdon et al. 1984) confirming the increased frequency of B7 in 42 Caucasoid Englilsh narcoleptic subjects, and revealing a 100% association with HLA-DR2 and DQwl in 37 Caucasoid English narcoleptic subjects. The other study in Tokyo (Juji et al. 1984) confirmed the increased frequency of HLA B35 and the decreased frequency of HLA Bw52, and showed a 100% association with HLA-DR2 and DQwl in 40 Japanese narcoleptic subjects. Subsequently the 100% association with HLA-DR2 and DQwl was reaffirmed by the French group (Billiard and Seignalet 1985) and a Canadian group (Poirier et al. 1986). However, there were some reports indicating that a fringe group of typical narcoleptic subjects with cataplexy and sleep onset REM (SOREM) episodes could be HLA-DR2 and DQwl negative (Andreas-Zietz et al. 1986; Guilleminault 1986; Langdon et al. 1986; Neely et al. 1986; Confavreux et al. 1987).

Subject Population

We performed HLA-DR and DQ typing in a total of 35 unrelated French Caucasoid narcoleptic subjects and 110 healthy French control subjects from the southern part of France. All patients had symptoms of fully developed narcolepsy, including excessive daytime somnolence, overwhelming sleep episodes, and attacks of cataplexy, with or without hypnagogic hallucinations and sleep paralysis, and two or more daytime SOREM episodes during 34 h continuous polysomnography beginning at 10:00 p.m. and ending at 8:00 a.m. The age of onset of the first symptom(s) varied from 5 to 45 years, median 16.5 years. Circumstances at onset were clearly identified in 24 of the 35 subjects (68.5%), severe psychological stress in 11, abrupt modification of the sleep-wake schedule in 8, significant medical disease in 3, head traumatism in 1, and pregnancy in 1. Family history was remarkable in five subjects (7%) having one or more relative(s) with excessive daytime somnolence and with either narcolepsy or narcolepsy and excessive daytime somnolence in six subjects (5.8%). We also performed HLA-DR and DQ typing in three further subjects, two of French origin and one of Jewish descent, who had incomplete narcolepsy characterized by excessive daytime somnolence, overwhelming sleep episodes, and two or more SOREM episodes during the 34-h polysomnography, but no history of cataplexy. Ages of onset were 17, 22, and 23 years. A circumstance at onset, namely a modification of the sleep-wake schedule, was found in one subject only.

Methods

Thirty-five HLA, A, B, C antigens were characterized by a standard one-stage lymphocytotoxicity technique, and 12 HLA-DR and DQ antigens also by a standard one-stage lymphocytotoxicity technique, after previous extraction of lymphocytes by differential centrifugation on Ficoll-mitrizoate and separation of B- and T-lymphocytes by the column method (Seignalet 1980).

In addition, HLA-Dw specificities restricted to DR2 subtypes Dw2, Dw12, and FJO were typed with the appropriate homozygous typing cells (Betuel et al. 1983) in 6 of our narcoleptic subjects and 16 from the Department of Neurology, Neurologic Hospital, Lyon.

In the same subjects DNA restriction fragment length polymorphism was analyzed (Marcadet et al. 1985). Genomic DNAs were extracted from the peripheral blood leukocytes (Cohen et al. 1983) and digested with the restriction endonucleases *Eco*RI and *Eco*RV. Restriction fragments were separated in agarose gel by electrophoresis, transferred from agarose gel to nitrocellular membranes (Southern 1975), and hybridized with a ^{32}P-labeled HLA-DQ beta cDNA probe (Larhammar et al. 1982).

Finally the transmission of HLA haplotypes was studied in two families with a narcolepsy proband and one or more members with either narcolepsy and excessive daytime somnolence.

Table 1. Frequencies of HLA antigens (classes I and II) among 35 French narcoleptic subjects

HLA antigens	Narcoleptic patients (*n*=35)		Controls (*n*=110)		X^2 (corrected)	Relative risk	P value
	n	%	*n*	%			
A3	10	28.5	25	22.7	0.22	1.36	
B7	18	51.4	16	14.5	18.12	6.22	<0.0001
DR1	0	0.0	18	16.3	5.12	0.07	<0.03
DR2	35	100.0	24	21.8	64.04	250.80	$<10^{-10}$
DR3	5	14.2	22	20.0	0.25	0.66	
DR4	5	14.2	22	20.0	0.25	0.66	
DR5	9	25.7	33	30.0	0.07	0.80	
DRw6	2	5.7	20	18.1	2.31	0.27	
DR7	4	11.4	33	30.0	3.89	0.30	<0.05
DRw8	1	0.02 (?)	4	3.6	-	-	
DRw9	0	0.0	5	4.5	0.56	0.70	
DRw10	1	0.02 (?)	1	0.9	-	-	
DQw1	35	100.0	60	54.5	46.30	58.4	$<10^{-10}$

(?) questionable antigen

Results

HLA Frequencies in Narcolepsy

DR2 was found in all narcoleptic subjects (100%) and in 24 controls (21.8%) and DQwl in all narcoleptic subjects (100%) and in 60 normal controls (54.5%); hence there was a relative risk of 250.8 for DR2 and 58.4 for DQwl. In addition HLA-B7 was present in 18 narcoleptic patients (51.4%) and in 16 controls (14.4%); hence there was a relative risk of 6.2 (Table 1). The DR2 antigen genotype frequencies among the 35 narcoleptic subjects were as follows: definite heterozygotes, 27; possible homozygotes, 8 (this class includes individuals who may be DR2 blank heterozygotes). HLA typing of the three subjects with incomplete narcolepsy gave the following results: the three subjects were DR2 and DQwl positive and one subject was B7 positive. The three subjects were heterozygotes for DR2.

HLA-D typing showed that the 6 subjects from our population and the 16 subjects from Lyon were all DR2-Dw2 (100%) against 19% of controls.

DNA Analysis

With the restriction enzyme *Eco*RV all subjects generated a 5.2-kb fragment and with the restriction enzyme *Eco*Rl all subjects generated a 2.7-kb fragment. These fragments correspond to a DQR2-6 positive subset of DR2 haplotypes - the other subset is a DQRl-positive subset - originally described by Cohen et al. (1984) after analysis of DQ restriction endonuclease fragments. This subset is associated with

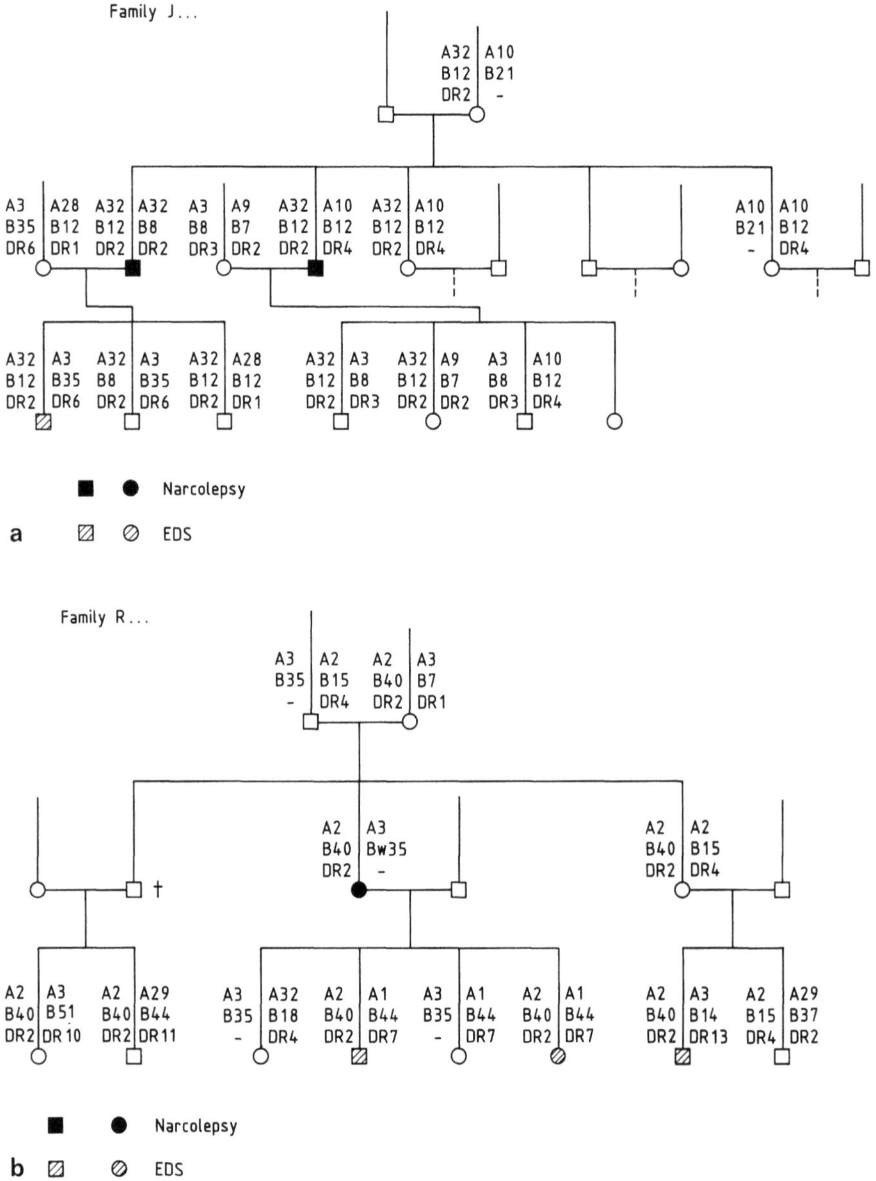

Fig. 1. Pedigrees of two families (J... and R...) with narcoleptic and excessive daytime somnolence (EDS) subjects

Dw2. Therefore all narcoleptic subjects were HLA DR2, Dw2, DQR2-6, DQwl positive.

In comparison the fragment cluster DQR2-6 was present in 63% of DR-matched controls only.

Family Studies

All narcoleptic and excessive daytime somnolence family members were DR2 DQwl positive. In the J... family the incriminated haplotype was A32, B12, DR2 and in the R... family A2, B40, DR2 (Fig. 1). Subjects with either narcolepsy or excessive daytime somnolence had the incriminated hapolotype but all the subjects with this haplotype were not necessarily narcoleptic or excessive daytime somnolence subjects. Furthermore, in the R... family, the three subjects, two boys and one girl, with alleged excessive daytime somnolence, underwent a multiple sleep latency test, which failed to show a mean sleep latency index of less than 5 min and two or more SOREM episodes typical of narcolepsy.

Discussion

A Clinical Variant of Narcolepsy

Our study identified a subgroup of three subjects who were all HLA-DR2 DQwl positive with excessive daytime somnolence, overwhelming sleep episodes, SOREM episodes, but no cataplexy. Duration of the condition was respectively 3, 20, and 28 years in these subjects. It is possible that some of these subjects may eventually develop cataplexy. It may also be that cataplexy never appears. A similar case was reported by Poirier et al. (1986).

DNA Restriction Fragment Length Polymorphism

Results obtained by Marcadet et al. (1985) deserve being compared with those by Inoko et al. (1986). Using restriction endonucleases *Eco*RI, *Bam*HI, and *Pst*I Japanese authors found significant differences in hybridation band patterns between narcoleptic subjects and controls. Moreover, with the restriction endonuclease *Eco*RI they obtained a 2.4-kb fragment whereas the French group obtained a 2.7-kb fragment. Now, in view of the difficulty of estimating the size of the fragments it is possible that results of both groups are in fact similar. This would confirm the same association with HLA-DR2, Dw2, in Mongoloids and Caucasoids, as predicted by Juji et al. (1985).

Possible Mechanism of HLA-DR2 Association with Narcolepsy

The fact that narcoleptic subjects of different ethnic groups are almost all HLA DR2 positive seems to imply a role of this molecule in the occurrence of the majority of narcolepsy cases.

1. According to a first hypothesis narcolepsy could depend on a susceptibility gene different from HLA-DR2 but linked and transmitted with it. In this instance genetic recombination between this susceptibility gene and HLA-DR2 could lead to typical cases of HLA-DR2 negative narcolepsy as already reported.
2. A second possibility would be that narcolepsy depends on a gene located outside the major histocompatibility complex and modified by the HLA-DR2 gene (epistasis effect).
3. Finally the narcolepsy susceptibility gene could be the HLA-DR2 molecule itself. Whether this molecule is modified or not in narcoleptic subjects has still to be investigated. If it is modified, HLA-DR2 negative narcolepsy should be either of a noninherited type or associated with other HLA antigens.

Immunity and Narcolepsy

At present clear evidence in favor of an autoimmune process at the origin of narcolepsy is still lacking. However, the hypothesis deserves being considered. Twenty-four of the narcoleptic subjects included in this study had clear circumstances, psychological stress, modification of the sleep-wake schedule, and so on at the onset of their condition. These factors could alter normal immune responses (Stein et al. 1985). Typical narcolepsy has been reported in association with multiple sclerosis and other immune-associated disorders (Bonduelle and Degos, 1976; Lascelles et al. 1976; Honda et al. 1986). Minor abnormalities including lymphocytosis and increase in the protein content have been pointed out in the cerebrospinal fluid of narcoleptic subjects (Parkes et al. 1986).

In this instance three stages could be proposed in the development of narcolepsy: In a predisposed HLA-DR2 subject, contact with an environmental agent, bacteria or virus, would trigger an abnormal immune response, either directly (by cross-reaction between heteroantigens of this agent and autoantigens probably located in the central nervous system) or indirectly (by inducing an abnormal immune response against these usually tolerated autoantigens). This immune response would result in either central nervous system lesions or metabolic disorders, such as an imbalance in the monoaminergic and cholinergic neuron dynamic equilibrium.

However, more evidence is needed to support an immune process. In a preliminary work in which we have tested 31 narcoleptic subjects for 22 different circulating antibodies, 14 subjects showed antistreptolysines characterized by titers above 200 IU and 23 antistreptodornases characterized by titers above 100 IU. Altogether only four subjects had normal titers of antibodies directed against streptococcus. Also of interest would be the search for antibodies directed against some brain structures involved in sleep mechanisms, by the indirect immunofluorescence method.

Family Study

Concerning the mode of inheritance of narcolepsy, our results are consistent with a dominant mode with an incomplete penetrance already suggested by Thomson (1985). Indeed all narcoleptic subjects had the DR2 antigen; there were eight (22.8%) possible homozygotes, which does not differ from the expected ratio (20%) - a recessive mode would be reflected in a high frequency of homozygotes; narcolepsy was always transmitted with a HLA haplotype including DR2 in our two pedigrees, and only a minority of subjects with the DR2 antigen do have narcolepsy. However, the question of why the penetrance is incomplete remains. Two hypotheses can be advanced: either the necessity of a second susceptibility gene (polygenic model) or of a contact with an environmental factor. However, multiple-case family studies are required to make possible the discrimination between a dominant model and various intermediate models (Day and Simons 1976). Another point of interest is the possibility of identifying in a given family those members at risk of narcolepsy. In the family R. the son in the second generation was a pilot; he had crashed during an airshow, now raising the question of a possible pathological fluctuation of alertness. In the same family the narcoleptic patient and her husband, a pilot, are concerned about their son, a DR2-positive subject, who would also like to become a pilot.

References

Andreas-Zietz A, Keller E, Scholz S, Albert ED, Roth B, Nevsimalova S, Sonka K, Docekal P, Ivaskova E, Schulz H, Geisler P (1986) DR2-negative narcolepsy. Lancet 2: 684-685

Baraitser M, Parkes JD (1978) Genetic study of narcoleptic syndrome. J Med Genet 15: 254-259

Betuel H, Gebuhrer L, Lambert J, Freidel AC, Farre A (1983) A possible new HLA-DR allele. Hum Immunol 8: 227-238

Billiard M, Seignalet J (1985) Extraordinary association between HLA-DR2 and narcolepsy. Lancet 1: 226-227

Bonduelle M, Degos C (1976) Symptomatic narcolepsies: a critical study. In: Guilleminault C, Dement WC, Passouant P (eds) Narcolepsy. Spectrum, New York, pp 313-332

Cohen D, Paul P, Font MP, Cohen O, Sayagh B, Marcadet A, Busson M, Mahouy G, Cann HM, Dausset J (1983) Analysis of HLA class I genes with restriction endonuclease fragments: implications for polymorphism of the human major histocompatibility complex. Proc Natl Acad Sci USA 80: 6289-6292

Cohen D, Le Gall I, Marcadet A, Font MP, Lalouel JM, Dausset J (1984) Clusters of HLA class II beta restriction fragments describe allelic series. Proc Natl Acad Sci USA 81: 7870-7874

Confavreux C, Gebuhrer L, Betuel H, Freidel C, Bastuji H. Aimard G, Devic M, Jouvet M (1987) HLA-DR2 negative narcolepsy. J Neurol Neurosurg Psychiatry 50: 635-636

Daly DD, Yoss RE (1959) A family with narcolepsy. Proc Staff Meet Mayo Clin 34: 313-320

Day NE, Simons MJ (1976) Disease susceptibility genes - their identification by multiple case family studies. Tissue Antigens 8: 109-119

Gelineau J (1880) De la narcolepsie. Gaz Hop (Paris) 53: 626-628; 54: 635-637

Guilleminault C (1986) Narcolepsy. Sleep 2: 99-101

Honda Y, Asaka A, Tanimura M, Furusho T (1983a) A genetic study of narcolepsy and excessive daytime sleepiness in 308 families with a narcolepsy or hypersomnia proband. In: Guilleminault C, Lugaresi E (eds) Sleep/wake disorders: natural history, epidemiology, and long-term evolution. Raven, New York, pp 187-199

Honda Y, Asaka A, Tanaka Y, Juji T (1983b) Discrimination of narcoleptic patients by using genetic markers and HLA. Sleep Res 12: 254
Honda Y, Doi Y, Ninomiya R, Ninomiya C (1986) Increased frequency of non-insulin dependent diabetes mellitus among narcoleptic patients. Sleep 9: 254-259
Inoko H. Ando A, Tsuji K, Matsuki K, Juji T, Honda Y (1986) HLA-DQ beta chain DNA restriction fragments can differentiate between healthy and narcoleptic individuals with HLA-DR2. Immunogenetics 23: 126-128
Juji T, Satake M, Honda Y, Doi Y (1984) HLA antigens in Japanese patients with narcolepsy. Tissue Antigens 24: 316-319
Kessler S (1976) Genetic factors in narcolepsy. In: Guilleminault C, Dement WC, Passouant P (eds) Narcolepsy. Spectrum, New York, 285-302
Krabbe E, Magnussen G (1942) Familial narcolepsy. Acta Psychiatr Neurol 17: 149-173
Langdon N, Welsh KI, Van Dam M, Vaughan RW, Parkes JD (1984) Genetic markers in narcolepsy. Lancet 2: 1178-1180
Langdon N, Lock C, Welsh KI, Vergani D, Dorow R, Wachtel H. Palenschat D, Parkes JD (1986) Immune factors in narcolepsy. Sleep 9: 143-148
Larhammar D, Schenning L, Gustaffson K, Wiman K, Claesson L, Rask L, Peterson PA (1982) Complete amino-acid sequence from an HLA-DR antigen-like β chain as predicted from the nucleotide sequence: similarities with immunoglobulins and HLA-A, B, and C antigens. Proc Natl Acad Sci USA 79: 3687-3691
Lascelles RG, Mohr PD, Peart I (1976) Unilateral cataplexy associated with systemic lupus erythematosus. J Neurol Neurosurg Psychiatr 39: 1023-1026
Marcadet A, Gebuhrer L, Betuel H, Seignalet J, Freidel AC, Confavreux C, Billiard M, Dausset J, Cohen D (1985) DNA polymorphism related to HLA-DR2 Dw2 in patients with narcolepsy. Immunogenetics 22: 679-683
Nevsimalova-Bruhova S, Roth B (1972) Heredofamilial aspects of narcolepsy and hypersomnia. Schweiz Arch Neurol Neurochir Psychiatr 110: 45-54
Neely SE, Rosenberg RS, Spire JP, Antel J, Arnason BGW (1986) HLA antigens in narcolepsy. Neurology 36 [Suppl 1]: 299
Parkes JD, Langdon N. Lock C (1986) Narcolepsy and immunity. Br Med J 292: 359-360
Poirer G, Montplaisir J, Decary F, Momege D, Lebrun A (1986) HLA antigens in narcolepsy and idiopathic nervous system hypersomnolence. Sleep 9: 153-158
Seignalet J (1980) Recherche d'anticorps anti-cellules B et typage HLA-DR à Montpellier. Rev Fr Transfus 23: 411-425
Seignalet J, Billiard M (1984) Possible association between HLA-B7 and narcolepsy. Tissue Antigens 23: 188-189
Southern EM (1975) Detection of specific sequences among DNA fragments separated by gel electrophoresis. J Mol Biol 98, 503-517
Stein M, Keller SE, Schleifer SJ (1985) Stress and immunomodulation: the role of depression and neuroendocrine function. J Immunol 135 [Suppl 2]: 827s-833s
Thomson G (1985) The mode of inheritance of the HLA-linked gene predisposing to narcolepsy. Tissue Antigens 26: 201-203
Westphal C (1877) Eigentümliche mit Einschlafen verbundene Anfälle. Arch Psychiatr Nervenkr 7: 631-635

Chapter 6

HLA in Narcolepsy in Canada

J. MONTPLAISIR and G. POIRIER

HLA Study in a Patient Population

Introduction

Four years ago we postulated, on the basis of our observations of nearly 100 narcoleptics and those of other researchers, the existence of two types of narcolepsy. Primary narcolepsy was thought to be characterized by an early onset (in adolescence or the 3rd decade), a high prevalence of afflicted individuals in the family, and the absence of precipitating factors associated with the onset of the illness. Secondary narcolepsy was characterized by a late onset of narcoleptic symptoms, the absence of other afflicted members in the family, and the presence of possible precipitating factors like head trauma, CNS infectious diseases, affective disorders, or other factors such as shift work likely to disrupt the sleep-wake cycle.

Because of its polymorphism, the HLA system has been extensively used to search for genetic markers in several diseases (Décary 1981). We therefore thought that it might be an appropriate method to differentiate primary from secondary narcolepsy. Honda et al. (1983) first reported an association between narcolepsy and HLA-Bw35 in Japanese patients and Seignalet et al. (1984) later reported a possible association between this disease and HLA-B7 in French Caucasoids. These conflicting results have been attributed to the different ethnic origins of the populations studied. However, only HLA-A, B, and C were typed in these early studies. We accordingly typed narcoleptics for HLA antigens of loci A, B, C, and DR.

In this chapter, we will summarize our recent findings on HLA antigens in narcoleptics, and in families of patients afflicted with this disease.

Methods

Patient Selection

Several fundamental criteria are needed for a study of the association between HLAs and a disease. First, subjects have to be unrelated and from the same ethnic origin. Second, the clinical population should be as homogeneous as possible with regard to the condition studied.

We investigated 48 unrelated Caucasoid narcoleptics. Patients were diagnosed by two independent evaluators unaware of the results of HLA typing. In all cases, the diagnosis was made on the basis of an unequivocal history of excessive daytime sleepiness (EDS), sleep attacks, and cataplexy. All patients were recorded during at least five consecutive naps [multiple sleep latency test (MSLT) (Richardson et al. 1978; Mitler 1982)] and all had sleep onset rapid eye movement period(s) and short sleep latencies during this procedure. The control group consisted of 158 unrelated Caucasoid subjects. All of them had already been typed for their HLA-A, B, and C, and 150 of them for their HLA-DR antigens during a previous genetic study conducted by the Canadian Red Cross.

HLA Typing

Antigens of loci A, B, and C were detected by the standard microlymphotoxicity technique (Terasaki and McClelland 1964). DR antigens were detected using the same technique (Terasaki et al. 1978) after B-cell enrichment performed by rosetting of T cells with sheep red blood cells treated with neuraminidase. National reference laboratory plates (Red Cross Toronto, Canada) were used for all typings. HLA typings were made blind with regard to the clinical and polygraphic findings. The Yate's corrected chi-square with one degree of freedom was used to compare frequencies of each antigen in narcoleptics and controls, and the relative risk was calculated for each antigen. In the case of an antigen frequency of 100%, the relative risk was calculated assuming that the next patient would not carry this antigen.

Results

Frequencies of each antigen for narcoleptics and controls are listed in Tables 1 and 2, and significant differences between the two groups are indicated. All narcoleptics were HLA-DR2 positive compared with 22% of controls; 12.50% ($n=6$) were possibly homozygotic for HLA-DR2. Frequency of HLA-B7 was also significantly increased in narcoleptics, and there was a non-significant increased frequency of HLA-A3. These two antigens, A3 and B7, are known to be in linkage disequilibrium with HLA-DR2 in Caucasoids (Dausset et al. 1985). HLA-Cw2 frequency was also significantly increased in narcoleptics and HLA-DRw6 and DR7 were decreased in these patients.

In addition to these results, one black narcoleptic woman was typed and found to be HLA-DR2 positive. Five other narcoleptic relatives of those included in the statistics were also typed and found to carry HLA-DR2.

Atypical Cases

In the course of this study, two atypical cases of narcolepsy were also investigated. One patient, aged 56 years, had a medical history of head trauma and possibly of encephalitis. Clinically, he had the full narcoleptic tetrad and no family history of this condition. No sleep onset rapid eye movement periods (SOREMPs) were observed during the standard MSLT. He was consequently excluded from the study. His HLA typing showed that he was not HLA-DR2. Further polygraphic investi-

Table 1. HLA-A, B, and C antigens in 48 Canadian Caucasoid narcoleptic patients and 158 controls

Antigen	Narcoleptics					Controls
	n	*f* (%)	*RR*	Ychi	*P*[a]	*f* (%)
Al	10	20.83	0.86	0.031	NS	23.42
A2	19	39.58	0.59	1.977	NS	52.53
A3	16	33.33	1.47	0.823	NS	25.32
A11	8	16.66	1.23	0.057	NS	13.92
A23	2	4.16	1.33	0.013	NS	3.16
A24	8	16.66	0.92	0.002	NS	17.72
A25	5	10.41	3.56	2.775	NS	3.16
A26	3	6.25	2.56	0.625	NS	2.53
A28	2	4.16	0.48	0.398	NS	8.23
A29	3	6.25	0.45	0.947	NS	12.66
A30+31	6	12.50	1.26	0.039	NS	10.13
B7	20	41.66	2.92	8.459	<0.005	19.62
B8	8	16.66	0.85	0.022	NS	18.99
B13	2	4.16	0.71	0.002	NS	5.70
B14	4	8.33	0.59	0.447	NS	13.29
B15	0	0.00	0.00	3.271	NS	8.86
B16	1	2.08	0.18	2.174	NS	10.13
B17	0	0.00	0.00	2.286	NS	6.96
B18	6	12.50	1.18	0.005	NS	10.76
B21	0	0.00	0.00	1.970	NS	6.33
Bw22	1	2.08	0.25	1.072	NS	7.59
B27	4	8.33	0.80	0.008	NS	10.13
B35	5	10.41	0.59	0.632	NS	16.46
B37	0	0.00	0.00	0.002	NS	1.27
B40	4	8,33	1.21	0.000	NS	6.96
B44	13	27.08	0.93	0.000	NS	28.48
B45	0	0.00	0.00	0.405	NS	0.63
B49	0	0.00	0.00	0.775	NS	3.80
Bw50	0	0.00	0.00	0.265	NS	2.53
B51	10	20.83	1.46	0.490	NS	15.19
Bw52	0	0.00	0.00	0.002	NS	1.27
Bw53	3	6.25	5.18	2.036	NS	1.27
Bw55	0	0.00	0.00	0.505	NS	3.16
Bw56	0	0.00	0.00	0.002	NS	1.27
Bw60	0	0.00	0.00	1.660	NS	5.70
Bw63	0	0.00	0.00	0.405	NS	0.63
Cw2	11	22.91	4.91	10.559	<0.005	5.70
Cw3	2	4.16	0.28	2.238	NS	13.29
Cw4	5	10.41	0.40	2.532	NS	22.15
Cw6	5	10.41	1.19	0.001	NS	8.86

n, number of subjects; *f*, frequency; *RR*, relative risk; NS, nonsignificant
[a] *P* value with Yate's corrected chi square (*Y*chi)

gation showed the presence of one SOREMP over 15 nap recordings. This case raised the possibility of a nongenetic form of narcolepsy, with a low propensity to SOREMPs, secondary to brain injury.

We also investigated a man aged 43 years who had a narcoleptic sister aged 50 years. The woman had the full narcoleptic tetrad in addition to polygraphic

Table 2. HLA-DR antigens in 48 Canadian Caucasoid narcoleptic patients and 150 controls

Antigen	Narcoleptics					Controls
	n	*f* (%)	*RR*	*Ychi*	*P*[a]	*f* (%)
DR1	10	20.83	0.77	0.192	NS	25.33
DR2	48	100.00	170.18	88.321	<0.0001	22.00
DR3	10	20.83	0.52	2.129	NS	33.33
DR4	8	16.66	0.53	1.684	NS	27.33
DR5	8	16.66	1.16	0.010	NS	14.67
DRw6	1	2.08	0.06	9.653	<0.005	23.33
DR7	3	6.25	0.22	5.416	<0.025	22.67
DRw8	2	4.16	1.58	0.001	NS	2.67
DRw9	0	0.00	0.00	0.852	NS	4.00
DRw10	0	0.00	0.00	0.357	NS	0.67

n, number of subjects; *f*, frequency; *RR*, relative risk; NS, non significant
[a] *P* value with Yate's corrected chi square (*Ychi*)

and immunogenetic features of narcolepsy. The man reported sleep attacks, sleep paralysis, and hypnagogic hallucinations. Cataplexy in this patient was atypical since most attacks were not associated with emotions, and on many occasions he experienced an alteration of consciousness during the attack with partial retrograde amnesia. The sleep laboratory study revealed short sleep latencies during MSLT and during two all-night polygraphic recordings. Rapid eye movements were also seen during stage 2 sleep (intermediate sleep) shortly after sleep onset but no SOREMP was observed. Epilepsy, sleep apnea syndrome, and periodic movements in sleep were ruled out during these recordings. HLA determination showed that the narcoleptic woman was HLA-A3, A24, B53, BY, DR2, and DR8 and that her hypersomniac brother was HLA-A2, A30/31, B21, B40, DR4, and DR5. These two siblings, therefore, one narcoleptic and one hypersomniac, inherited different alleles from each parent. This case illustrates the complexity of the association between clinical, polygraphic, and immunogenetic findings. It suggests that some features of narcolepsy may be associated with a non-DR2 linked genetic factor.

HLA Study in Familial Narcolepsy

Introduction

Probably the most characteristic feature of a genetic disorder is its familial occurrence. Several studies have shown that siblings of patients afflicted with narcolepsy have 60 and 200 times more risk of developing this disease than do other individuals (Kessler et al. 1974; Kessler 1976; Nevsimalova-Bruhova and Roth 1972). In our own population of narcoleptic patients, a recent survey indicated that 23% of them presented a positive family history for this disease, and that 44% of them had at least one other relative suffering from EDS (personal unpublished data).

The genetic mode of transmission for narcolepsy has not yet been clearly understood. While some authors proposed that narcolepsy was inherited according to a dominant mode of transmission, others suggested a two-threshold multifactorial model of inheritance. The use of HLA typing in families with multiple cases of narcolepsy may provide additional data with regard to the genetic transmission of this disease. HLA typing was thus carried out in families with two or more well-defined cases of narcolepsy and other cases of hypersomnolence.

Methods

Family Selection

Three families with multiple cases of narcolepsy were studied. All narcoleptics in these families presented severe EDS, sleep attacks, and a nonequivocal history of cataplexy. All experienced SOREMPs during the MSLT (one subject has not yet been recorded).

HLA Typing

Human leukocyte antigens were detected by the same technique described previously. All diagnostic tests and typings were made blind with regard to each other.

Results

Results of the family study will only be summarized here. A total of 52 persons were typed for the HLA-A, B, C, and DR in these three families. All seven narcoleptics were HLA-DR2 positive. However, 19 other members of these families had the same HLA haplotype as their narcoleptic relatives altough they were not narcoleptic; 6 were identical to their narcoleptic siblings in all their A, B, C, and DR antigens but did not have narcoleptic symptoms.

Three cases of genetic crossing-over, one of whom was narcoleptic, were found in one of these families. All involved the HLA-DR2 antigen, indicating that the site of rupture of the sixth chromosome was between the B and the D loci of the HLA region.

Twin Study

Cases of monozygotic twins in which narcolepsy was diagnosed are often cited as evidence supporting a genetic contribution to this disease (Imlah 1961; Mamelak et al. 1979; Schrader et al. 1980). However, an attentive reading of these reports may leave the reader unconvinced. In the first case (Imlah 1961), sleepiness in both twins was atypical since they experienced difficulty in getting up in the morning and remained in a dazed state after awakening. These twins reported cataplexy only during their military service and this symptom never recurred. In addition, cataplexy was not closely associated with emotion, as is usually the case in narcolepsy. No polygraphic recording was done in either twin. It therefore remains uncertain whether either actually suffered from narcolepsy.

Mamelak et al. (1979) also reported a case of monozygotic twins both afflicted with narcolepsy. The diagnosis was well established both clinically and polygraphically in the propositus. Altough her twin sister had complained of sleep attacks and cataplexy, at the time of laboratory investigation she had only mild daytime drowsiness and fatigue, but no cataplexy. In addition, no SOREMP was recorded during a 48-h polygraphic monitoring.

A case of monozygotic twins discordant for narcolepsy was also reported (Schrader et al. 1980). The hypothesis in this case was that narcolepsy in the propositus was secondary to multiple sclerosis (MS), which had appeared several years before. HLA-DR antigens were not typed in these subjects, but these twins both carried HLA-Dw2, a specificity known to be closely linked to DR2 in Caucasoids. We believe that MS and narcolepsy may appear independently in the same individual, since both diseases are associated with HLA-DR2 (Poirier et al. 1986; Duquette et al. 1985; Govaerts et al. 1985). Thus, in the case reported here narcolepsy may not be secondary to brain damage associated with MS. This assertion is supported by one of our patients, who developed MS several years after narcolepsy.

Case Report

We recently studied a case of monozygotic twins one of whom was afflicted with narcolepsy. Both twin brothers were investigated clinically, polygraphically, and immunogenetically (Montplaisir and Poirier 1987).

These twins were born in 1934. One of them, the second born, developed excessive daytime sleepiness at age 14, and sleep attacks at age 28 without any precipitating factor. He reported onset of cataplectic attacks at age 34 and typical episodes of sleep paralysis, hypnagogic hallucinations, and automatic behaviors. All-night polygraphic recordings were performed when the patient was 51 years old. His sleep was typical of narcolepsy, with REM fragmentation and frequent nocturnal awakenings (Montplaisir and Godbout 1986). He also experienced periodic movements in sleep. No sleep apnea was observed in this patient. Daytime nap recordings (MSLT) (Richardson et al. 1978; Mitler 1982) showed a mean sleep latency of 4 min and the presence of two SOREMPs. This narcoleptic patient was successfully treated with methylphenidate and chlorimipramine.

A clinical interview made with his twin brother at age 52 did not show any narcoleptic symptoms. His mean sleep latency during the MSLT was 16.4 min, and he fell asleep during only two of the five naps. No SOREMP was observed. There was, therefore, no clinical or polysomnographic evidence of narcolepsy or hypersomnia.

HLA-A, B, C, and DR typings, done by the standard method (Terasaki and McClelland 1964; Terasaki et al. 1978), revealed that both twins were HLA-All, A24, B51, BY, Cw4, Cw6, DR2.1, DRX, confirming the monozygoticity.

A second pair of monozygotic twins discordant for narcolepsy was recently studied in our laboratory. Results of the investigations were essentially the same as in the case reported above.

These cases, and the critical review of other twin cases previously published, lead to the conclusion that there are no unquestionable monozygotic twins concordant for narcolepsy reported so far. This strongly suggests that, in addition to genetic factors responsible for the high family incidence of the disease, nongenetic factors may be necessary for narcolepsy to develop.

General Discussion

Mode of Transmission

Our results show a perfect association between narcolepsy and the presence of the HLA-DR2 in 48 Caucasoid patients and one black patient. These findings and others in Mongoloid and Caucasoid narcoleptics (Juji et al. 1984; Langdon et al. 1984; Billiard and Seignalet 1985; Billiard et al. 1986; Honda et al. 1986; Langdon et al. 1986) strongly suggest the universality of the link between narcolepsy and HLA-DR2. In addition, only six patients were possibly homozygotic for the DR2 antigen, showing that only one DR2 antigen is sufficient for development of narcolepsy. The clinical history and polygraphic findings of these six patients homozygous for DR2 antigen do not show to be clinically or polygraphically different from the entire narcoleptic population. Observation of relatives of narcoleptic patients showed that the simple presence of HLA-DR2 in families at risk is not sufficient for development of the disease. Additional genetic and/or environmental factors must be present for narcolepsy to develop. Moreover, the narcolepsy susceptibility gene must have an incomplete penetrance.

Genetic crossing-over events, all involving HLA-DR2, were observed in one family. The presence of narcolepsy in one of these recombination cases indicates that the narcolepsy susceptibility gene was conserved after the crossing-over, strongly suggesting that this gene (if it is not DR2 itself) is centromeric to the B locus of the HLA region.

Is HLA-DR2 Directly Involved in Narcolepsy?

Since HLA-DR2 is observed in narcoleptic patients of all ethnic groups, can we hypothesize that this antigen is specifically involved in the pathophysiology of narcolepsy? Although the HLA-DR2 molecule is serologically identical in patients and controls, the HLA-DR2 DNA chain is possibly modified in narcoleptics. Marcadet et al. (1985) tried to answer this question in a DNA restriction fragment length polymorphism study. They did not find any modification of the DR2 DNA chain with the enzymes used, but Honda et al. (1986), using other restriction enzymes, found significant differences between the HLA-DR2 DNA bands of narcoleptic Mongoloid patients and controls.

Observations of families of narcoleptic patients in our study did not support the hypothesis of a modification of the HLA-DR2 molecule in narcoleptics. Since HLA genes are transmitted as a whole from parents to offspring, the HLA-DR2 molecule is probably identical in all family members who inherit this antigen. It is unlikely that only one of two monozygotic twins would have a modified HLA-DR2 antigen. In addition, 30 members of the 3 families previously reported carried HLA-DR2; 7 were afflicted with narcolepsy. It is also unlikely that only 7 of these 30 relatives had a modified HLA-DR2 antigen and developed narcolepsy. More studies are needed to clarify this issue but, even if one finds DNA chain modification, this antigen is probably not the only factor involved in narcolepsy. Narcolepsy could thus be considered a polyfactorial disease.

Is Narcolepsy Associated with a Gene Adjacent to DR2?

Narcolepsy may not be associated with HLA-DR2 itself but instead with a gene adjacent to DR2 and always transmitted with it. In Caucasoids, HLA-DR2 has two linked specificities, namely Dw2 and DQw1. Narcoleptic patients of different ethnic origins were all found to be HLA-DR2, DQw1, Dw2 positive (Marcadet et al. 1985; Honda et al. 1986). Consequently, narcolepsy may be linked with the HLA-DR2-DQw1-Dw2 haplotype, with one of these three specificities, or with a combinatin of them.

If the narcolepsy susceptibility gene is not the DR2 itself, it is most likely located in the HLA-D region and always transmitted with the DR2. If such is the case, a few cases of narcoleptic patients would probably not be HLA-DR2 positive as a result of a crossing-over event taking place between the narcolepsy susceptibility gene and the DR2 gene. A case of narcolepsy following cerebral ischemia was recently reported and said to be non-DR2 (Riviera et al. 1986), but only results of HLA-A, B, and C typings were given. Langdon et al. (1986) have shown that a negroid narcoleptic woman was not HLA-DR2 positive, but no objective finding of narcolepsy was reported. In a recent paper, Neely et al. (1986) described a family with EDS in members of three generations. Narcolepsy was diagnosed in a man who was HLA-DR2 positive and in his daughter who was not. This could be an instance of genetic crossing-over taking place between the narcolepsy susceptibility gene and the HLA-DR2 gene, but details of all HLA typings in other members of this family, which could confirm this possibility, are lacking. More typings should be done to clarify the existence of non HLA-DR2 narcoleptics and therefore the existence of a DR2-linked narcolepsy susceptibility gene.

Is Narcolepsy a Disease Linked to the Immune System?

As noted above, narcolepsy is probably a polyfactorial or a polygenic disease. It is probable that environmental and/or other genetic factors must be present for narcolepsy to occur. Parkes et al. (1986) estimated that in 15% of narcoleptics the onset is sudden, sometimes after a febrile, viral, or respiratory illness, suggesting that "narcolepsy may be caught". This figure seems quite high, although sudden onset of narcolepsy was observed in 6% of our patients. In one case a 50-year-old man with no history of medical illness, surgical intervention, or head injury, who had never complained of hypersomnolence, sleep attacks, or cataplexy previously, was bitten by a fly *(Tabanus sp.)* common in Québec (this fly is not infectious). On the same day, he experienced sudden loss of vision lasting approximately 30 min, and when he recovered he could not hear for an additional 15 min. He then recuperated completely. Approximately 2 h later, the same symptoms reoccurred. During the 1st day, he developed a major local reaction to the bite. His hand and arm swelled markedly, the edema extending to his shoulder. During the evening, his mouth and upper lip also swelled. The patient had several bouts of shivering as if he had a fever; however, his temperature remained normal. Approximately 1 week after this event, the patient suddenly developed excessive daytime sleepiness and cataplexy. Symptoms in this patient were severe from the beginning. He had several daily sleep attacks and marked daytime somnolence. Cataplexy started the same day as excessive daytime sleepiness and was triggered by laughing, startling stimuli, or catching a fish. This patient was seen in the sleep laboratory 4 years later and the MSLT revealed five SOREMPs. HLA typing showed the presence of the DR2 antigen. There was no family history and the patient was convinced that this condition was closely related to the fly bite. This case report suggests that narcolepsy can be triggerred by a specific environmental factor in a genetically predisposed individual.

We have seen several other narcoleptic patients who complained of excessive daytime sleepiness for more than 20 years before developing cataplexy, patients in whom the onset of cataplexy was closely associated with environmental factors. For example, cataplexy occasionally developed in a hypersomnolent patient after sleep deprivation or a psychological shock. We already know from the works by Palmbald et al. (1976, 1979) that the immune response can be lowered by sleep deprivation. In addition, recent studies (Gachelin 1986) suggest decreased immune response during grief, psychic suffering, or depression. Finally, some authors consider that the immune response is already lower in HLA-DR2 (and Dw2)-positive subjects (Hors 1985; Ilonen et al. 1986). Thus, it is quite possible that low immune response individuals, carrying a narcolepsy susceptibility gene, could develop the disease if they are exposed to a situation that further lowers their immune response, such as sleep deprivation or grief. Narcolepsy could then be considered as a disease of immunological origin involving a environmental agent responsible for its development.

There is some evidence for the presence of immune factors in narcolepsy in the work of Parkes et al. (1986), who noted the presence of lymphocytosis and an increase in the protein content of the CSF in approximately 25% of narcoleptics. However, CSF analysis of 40 narcoleptic patients done in our laboratory did not shown such abnormalities.

The association of a neurological disease like narcolepsy with the immune system seems surprising. However, it must be remembered that the nervous and immune systems are closely related, implicating classical hormones, neurotransmitters, and neurohormones (Gachelin 1986). Lymphoid cells of the thymus, which receive nervous endings, integrate signals produced by the nervous system in response to external information and modulate the physiological activity of immune cells (Gachelin 1986). This could explain how psychological or environmental factors trigger the development of narcolepsy.

References

Billiard M, Seignalet J (1985) Extraordinary association between HLA-DR2 and narcolepsy. Lancet 1: 226-227
Billiard M, Seignalet J, Besset A, Cadilhac J (1986) HLA-DR2 and narcolepsy. Sleep 9: 149-152
Dausset J, Pla M (eds) (1985) HLA, complexe majeur d'histocompatibilité de l'homme. Flammarion Médecine-Science, Paris
Décary F (1981) HLA et maladies. Union Med Can 110: 325-328
Duquette P, Décary F, Pleines J. Boivin D, Lamoureux G, Cosgrove JBR, Lapierre Y (1985) Clinical sub-groups of multiple sclerosis in relation to HLA: DR alleles as possible markers of disease progression. Can J Neurol Sci 12: 106-110
Gachelin G (1986) Emotions et immunité. Recherche 17: 662-666
Govaerts A, Gony J, Martin-Mondière C, Poirier JC, Schmid M, Schuller E, Degos JD, Dausset J (1985) HLA and multiple sclerosis: population and families study. Tissue Antigens 25: 187-199
Honda Y, Asaka A, Tanaka Y, Juji T (1983) Discrimination of narcoleptic patients by using genetic markers and HLA. Sleep Res 12: 254
Honda Y, Juji T, Matsuki K, Naohara T, Satake M, Inoko H. Someya T, Harada S, Doi Y (1986) HLA-DR2 and Dw2 in narcolepsy and in other disorders of excessive somnolence without cataplexy. Sleep 9: 133-142
Hors J (1985) HLA et maladies. In: Dausset J, Pla M (eds) HLA, complexe majeur d'histocompatibilité de l'homme. Flammarion Médecine-Science, Paris, pp 227-256
Ilonen J, Hyypia T, Lankinen K, Karttunen R, Salmi A (1986) Immune function in healthy blood donors with HLA-Dw2 and -Dw3 antigens. Immunobiology 171: 388-399
Imlah NW (1961) Narcolepsy in identical twins. J Neurol Neurosurg Psychiatry 24: 158-160
Juji T, Satake M, Honda Y, Doi Y (1984) HLA antigens in Japanese patients with narcolepsy: all the patients were DR2 positive. Tissue Antigens 24: 316-319
Kessler S, Guilleminault C, Dement WC (1974) A family study of 50 REM narcoleptics. Acta Neurol Scand 50: 503-512
Kessler S (1976) Genetic factors in narcolepsy. In: Guilleminault C, Dement WC, Passouant P (eds) Narcolepsy. Spectrum, New York, pp 285-302
Langdon N, Welsh KI, Van Dam M, Vaughan RW, Parkes D (1984) Genetic markers in narcolepsy. Lancet 2: 1178-1180
Langdon N. Lock C, Welsh K, Vergani D, Dorow R, Wachtel H, Palenschat D, Parkes JD (1986) Immune factors in narcolepsy. Sleep 9: 143-148
Mamelak M, Caruso VJ, Stewart K (1979) Narcolepsy: a family study. Biol Psychiatr 14: 821-834
Marcadet A, Gebuhrer L, Betuel J, Seignalet J, Freidel AC, Confavreux C, Billiard M, Dausset J, Cohen D (1985) DNA polymorphism related to HLA-DR2 Dw2 in patients with narcolepsy. Immunogenetics 22: 679-683
Mitler MM (1982) The multiple sleep latency test as an evaluation for excessive somnolence. In: Guilleminault C (ed) Sleeping and waking disorders: Indications and techniques. Addison Wesley, Menlo Park, pp 145-153
Montplaisir J, Godbout R (1986) Nocturnal sleep of narcoleptic patients: revisited. Sleep 9: 159-161
Montplaisir J, Poirier G (1987) Narcolepsy in monozygotic twins. Neurology 37: 1089
Neely SE, Rosenberg RS, Spire JP, Antel J, Arnason BGW (1986) Familial narcolepsy and HLA antigens. Ann Neurol 20: 168
Nevsimalova-Bruhova S, Roth B (1972) Heredofamilial aspects of narcolepsy and hypersomnia. Schweiz Arch Neurol Neurochir Psychiatr 110: 45-54
Palmbald J, Cantell K, Strander H, Froberg J, Karlsson CG, Levi L, Granstrom M, Unger P (1976) J Psychosom Res 20: 193-199
Palmbald J, Petrini B, Wasserman J, Akerstedt T (1979) Psychosom Med 41: 273-278
Parkes JD, Langdon N, Lock C (1986) Narcolepsy and immunity. Br Med J 292: 359-360
Poirier G, Montplaisir J, Décary F, Momège D, Lebrun A (1986) HLA antigens in narcolepsy and idiopathic central nervous system hypersomnolence. Sleep 9: 153-158
Richardson GS, Carskadon MA, Flagg W, Van Den Hoed J, Dement WC, Mitler MM (1978) Excessive daytime sleepiness in man: multiple sleep latency measurement in narcoleptic and control subjects. Electroencephalogr Clin Neurophysiol 45: 621-627

Riviera VM, Meyer JS, Hata T, Ishikawa Y, Imai A (1986) Narcolepsy following hypoxic ischemia. Ann Neurol 19: 505-508
Schrader H, Gotlebsen OB, Skomedal GN (1980) Multiple sclerosis and narcolepsy/cataplexy in a monozygotic twin. Neurology (NY) 30: 105-108
Seignalet J, Billiard M (1984) Possible association between HLA-B7 and narcolepsy. Tissue Antigens 23: 188-190
Terasaki PI, McClelland JD (1964) Microdroplet assay of human serum cytotoxins. Nature 204: 998-1000
Terasaki PI, Bernoro D, Park MS, Ozturk G, Iwaki Y (1978) Microdroplet testing for HLA-A, B, C, and D antigens. Am J Clin Pathol 69: 103-120

Chapter 7

HLA-DR2 and the Narcolepsy Syndrome: The Stanford Experience

C. GUILLEMINAULT, J. HOLLOMAN, C. GRUMET, T. KILDUFF, H. O. MCDEVITT, W. C. DEMENT, and M. M. MITLER

Susceptibility to a wide variety of human diseases is now strongly associated with genes within the human major histocompatibility complex (MHC). This complex, found on chromosome six, encodes three classes of molecules that are central to immunological function: class I (HLA-B, -C and the differentiation antigens TL and TQ), class II (HLA-DR, -DQ, -DP), and class III molecules (C2-C4 and BF). In addition to these molecules, other proteins are encoded by genes in this region.

The first suggestion that genes within the MHC might be responsible for susceptibility to a specific disease came from the recognition that susceptibility to virally induced leukemia in mice was regulated by the MHC genotype (Lilly et al. 1964). The list of diseases for which MHC apparently affects suceptibility now numbers greater than 40 (Stastny et al. 1983). The majority of these diseases are autoimmune in character and therefore associated with circulating antibodies, immune complexes, or evidence of immune-mediated injury. Examples of diseases with strong association are ankylosing spondylitis (95% of patients have HLA-B27), juvenile-onset diabetes mellitus (95% of patients have DR3 or DR4), and celiac disease (95% of patients have DR3 or DR7 alleles). The most impressive HLA disease association reported to date, however, has been observed for a disease not commonly recognized to be autoimmune in nature: narcolepsy. Japanese (Honda et al. 1983; Juji et al. 1984) and, subsequently, French (Billiard and Seignalet 1985) and British (Langdon et al. 1984) researchers have reported that the DR2 allele, normally present in 33.8%, 21.8%, and 25.2% (British Caucasian) of their populations, respectively, is found in 100% of their patients with narcolepsy. It is thus currently hypothesized that the immune system may be involved in this disease. The observation that the same serologically defined allele is associated with narcolepsy among different races supports the hypothesis that the susceptibility gene may indeed be an MHC product rather than a linked gene encoding a non-HLA-related product.

In order to validate these preliminary findings, however, an important methodological issue must be addressed: the definition of narcolepsy.

Current Stanford Classification of the Narcolepsies

Classical narcolepsy (CN) is defined by presence of daytime napping, complaint of daytime sleepiness, presence of cataplexy, and presence of short mean sleep latency on the Multiple Sleep Latency Test (MSLT) <7 min (Richardson et al. 1982),

Table 1. Stanford criteria for the classification of narcolepsies

	CN	NWC	CNSH	AN		
EDS	+	+	+	+	+	+
Cataplexy	+	−	−	−	−/+	−/+
MSLT	<7	<7	<7	<7	<7	<9
SOREMP	>2	>2	0	1	0–1	0–2

EDS, excessive daytime sleepiness; MSLT, multiple sleep latency test; SOREMP, sleep-onset rapid eye movement period; CN, classical narcolepsy; NWC, narcolepsy without cataplexy; CNSH, central nervous system hypersomnia; AN, ambiguous narcolepsy

with the presence of at least two sleep-onset-REM periods on the MSLT. Cataplexy may be noted at examination or defined by a response of "3" or greater on a specific questionnaire [item #218 of the Sleep Questionnaire and Assessment of Wakefulness (SQAW; Miles 1983): "How often do you have episodes of sudden muscular weakness (paralysis or inability to move) when laughing, angry, or in other emotional situations?"].

Narcolepsy without cataplexy (NWC) is defined as no evidence of cataplexy

(a) at examination,
(b) from reports of patients and family members, and
(c) response not higher than "9" on item #218 of SQAW. Mean MSLT scores are less than 7 min, and at least two sleep-onset REM periods must be recorded.

Isolated excessive daytime sleepiness (EDS) is also called central nervous system hypersomnia (CNSH) and is defined by:

(a) complete absence of auxillary symptoms of narcolepsy at interviews,
(b) response not higher than "2" on item #218 of the SQAW questionnaire,
(c) presence of EDS clinically, confirmed by short mean sleep latency (<7 min) on the MSLT, and
(d) absence of sleep-onset REM periods.

Ambiguous narcolepsy (AN) is defined as the complaint of excessive daytime sleepiness and the report of daytime napping, the complaint of vague feelings of muscle weakness that cannot be confirmed as cataplexy by medical observation, and the absence of a convincing history for the disorder. At polygraphic examination, the MSLT shows various results:

(a) a mean sleep latency <7 min, with no more than one sleep-onset REM period or
(b) a mean sleep latency between 7 and 9 min, with one or two sleep-onset REM periods.

Our classification indicates that two entities are well identified: "classical narcolepsy" (CN) and "isolated EDS-CNS hypersomnia" (CNSH) [these correspond closely to B.6 and B.7 of the Disorders of Excessive Somnolence described in the Association of Sleep Disorders Centers nosology (1979)] and that two are difficult to define: "narcolepsy without cataplexy" (NWC) and "ambiguous narcolepsy" (AN). The relationship between clinical symptoms, clinical complaints, and polygraphic monitoring needs further investigation. For example, we have investigated the families of patients from group CN, the classical narcoleptics, and found that among those family members complaining of EDS there were representatives of all four categories. The use of HLA typing promises to focus some light on these somewhat murky relationships.

Relationship Between Serologic HLA-DR Typing and the Stanford Clinical Classifications

Blood samples from 20 index cases have been submitted for serological HLA-DR typing. Typing and sleep scoring were performed blindly. A total of 13 subjects were classified as "classical narcoleptics" (CN). One patient was classified as "ambiguous narcolepsy" (AN); three patients were classified as "narcolepsy without cataplexy" (NWC); and three patients were classified as "isolated EDS-CNS hypersomnia". The HLA-DR typing showed that 12 of our 13 subjects with "classical narcolepsy" were DR2 and none of the "isolated EDS-CNS hypersomnia" or "ambiguous narcolepsy" patients possessed the DR2 allele. One out of three patients classified "narcolepsy without cataplexy" was typed as DR2.

HLA-DR and Restriction Fragment Length Polymorphisms

A second technique was used to study the HLA typing of 12 of the above 20 subjects. Restriction fragment length polymorphisms (RFLPs) provide a means of subdividing DR haplotypes. Using homozygous cell lines and a DR beta 3' untranslated region probe, it has been possible to identify distinct patterns for the different DR haplotypes and the different subtypes of HLA-DR2. Nine out of 12 subjects were typed as having the DR2 pattern on RFLPs. These nine subjects were also DR2 at serologic typing and none of the last three were serologically DR2. The pattern obtained for the DR2 haplotype was identical in all the DR2-positive narcoleptics and was identical to the DR2, DW2 patterns seen in the homozygous consanguinous cell line called PGF. This was true with six different restriction enzymes typing line PGF.

In summary, the nine patients clinically classified as "classical narcoleptic" and presenting serologically with DR2 were similarly typed by RFLPs. The data obtained with this probe suggest that the DR2 allele associated with "classical narcolepsy" is not a variant allele, at least not at the level of RFLPs. It is possible, however, that the gene has some variation in nucleic sequence that is not reflected by restriction fragment.

Anomalous Findings

"Narcolepsy Without Cataplexy" with Positive DR2

This subject is a 12-year-old girl in the developing phase of narcolepsy so the apparent discrepancy is not surprising. In most cases cataplexy, as previously reported in several large narcoleptic population studies, appears several months or even years after development of daytime sleepiness. One can still anticipate the appearance of cataplexy in this case.

"Cataplexy Without Daytime Sleepiness"

This subject is a 33-year-old woman who has experienced cataplctic attacks since adolescence. Her cataplexy is induced by various emotions, such as surprise and laughter. The condition has been a considerable handicap in her professional life where contact with the public is required. She has never complained of daytime sleepiness, does not take naps during the day, and feels fully alert for long hours. Monitored polygraphically for two 24-h periods with two successive days of MSLT, she has had no sleep-onset REM period and a mean sleep latency of 9.4 min - considered within the normal range. Her phenotype was DR1, DR2, DQW1, DRW52.

"Classical Narcolepsy" Without DR2

Until now, all reports have emphasized the 100% correlation between HLA-DR2 and narcolepsy-cataplexy. For 2½ years, we have followed a 52-year-old Caucasian woman who developed narcoleptic symptoms at 46 years of age, at onset of menopause. Within a year of the onset of her symptoms, she presented a complete clinical picture: a minimum of three short naps daily, intermittent irresistible sleep attacks, daily cataplectic attacks of variable intensity (ranging from loss of muscle tone in the head, neck, and shoulder to complete attacks during which she collapses on the floor) and variable duration (ranging from a few seconds to up to 8 min), sleep paralysis, and hypnagogic hallucinations occurring at least weekly. The patient has undergone six different nocturnal polygraphic monitoring sessions with MSLTs the following day. She had a mean total nocturnal sleep time of 416 min. The mean sleep latency on the MSLTs was 2 min 5 s (with standard error of the mean = 10 s) with between three and five sleep onset REM periods at each MSLT. Regardless of the clinical criteria used, this patient will be classified as having narcolepsy-cataplexy. Despite her bona fide narcolepsy, in two different HLA-DR typings conducted 3 months apart on different blood samples and in a blind fashion, her phenotype was DR1, DR4, DRW53, DQW3. Since the identification of this patient, which was in itself surprising given our small (20) group of subjects, a second case, a 24-year-old Caucasian woman, has been identified by Mitler et al. (1986). She has clear classical narcolepsy of 6 years' duration and clinically verified cataplexy. She exhibits four sleep-onset REM periods on the MSLT. This patient is also not DR2, but DR4-DR7, DQWZ, DQW3.

In Conclusion

It appears, therefore, that the association between HLA-DR2 and narcolepsy - at least in its classical form - is not universal, suggesting either that there are subsets of this disorder, or that DR2 is an associated marker rather than the disease susceptibility gene itself (at least in Caucasians). Further investigation of these DR2-negative patients, who are clinically and polygraphically indistinguishable from other cases of classical narcolepsy, may enlarge our understanding of the causes of the syndrome.

Findings by Other US Research Teams

Scripps Clinic and Research Foundation (San Diego) Findings
(M. Mitler, R. L. Rubin et al., personal communication)

The Scripps Clinic researchers have determined HLA phenotypes at the A, B, C, and D loci in a group of Caucasian narcoleptics. Considering that excessive daytime sleepiness is a common finding in obstructive sleep apnea syndrome, these authors made a comparison with a group of Caucasian patients with this disorder. The subjects were 11 patients with clinical diagnoses of narcolepsy based on complaints of daytime sleep attacks, cataplexy, and objective evidence of REM sleep abnormalities on the MSLT with at least two sleep-onset REM periods. They included three men and eight women, with a mean age of 44 years. The obstructive sleep apnea group included ten patients, eight men and two women, with a mean age of 53 years. The sleep apneic patients had a clinical complaint of daytime sleepiness and inappropriate daytime sleep. Polygraphic monitoring during nocturnal sleep detected obstructive events lasting longer than 10 s at a rate greater than 30/h. They were free of major REM sleep abnormalities, characteristics of narcolepsy such as cataplexy, sleep paralysis, and hypnagogic hallucinations. HLA phenotypes were determined by the immunocytotoxicity method of Terasaki: on cryopreserved lymphocytes. Additionally levels of circulating antibodies associated with systemic lupus erythematosus (SLE) and rheumatoid arthritis (RA) including anti-DNA, antihistone, anti-Sm, anti-SS-B, and rheumatoid factors were determined by solid phase immunoassays. These researchers also screened for antibodies to brain tissues, antineuronal antibodies, and antinuclear antibodies by immunofluorescence and cytotoxic assays as well as general indices of inflammation.

The narcoleptic population had a mean of 3.9 sleep-onset REM periods on the MSLT versus 0.7 for sleep apnea, with a nocturnal REM sleep percentage of 23.40% for narcoleptics versus 13.30% for sleep apneics.

In a Caucasian control group, they found a frequency of HLA-DR2 of 25.2%. Nine narcoleptics were HLA-DR2, while three sleep apneics (30%) were DR2 positive (Chi-square = 18.8, df = 1 $p < 0.001$). When considering HLA DQw1, 54.5% of the control group were DQw1 positive, while 91% of the narcoleptics (i.e., 10 out of 11 patients) and 30% of the sleep apneics (i.e., 3 out of 10 subjects) were positive for DQw1.

The two groups were distinctly different on each of the tabulated polygraphic and HLA parameters (all $p < 0.01$). However, there were two patients - one with a clear history of cataplexy and sleep attacks, the other with a history of cataplexy more difficult to assess at the time of the evaluation - that exhibited three and four sleep-onset REM periods at MSLT and who were not DR2. Their respective phenotypes were DR1-DR3-DQw1, DQw2 and DR4-DR7, DQw2, DQw3.

University of Chicago Sleep Laboratory Findings

Neely and collaborators (1986) have evaluated 11 black Chicagoans. Two patients had a strong history of cataplexy and daytime sleepiness and were DR2 positive. The two, however, were not studied polygraphically. Nine other patients had a history of cataplexy and daytime sleep attacks. After polygraphic monitorings, three of the patients exhibited one sleep onset REM period on the MSLT and were DR2 positive. The six remaining patients had two or more sleep-onset REM periods on the MSLT and were DR2 positive. The gene frequency of DR2 in a local black control group totaling 99 subjects was 27%. As emphasized by the authors, the DR2 gene frequency was highly statistically different by chi-square test ($p < 0.01$) in this black narcoleptic population, confirming the multiracial validity of the Japanese team findings. However, the finding that two patients were DR2 negative indicates that DR2 is not invariably present in black narcoleptics either.

References

Association of Sleep Disorders Centers (1979) Diagnostic classification of sleep and arousal disorders, 1st edn. Prepared by the Sleep Disorders Classification Committee. Sleep 2: 1-137

Billiard M, Seignalet J (1985) Extraordinary association between HLA-DR2 and narcolepsy. Lancet I: 226-227

Honda Y, Asaka A, Tanaka A, Juji T (1983) Discrimination of narcoleptic patients using genetic markers and HLA. Sleep Res 12: 254

Juji T, Satake M, Honda Y, Doi Y (1984) HLA antigens in Japanese patients with narcolepsy. Tissue Antigens 24: 316-319

Langdon N. Welsh K, van Dam M, Vaugham RM, Parkes JD (1984) Genetic markers in narcolepsy. Lancet I: 226-227

Lilly F, Boyse EA, Old LJ (1964) Genetic basis for susceptibility to viral leukemogenesis. Lancet II: 1207-1209

Miles L (1983) Sleep questionnaire and assessment of wakefulness [SQAW]. In: Guilleminault C (ed) Sleeping and waking disorders: indications and techniques. Addison Wesley, Menlo Park, appendix

Mitler MM, Shafor R, Sobers M, Hajdukovich RM, Rubin RL (1986) Human leukocyte antigen [HLA] studies in excessive somnolence: narcolepsy vs. sleep apnea (abstract). Sleep Res 15

Neely SE, Rosenberg AS, Spire JP, Antel J, Arnasson BEW (1986) HLA, antigens in narcolepsy. Neurology 36 [Suppl I]: 299

Richardson G, Carskadon M, Flagg W, Van den Hoed J, Dement W, Mitler M (1982) Excessive daytime sleepiness in man: multiple sleep latency measurements in narcoleptics vs. control subjects. Electroencephalogr Clin Neurophysiol 45: 621-627

Stasny P, Ball EJ, Day PJ (1983) The human immune response region (HLA-D) and disease susceptibility. Immunol Rev 70: 113-152

Chapter 8

Narcolepsy and HLA in the Federal Republic of Germany: Population and Family Data

K. MEIER-EWERT, G. MUELLER-ECKHARDT, and D. J. SCHENDEL

Fifty-nine unrelated narcolepsy patients as well as 14 families (01-14), including 16 patients and 44 healthy relatives, were investigated for MHC class I (HLA-A, B, C), class II (HLA-DR, DQ), and class III (BF, C4A, C4B) alleles. Glyoxalase-1 (GLO) was determined as an additional marker in family studies. For the population study, unrelated healthy individuals (class I, $n=1329$; class II, $n=418$; class III, $n=408$) served as normal controls. All methods used were described recently (Mueller-Eckhardt et al. 1986). Statistical evaluations were made with the X^2 test with Yates' correction. *P*-values were corrected for the number of antigens tested. Some of these results have been published elsewhere (Mueller-Eckhardt et al. 1986). They are presented here in more detail for comparison with data from other populations.

Diagnostic Criteria

The diagnosis of narcolepsy was based on the following criteria (Honda et al. 1983; Meier-Ewert 1983; Honda et al. 1986; Matsuki et al. 1985):

1. Recurrent daytime naps occurring almost every day and persisting for at least 6 months.
2. Clinical confirmation of cataplexy in the patient's history. We adopted the following definition of cataplexy: "Sudden loss of muscle tone bilaterally on unexpected strong emotion, such as laughter, feelings of pride, anticipation just prior to showing off in front of others, anger or surprise, without marked sleepiness or loss of consciousness" (Juji et al. 1986).
3. Presence of a sleep onset REM period (defined as REM sleep within 15 min after onset of NREM stage I) in an all night polysomnography or in a multiple sleep latency test, performed in our hospital.

Patients

These criteria have been fulfilled by 59 unrelated Caucasian narcolepsy patients (36 males, 23 females, average age 50,7 years, range 11-72 years, average age at onset of narcolepsy 20.8 years). In one patient narcolepsy was considered to be of symptomatic origin, appearing shortly after an infection of malaria tertiana. One male patient, 46 years of age, was HLA-DR-2 negative. He gave the following history: At the age of 23 he did nightshift work for 1 year. At the age of 24, within a few weeks both irresistible sleep attacks and cataplectic attacks appeared. The latter were elicited by special emotions which were triggered by dry jokes. While the sleep attacks persisted without much change, the cataplectic attacks were successfully suppressed for several years by tricyclics. On one occasion when this medication was stopped, recurrent cataplectic attacks appeared for many days. Sleep onset REM periods with persisting tonus of the musculus mentalis (Raynal 1976) and frequent appearance of "signs of REM prior to REM" were documented in three sequential all night recordings. Three further sequential all night recordings showed suppression of sleep onset REM by 75 mg clomipramine p.d. Apart from cataplectic and sleep attacks this patient suffered from hypnagogic hallucinations, sleep paralysis, and disturbance of night sleep. At the time of clinical observation (1981) he was 9 kg overweight. This patient has since been examined by Andreas-Zietz et al. (1986).

Population Studies

Phenotype frequencies of class I, II, and III alleles were compared with those of normal controls (Tables 1-3). Among class I antigens (Table 1) no significant deviations were found in narcolepsy patients except for HLA-B7 which is concordant with other reports on Caucasian patients and probably due to the known linkage disequilibrium with HLA-DR-2 in these populations (Billiard and Seignalet 1985; Billiard et al. 1986; Langdon et al. 1984; Marcadet et al. 1985; Poirier et al. 1986).

Als expected from all other reports (Billiard and Seignalet 1985; Billiard et al. 1986; Honda et al. 1986; Juji et al. 1984, 1985; Langdon et al. 1984; Marcadet et al. 1985; Matsuki et al. 1985; Mueller-Eckhardt et al. 1986; Poirier et al. 1986; Seignalet and Billiard 1984) the associations with the highest strength and significance were with the class II antigens (Table 2) DR2 and DQw1. Surprisingly, however, in our population the association between these two markers and the disease was not complete. One patient (F.H.) with unequivocal symptoms of narcolepsy (see above) was found to be DR2/DQw1 negative. He was typed HLA-A11, 24; Bw55,-; Cw3,-; DR4, 5; DQw3,-; BF F, F; C4A3, 3; C4B1, 1.

In 11 of 59 patients (18.6%) DR2 was the only DR antigen found. Genotyping was possible in five cases (Fig. 2). Homozygosity for DR2 (and DQw1) was proven by segregation in three families (02, 04, 06) and appeared most probable in one case (family 03). In contrast to DR2, two other DR alleles in linkage disequilibrium with DQw1, i.e., DR1 and DRw6, were found to be significantly decreased. The same was true for DRw52 and DQw2.

Complement allotype frequencies (Table 3) were not significantly different from normal controls. However, C4BQ0 was found decreased in the patient group. Whether this difference is important for disease susceptibility is uncertain until it is confirmed by other studies in Caucasian patients. Frequency deviations as reported for Japanese patients, i.e., for BF S, BF F, C4A2, and C4B2, respectively, were not observed in our German group of narcoleptics.

Table 1. Comparison of class I phenotype frequencies (%) in unrelated narcolepsy patients (P) and normal controls (C)

HLA	P (n=59)	C (n=1329)	x^2y	*P*-value	*Pc*	*RR*
A 1	22.0	29.4	1.16			
2	35.6	50.3	4.34			
3	42.4	27.9	5.10	0.0239	NS	1.9
11	15.3	10.1	1.08			
23(9)	1.7	4.9	0.67			
24(9)	18.6	16.9	0.03			
25(10)	3.4	4.5	0.01			
26(10)	5.1	7.4	0.17			
28	8.5	7.6	0.00			
29	8.5	5.3	0.59			
30(w19) 31(w19)	6.8	6.5	0.03			
32(w19)	6.8	6.6	0.05			
w33(w19)	0.0	1.9	0.35			
w34(10)	0.0	0.3	0.67			
B 7	57.6	23.3	33.84	$<10^{-8}$	$<10^{-6}$	4.47
8	13.6	20.8	1.42			
13	6.8	6.3	0.02			
14	3.4	5.8	0.24			
18	15.3	10.4	0.95			
27	10.2	7.2	0.33			
35	20.3	17.8	0.10			
37	0.0	2.9	0.87			
38(16)	0.0	4.3	1.75			
39(16)	3.4	3.4	0.13			
w41	0.0	1.1	0.04			
44(12)	15.3	26.7	3.26			
45(12)	1.7	0.6	0.04			
w47	0.0	0.6	0.08			
49(21)	0.0	2.2	0.46			
50(21)	1.7	1.4	0.15			
51(5)	8.5	8.9	0.01			
w52(5)	0.0	0.9	0.00			
w53	1.7	1.0	0.02			
w55(w22)	3.4	4.1	0.00			
w56(w22)	3.4	1.6	0.24			
w57(17)	5.1	7.3	0.17			
w58(17)	0.0	1.3	0.07			
w60(40)	3.4	9.1	1.63			
w61(40)	1.7	2.5	0.00			
w62(15)	8.5	15.9	1.83			
w63(15)	0.0	1.2	0.05			
Cw1	5.1	4.6	0.02			
2	10.2	9.3	0.00			
3	17.0	27.4	2.62			
4	17.0	18.7	0.42			
5	3.4	12.3	3.44			
6	15.3	18.0	0.14			
7	35.6	27.3	1.38			
8	3.4	3.4	0.14			

x^2y, x^2 with Yates' correction; *Pc*, *P*-value corrected for the number of antigens tested; *RR*, relative risk; NS, not signifikant

Table 2. Comparison of class II phenotype frequencies (%) in unrelated narcolepsy patients (P) and normal controls (C)

HLA	P (n=59)	C (n=418)	x^2y	P-value	Pc	RR
DR 1	1.7	21.8	12.13	0.0005	0.0074	0.1
2	98.3	23.9	125.79	$<10^{-10}$	$<10^{-10}$	184.4
3	8.5	19.6	3.62			
4	23.7	21.5	0.05			
5	22.0	27.8	0.61			
w6	3.4	24.5	12.28	0.0005	0.0067	0.1
7	15.3	25.8	2.58			
w8	1.7	3.1	0.04			
w9	3.4	1.0	0.47			
w10	1.7	1.4	0.18			
w52	37.3	65.3	16.04	$<10^{-4}$	0.0009	0.3
w53	42.4	45.2	0.07			
DQw1	98.3	65.8	24.42	$<10^{-6}$	$<10^{-4}$	30.2
2	23.7	44.3	8.14	0.0043	NS	0.4
3	49.2	43.3	0.50			

x^2y, x^2 with Yates' correction; ,Pc, P-value corrected for the number of antigens tested; RR, relative risk; NS, not significant

Table 3. Comparison of class III and GLO phenotype frequencies (%) in unrelated narcolepsy patients (P) and normal controls (C)

	P (n=48)	C (n=408)	x^2y	P-value	Pc	RR
C4 A6	4.2	8.1	0.46			
A5	0.0	2.0	0.16			
A4	18.8	15.0	0.23			
A3	83.3	88.0	0.48			
A2	8.3	14.0	0.74			
A1	0.0	2.0	0.16			
AQ0	12.5	23.0	2.20			
C4 B1	95.8	92.9	0.21			
B2	16.7	16.9	0.03			
B3	2.1	2.0	0.24			
Bvar	0.0	3.9	0.96			
BQ0	6.3	26.0	8.14	0.0043	NS	0.2
	(n=45)					
BF F	28.9	33.1	0.16			
S	97.8	96.1	0.02			
F_1	0.0	2.0	0.12			
S_1	2.2	2.0	0.20			
	(n=36)					
GLO 1	58.3	67.6	2.60			
2	72.2	81.4	2.61			

x^2y, x^2 with Yates' correction; Pc, P-value corrected for the number of antigens tested; RR, relative risk; NS, not significant

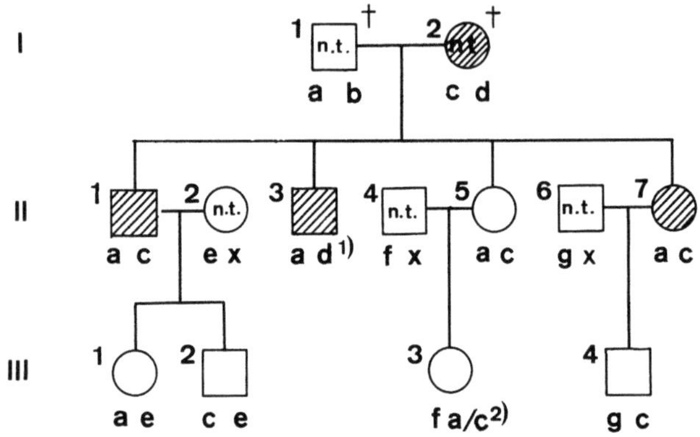

Fig. 1. Pedigree of family 01. (Mueller-Eckhardt et al. 1986). Designation of haplotypes: *a*, GLO2, DQw2, DR7, BFS, C4B1, A3, HLA B18, Cw6, A1; *c*, GLO2, DQw1, DR2, BFS, C4B1, A3, HLA B51, Cw3, A11; *a/c*, GLO2, DQw2, DR7, BFS, C4B1, A3, HLA B51, Cw3, A11; *d*, GLO2, DQw1, DR2, BFS, C4B1, A3, HLA B7, Cw7, A24; *e*, GLO2, DQw1, DR2, BFS, C4B1, A3, HLA B35, Cw4, A2; *f*, GLO1, DQw3, DR4, BFS, C4B0, A3, HLA Bw55, C-, A32; *g*, GLO1, DQw1, DR2, BFS, C4B1, A3, HLA B7, Cw4, A2; *x*, undefined; *1*, possibly B/DR recombinant haplotype *(c/d)*; *2*, B/DR recombinant

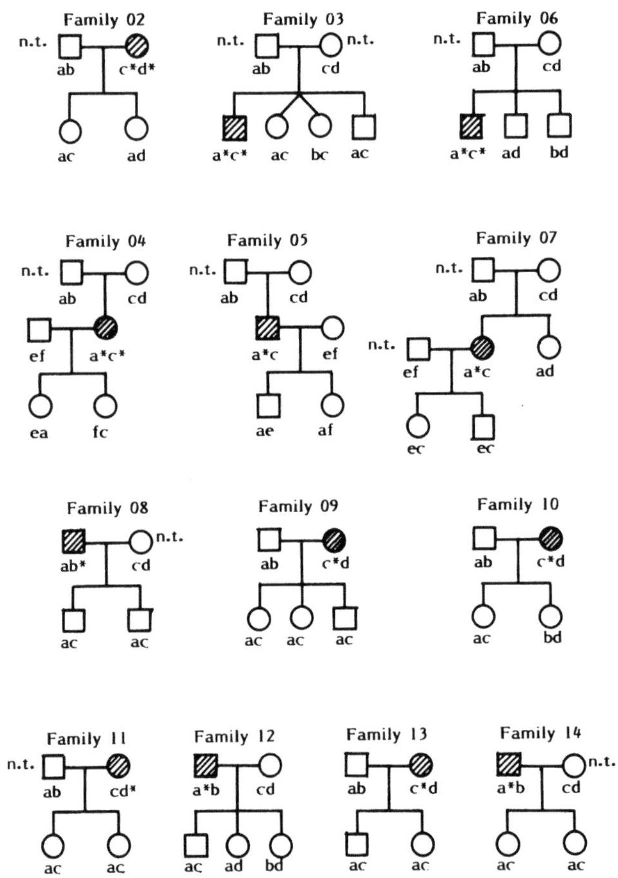

Fig. 2. Pedigrees of families 02–14. * DR2-linked haplotypes of patients (see Table 4)

Family Studies

Among the 14 families used for segregation analysis there was one multicase family in which narcolepsy could be traced from the mother to three of four children (family 01, Fig. 1). Of the three genotypically identical (DR2-positive) siblings only two had developed the disease. Interestingly, the haplotype shared by all three patients (II: 1, 3, 7) is not the DR2- (c) but a DR7-linked haplotype (a). In patient II: 3, however, a different DR2-bearing haplotype (d) from the same parent (presumably the mother) was detected. Since both parents were deceased the question could not be answered whether the DR2 antigen in all three patients is genotypically identical due to a maternal crossing over in patient II: 3. The same was recently found in a Canadian family (Poirier et al. 1986). Our data from family 01 are concordant with those from multicase families published by two other groups (Honda et al. 1986; Matsuki et al. 1985; Poirier et al. 1986), favoring a dominant mode of inheritance with incomplete penetrance of an HLA-linked disease susceptibility gene.

Nevertheless, familial occurrence of narcolepsy is seen only for a minority of patients. In our families 02-14 (Fig. 2) no narcolepsy symptoms were observed in any individuals other than the patients, although the DR2-linked haplotypes identified in the patients (Table 4) were also observed in healthy relatives of all but two families (08, 11, Fig. 2).

Analysis of these extended haplotypes revealed interesting differences from those reported from Japanese narcoleptics. While Matsuki et al. (1985) have calculated a significantly higher frequency of particularly rare haplotypes than in nor-

Table 4. Extended DR-2-linked haplotypes involved in 16 narcolepsy patients as deduced from 14 families (for pedigrees see Figs. 1, 2)

Family No.	haplotype	GLO	HLA DQ	HLA DR	BF	C4 B	C4 A	HLA B	HLA C	HLA A
01	c	2	wl	2	S	1	3	51	w3	11
	d	2	wl	2	S	1	3	7	w7	24
02	c	1	w1	2	F	1	3	8	-	1
	d	(1)	w1	2	S	1	3	7	w7	11
03	a	1(2)	w1	2	S	1	3	w56	w1	26
	c	2(1)	w1	2	S	1	3	8	w7	24
04	a	1	w1	2	F	1	3	w62	w3	3
	c	1	w1	2	S	1	3	7	-	2
05	a	1	w1	2	F	1	3	7	w7	24
06	a	1	w1	2	S	1	3	w55	-	2
	c	1	w1	2	S	1	3	7	w7	3
07	a		w1	2	S	1	3	44	w5	1
08	b		w1	2	S	1	3	7	-	2
09	c	2	w1	2	S	1	3	7	-	3
10	c		w1	2	S	0	0	7	w7	3
11	d		w1	2	S	1	3	7	w7	24
12	a	1	w1	2	S	1	3	7	w7	3
13	c		w1	2	S	1	3	7	-	2
14	a	1	w1	2	S	1	3	7	w7	2

mal controls, we observed DR2 haplotypes with the typical linkage disequilibrium known for European Caucasians: 10 of 20 haplotypes included HLA DQw1, DR2, BFS, C4B1, C4A3, HLA B7, (Cw7), while 16/20 had DQw1, DR2, BFS, C4B1, C4A3 in common.

In conclusion, population and family studies in German narcoleptics have shown associations with HLA DR2 and DQw1 which are concordant with those of all other investigators, with the exception of one DR2-negative patient. However, frequency deviations for class I and class III markers as well as the composition of DR2-linked extended haplotypes in Caucasian patients are clearly different from those in Orientals.

References

Andreas-Zietz A, Keller E, Scholz S, Albert ED, Roth B, Nevsimalova S, Sonka K, Docekal P, Ivaskova E, Schulz H, Geisler P (1986) DR2-negative narcolepsy. Lancet II: 684-685

Billiard M, Seignalet J (1985) Extraordinary association between HLA-DR2 and narcolepsy. Lancet I: 226-227

Billiard M, Seignalet J, Besset A, Cadilhac J (1986) HLA-DR-2 and narcolepsy. Sleep 9: 149-152

Guilleminault C (1986) Narcolepsy 1985 (editorial). Sleep 9: 99-101

Honda Y, Asaka Y, Tanimura M, Furusho T (1983) A genetic study of narcolepsy and excessive daytime sleepiness in 308 families with a narcolepsy or hypersomnia proband. In: Guilleminault C, Lugaresi E (eds) Sleep wake disorders. Raven, New York

Honda Y, Juji T, Matsuki K, Naohara T, Satake M, Inoko H, Someya T, Harada S, Doi Y (1986) HLA-DR2 and Dw2 in narcolepsy and in other disorders of excessive somnolence without cataplexy. Sleep 9: 133-142

Juji T, Satake M, Honda Y, Doi Y (1984) HLA antigens in Japanese patients with narcolepsy. Tissue antigens 24: 316-319

Juji T, Matsuki K, Naohara T, Satake M, Honda Y (1985) Extraordinary association between HLA-DR2 and narcolepsy. Lancet I: 227

Juji T, Honda Y, Matsuki K, Bashir H (1986) Narcolepsy: joint report. In: Aizawa M, Tatsri T, Wakiaka A, Konoeda Y (eds) Proc III Asia-Oceania histocompatibility workshop, Sapporo, 1986, pp 346-348

Langdon N. Welsh K, van Dam M, Vaughan RW, Parkes D (1984) Genetic markers in narcolepsy. Lancet II: 1178-1180

Marcadet A, Gebuhrer L, Betuel H, Seignalet J, Freidel AC, Confavreux C, Billiard M, Dausset J, Cohen D (1985) DNA polymorphism related to HLA-DR2 Dw2 in patients with narcolepsy. Immunogenetics 22: 679-683

Matsuki K, Juji T, Tokunaga K, Naohara T, Satake M. Honda Y (1985) Human histocompatibility leucocyte antigen (HLA) haplotype frequencies estimated from the data on HLA class I, II, and III, antigens in 111 Japanese narcoleptics. J Clin Invest 76: 2078-2083

Meier-Ewert K (1983) Zur Begutachtung der Narkolepsien. Öff Gesundh Wes 45: 488-493

Mueller-Eckhardt G, Meier-Ewert K, Schendel DJ, Reinecker FB, Multhoff G, Mueller-Eckhardt C (1986) HLA and narcolepsy in a German population. Tissue Antigens 28: 163-169

Poirier G, Montplaisir J, Décary F, Momège D, Lebrun A (1986) HLA antigens in narcolepsy and idiopathic central nervous system hypersomnolence. Sleep 9: 153-158

Raynal D (1976) Polygraphic aspects of narcolepsy. In: Guilleminault C, Dement WC, Passouant P (eds) Narcolepsy. Spectrum, New York

Seignalet J, Billiard M (1984) Possible association between HLA-B7 and narcolepsy. Tissue Antigens 23: 188-189

Chapter 9

Positive HLA-Dw2 in Narcolepsy

T. Naohara, Y. Honda, and T. Juji

Some authors reported that all the narcoleptic patients studied were positive for HLA-DR2 and DQw1 (Honda et al. 1984; Juji et al. 1984; Langdom et al. 1984; Billiard and Seignalet 1985). These findings prompted us to investigate HLA-D specificities of narcoleptics, because, in the Japanese population, HLA-D specificities that associate with HLA-DR2 have been reported to be HLA-Dw12 and less frequently Dw2, which is in contrast to the high correlation of HLA-DR2 and HLA-Dw2 (*r* value is approximately 0.9) in Caucasoid populations (Jaraquemada 1984).

The mixture of lymphocytes from two different individuals, known as the mixed lymphocyte reaction (MLR), usually results in a blastogenic response with cell proliferation (Schrek and Donelly 1961) and this in vitro response is now generally accepted to be the in vitro cellular immune response to allogeneic determinants of the major histocompatibility complex.

In the 1960s, when lymphocytes from two genetically different individuals were cultured together in vitro, a proliferative response was observed and pairs of monozygotic twins always resulted in the lack of the proliferation of lymphocytes (Bain et al. 1964). In the late 1960s, there were strong reactions in MLR between serologically identical siblings in some instances, and, conversely, negative MLR or unidirectional nonstimulation between HLA-A and B disparity individuals were demonstrated (Amos and Bach 1968). In the early 1970s, some reports were shown that MLR tests between randomly selected unrelated individuals almost always gave strongly positive MLR. However, approximately 10% of serologically identical individuals did not stimulate each other in MLR (Mempel et al. 1973). These studies indicated that a linkage disequilibrium might exist between the genetic determinant(s) of the lymphocyte activation in MLR and HLA-SD (serologically defined) determinant(s). In 1971, Yunis and Amos demonstrated that the cell surface determinant(s) responsible for MLR, later designated HLA-D determinant(s), was independent of, although closely linked with, serologically defined antigens in the study of some recombinant families. The following studies showed that the genes of HLA-D determinant(s) were encoded in the genetic region centrometric to the HLA-B locus for about 0.7 centimorgans and telemetric to the locus controlling the red cell antigen glyoxylase, GLO, on the short arm of chromosome 6. HLA-D determinant(s) is predominantly expressed on B-lymphocytes and monocytes as well as other HLA-D region products and controls lymphocyte recognition and T-cell proliferation under the existence of antigen-presenting cells in MLR experiments. Identification of specificities of allogeneic HLA-D determinant(s) is still an area of intensive investigation. Nineteen HLA-D specificities, Dw1 through Dw19, have been established after the 9th International Histocompatibility Workshop in 1984; however, the gene frequency of HLA-D "blank" (undefined) was estimated to be approximately 20% in Caucasoid populations (Bauer et al. 1984). This finding suggests that some HLA-D specificities remain unknown.

Although there are still disagreements on the molecular basis of the determinant(s), some hypotheses have been suggested. One is that HLA-D is independent of DR or DQ but the determinant(s) is encoded by genes in the HLA-DR subregion (Jaraquemada et al. 1986). Another is that the HLA-D determinant(s) is the summation of stimulatory effects of whole antigenic products that are encoded in HLA genes on chromosome 6 (Bach 1985). Some authors speculate the additive effect of HLA-D region products on the haplotype instead of the whole HLA gene products, i.e., HLA-D = DR+DQ+X, where X stands for the further splitting products of HLA-DR or DQ genes and/or unknown gene products (Bauer et al. 1984). As the relationship between serological and cellular typing specificities of DR2-positive cells will be discussed later, however, HLA-DQ molecules do not seem to play an important role in MLR.

The history, methodology, genetics, and biological implications of MLR were reviewed by Dupont et al. (1976).

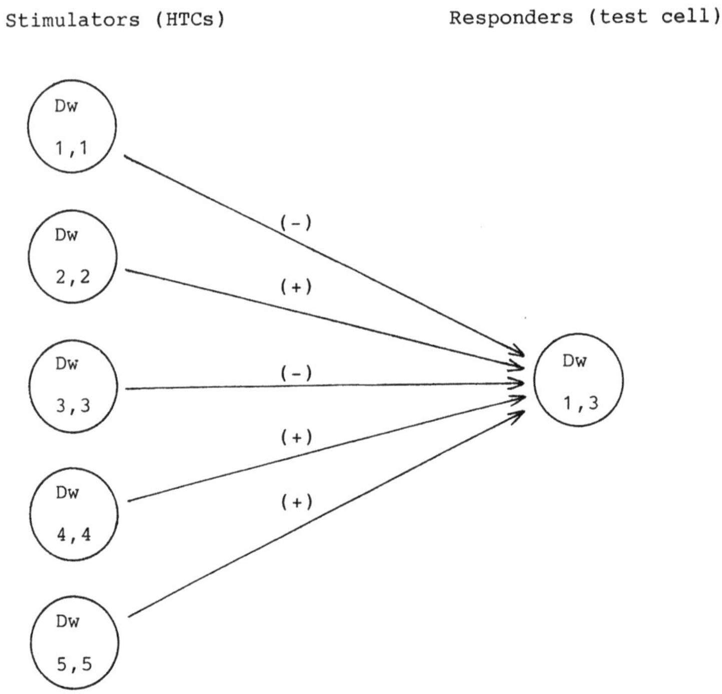

Fig. 1. The assignment of HLA-D specificities of a test cell by an MLR test using HTCs as stimulating cells. The proliferation of responding cells against either Dw1 or Dw3 determinant is indicated by a plus sign *(+)*. The lack of proliferation (typing response) is indicated by a minus sign *(−)*. When HLA-D specificities of stimulating cells are a part of those responders, the proliferation does not ensue

Assignment of HLA-D Specificities

The DNA synthetic rate for the proliferation of responding T-lymphocytes (the responding cells) is usually measured by the degree of radiolabeled [^{3}H]thymidine uptake after culturing with stimulating cells for about 96–144 h. Stimulating cells are inactivated with antimitotic agents such as irradiation or mitomycin C (one-way MLR). Stimulating cells are obtained from individuals who are homozygous at the HLA-D specificities (homozygous typing cell, HTC) in order to identify HLA-D specificities. The example of the interpretation of the results of the MLR test and of the identification of HLA-D specificities of the test cell against stimulating cells (HTCs), which depend on whether the proliferation of the responding cells ensues or not, is shown in Fig. 1.

Materials and Methods

Stimulating and responding lymphocytes were stored in liquid nitrogen and thawed just before use. Cells were resuspendend at a concentration of 5×10^5/ml in RPMI 1640 supplemented with 20% human AB serum; then 5×10^4 stimulating cells, inactivated by irradiation (3000 rad), were cultured with the same number of responding cells in triplicate for 6 days in microtiter plates. Eighteen hours before the end of incubation, 1 μCi [^{3}H]thymidine was added to each well. [^{3}H]Thymidine-incorporated cells were harvested onto glass fiber papers and counts per minute *(cpm)* were measured by a liquid scintillation counter. The definition of narcolepsy and serological HLA typing will be dicussed in other chapters (chap 2, 3). HTCs used in this study were either kindly supplied by Dr F. H. Bach or locally obtained.

Data Editing

As mentioned above, it is essential to discriminate negative or weak MLR (typing response) from a positive one (strong lymphocyte proliferation) to identify HLA-D specificities. Evaluation of response differences in the weak intermediate range, however, remains the major problem. Factors that influence the variation in the result of MLR experiments are:

(1) various technical factors,
(2) responsive abilities of responding cells,
(3) stimulatory abilities of stimulating cells, and
(4) the genetic disparity between stimulating and responding cells.

In order to normalize abilities of responding and stimulating cells, we employed 75th percentile double normalization introduced by Ryder et al. (1975) with minor modification. The data were prepared as follows:

1. Calculate the responder normalized values (*RNVs*)

$$RNV = \frac{\text{median } cpm}{\text{75th percentile of } cpm} \times 100$$

for all responding cells.
2. Calculate the double normalized values (*DNVs*) for each stimulating-responding cell combination

$$DNV = \frac{RNV}{\text{75th percentile of the } RNV} \times 100$$

3. *DNVs* were converted into logarithms (log-*DNVs*)
4. In the frequency distribution of log-*DNVs*, distributions greater than the value that gave the maximum frequency were considered to be normal distributions; standard deviation *(SD)* was then calculated in that group.
5. Log-*DNVs* less than 3 SD in stimulating-responding cell combinations were identified as "typing responses" and combinations between 2 SD and 3 SD were identified as doubtful ("gray zone").

Results

As shown in Table 1, all nine narcoleptic patients showed typing responses ($DNV < 55$ in this experiment) against HLA-Dw2 HTCs. Although four patients (SN, TA, MO, and KA) showed a typing response or "gray zone" ($55 < DNV < 67$ in this experiment) against Dw12 HTCs, we assigned these patients as positive for Dw2 because they showed typing responses against both Dw2 HTCs. One (patient HT) out of nine patients could not be clearly assigned to Dw2. All responders except one control were identified to be either Dw2 or Dw12 or both. This result indicates that the HLA-D specificity which is in association with narcoleptics' DR2 and DQw1 is, so far as HLA-D specificities are identified with certainty, HLA-Dw2. In other experiments of HLA-D typing of other narcoleptic patients, 22 more patients have been confirmed to be positive for Dw2 (Tables 2-5). Three patients were unable to be identified clearly as Dw2 as shown in Table 1 (patient HT) and in Table 3 (patient AN, TN) due to discrepant results against Dw2 HTCs; however, we could not deny the positiveness of Dw2. Several HLA-D specificities which are in association with HLA-DR2 have been reported such as HLA-Dw2, Dw12, FJO, BAS, REM, and AZH. In the Japanese population, however, HLA-D specificities that associate with DR2 have been known to be Dw12 and Dw2. Although there is not report yet identifying HLA-D specificities with a large sample of the Japanese population, some investigators have reported that the gene frequencies of HLA-Dw2 and Dw12 in the Japanese population are about 0.04 and 0.1, respectively (Sasazuki et al. 1977, 1980). In our data concerning HLA-D typing of 60 panels, there were 6 Dw2-positive individuals out of 23 DR2 positives. Table 6 shows the chi square testing in a 2×2 contingency table between 30 HLA-D-confirmed narcoleptics and 60 normal healthy controls whether they were assigned as positive for HLA-Dw2 or not. HLA-Dw2 was significantly increased in

Table 1. HLA-D clusters of nine narcoleptic patients

Responders			Stimulators						Dw assignment
	Class II		HTCs				Controls		
	DR	DQw	Dw2		Dw12		DR4	DRw8,w11	
			AMG	MIF	KAW	TOK	NT	HK	
Narcoleptics									
HA	2,w6	1	3	3	1	1	1	1	2
KK	2,w11	1,3	3	3	1	1	1	1	2
HO	2	1	3	3	1	1	1	1	2
SN	2	1	3	3	1	2	1	1	2
TA	2	1	3	3	1	2	1	1	2
MO	2,w8	1,3	3	3	1	3	1	1	2
KA	2	1	3	3	1	3	1	1	2
TN	2,4	1	3	nt	1	1	1	1	2
HT	2,4	1	3	1	1	1	1	2	2?
Controls									
#1.	2	1	2	2	3	3	1	1	2,12
#2.	2	1	3	3	1	1	1	1	2
#3.	w9,w12	1,3	1	1	1	1	1	1	

Results are expressed as follows: score 3, typing response ($DNV < 55$ in this experiment); score 2, "gray zone" ($55 \leq DNV \leq 67$); score 1, positive MLR ($DNV > 67$); *nt*, not tested

Table 2. HLA-D clusters of nine narcoleptic patients

Responders			Stimulators						Dw assignment
	Class II		HTCs				Controls		
	DR	DQw	Dw2		Dw12		DR1,4	DR4,w8	
			Len-2	AMG	KAW	TOK	KM	KW	
Narcoleptics									
SN	2	1	3	3	3	3	1	1	2,12
YS	2	1	3	3	1	1	1	1	2
TS	2,w9	1,3	3	3	1	1	1	1	2
MS	2,w9	1,3	3	3	1	1	1	1	2
KK	2,4	1	3	3	1	1	1	1	2
IS	2,w13	1	3	3	2	1	1	1	2
MN	2,w9	1,3	3	3	2	1	1	1	2
HH	2,w13	1	3	3	1	3	1	1	2
TS	2	1	3	2	3	1	1	1	2
Controls									
#1.	1,4	1	1	1	1	1	3*	1	
#2.	4,w8	1,3	1	1	1	1	1	3*	

Results are expressed as follows: score 3, typing response ($DNV < 32$ in this experiment); score 2, "gray zone" ($32 \leq DNV \leq 40$); score 1, positive MLR ($DNV > 40$); *, autologous MLR

Table 3. HLA-D clusters of six narcoleptic patients

Responders			Stimulators						Dw assignment
	Class II		HTCs				Controls		
	DR	DQw	Dw2		Dw12		DRw12,w13	DRw8	
			Len-2	AMG	KAW	TOK	TK	HY	
Narcoleptics									
MS	2	1	3	3	3	3	1	2	2,12
TI	2	1	3	3	3	3	1	nt	2,12
MT	2,1	1	3	2	1	1	2	1	2
SY	2,w9	1,3	3	2	3	1	1	nt	2
AN	2,1	1	3	1	1	1	1	1	2?
TN	2,w9	1,3	1	3	2	1	1	1	2?
Controls									
#1.	w12,w13	3	1	1	1	1	3*	1	
#2.	4,w8	1,3	1	1	1	1	1	1	

Results are expressed as follows: score 3, typing response ($DNV < 39$ in this experiment); score 2, "gray zone" ($39 \leq DNV \leq 52$); score 1, positive MLR ($DNV > 52$); *, autologous MLR; nt, not tested

Table 4. HLA-D clusters of five narcoleptic patients

Responders			Stimulators						Dw assignment
	Class II		HTCs				Controls		
	DR	DQw	Dw2		Dw12		Pooled Lymph	DR4,w8	
			Len-2	AMG	KAW	TOK		KW	
Narcoleptics									
SM	2	1	3	3	1	1	1	1	2
IS	2,w9	1,3	3	2	1	1	1	1	2
KS	2,w9	1,3	3	3	1	1	1	2	2
TO	2,4	1	3	3	2	1	1	1	2
KO	2,w9	1,3	3	3	1	1	1	3	2
Controls									
#1.	2,w12	1,3	3	3	1	1	1	1	2
#2.	4,w8	1,3	1	1	1	1	2	3*	

Results are expressed as follows: score 3, typing response ($DNV < 43$ in this experiment); score 2, "gray zone" ($43 \leq DNV \leq 62$); score 1, positive MLR ($DNV > 62$); *, autologous MLR. Pooled lymphocytes were obtained from 20 unrelated individuals

narcoleptic patients compared with healthy controls (chi square value = 67.5, corrected $P < 10^{-9}$) and the relative risk of narcolepsy in patients who were assigned as Dw2 was very high (relative risk = 511). This value implies that narcolepsy is 511 times more frequent in the individuals positive for Dw2 than individuals negative for Dw2 in the Japanese population. As for the frequency of Dw12 in narcoleptics, compared with normal persons, it showed a tendency to decrease, although this was not significant (Table 7).

Table 5. HLA-D clusters of four narcoleptic patients

Responders			Stimulators (HTCs)					Dw assignment
	Class II		Dw2			Dw12	Dw4	
	DR	DQw	Len-2	AMG	MS-7	TOK	MJ-4	
Narcoleptics								
TS	2,w12	1,3	3	3	3	1	1	2
YO	2,4	1,3	3	3	3	1	1	2
KK	2,4	1	3	3	2	1	1	2
TT	2,w9	1,3	3	3	1	1	1	2
Controls								
#1.	w9,w12	3	1	1	1	1	1	

Results are expressed as follows: score 3, typing response ($DNV < 44$ in this experiment); score 2, "gray zone" ($44 \leq DNV \leq 61$); score 1, positive MLR ($DNV > 61$)

Table 6. 2 × 2 table analysis of HLA-Dw2 in narcoleptics

	Dw2	
	+	−
Narcoleptics	30	0
Controls	6	54

Chi square value = 67.5 (corrected $P < 10^{-9}$)
Relative risk ≒ 511 (calculated with Haldane's formula)

Table 7. 2 × 2 table analysis of HLA-Dw12 in narcoleptics

	Dw12	
	+	−
Narcoleptics	3	27
Controls	8	52

Chi square value = −0.207 (not significant)

It was demonstrated that FJO, BAS, and REM were not stimulated mutually, or weakly if they were, in MLR experiments (Cohen et al. 1984; Ollier et al. 1984). Therefore, HLA-D specificities of these three HTCs might be within the same cluster and this specificity is designated to DB9. At present, it is known that there are at least four HLA-D specificities in association with DR2, i.e., Dw2, Dw12, DB9, and AZH. Serological characterizations of these HTCs have been demonstrated which are more complicated in form: Regarding DR specificities, Dw2 and Dw12 are associated with DR2, whereas DB9 and AZH are associated with DR2 short. As for DQ specificities, Dw2, Dw12, and FJO (DB9) are positive for DQw1, and DB9 cells except FJO are positive for both DQw3 and a probable short component of DQw3 antigen, TA10 (Schreuder and Degos 1984). As mentioned previously, in a Caucasian population, almost all the HLA-D specificities that associate with HLA-DR2 have been demosntrated to be Dw2. In fact, it has been identified that all 22 French Caucasian narcoleptic patients who were serologically typed for HLA-DR2 and DQw1 were positive for HLA-Dw2 (Marcadet et al. 1985). These data show that all the narcoleptic patients are Dw2 positive along with HLA-DR2 and DQw1 over ethnic differences. This striking finding may support the hypothesis that, rather than the HLA-D region genes or molecules themselves having a direct relationship with the pathogenesis of narcolepsy, a susceptible gene to narcolepsy, if present, is closely linked with HLA-DR2, DQw1, and Dw2 genes in all ethnic groups. In cases where genetic factors appear to play a role in the pathogenesis and/or the development of the disease, these results of HLA typing of narcoleptic patients will offer a good model to study the relationship between the disease and its genetic background.

HLA-DP locus determinants, one of the genetic products of HLA-D subregion genes, can be identified with a cellular technique, named primed lymphocyte typing (PLT). In brief, while the primary MLR is cultured for a longer period than usuall MLR aiming at typing of HLA-D specificities, responding cells are subject to be primed with HLA-D region products, particularly HLA-DP determinants, of stimulating cells. When these primed cells are then used as responding cells in secondary MLR culture with allogeneic stimulating cells, proliferative responses will result in primed cells and stimulating cells sharing the same HLA-DP determinants. Little is known about frequencies of DP specificities, DPw1 through DPw6, in the population and its association, if present, with the other HLA-D subregion products. The recent study of mapping the HLA-D subregion genes suggests the existence of a recombination hot spot between DP and DR-DQ genes (Hardy et al. 1986); however, on the basis of the speculation that there may be some relationships between narcolepsy and HLA-DP locus products as well as other HLA-D subregion products, such as DR2, DQw1, and Dw2, investigations are now in progress.

References

Amos DB, Bach FH (1968) Phenotypic expressions of the major histocompatibility locus in man (HL-A): leukocyte antigens and mixed leukocyte culture reactivity. J Exp Med 128: 623-637

Bach FH (1985) The HLA class II genes and products: the HLA-D region. Immunol Today 6: 89-94

Bain B, Vas MR, Lowenstein L (1964) The development of large immature mononuclear cells in mixed leukocyte culture. Blood 23: 108-116

Bauer MP, Neugebauer M, Deppe H, Sigmund M, Luton T, Mayr WR, Albert ED (1984) Population analysis on the basis of deduced haplotypes from random families. In: Albert ED, Baur MP, Mayr WR (eds) Histocompatibility testing 1984. Springer, Berlin Heidelberg New York, pp 333-341

Billiard M, Seignalet J (1985) Extraordinary association between HLA-DR2 and narcolepsy. Lancet i: 226-227

Cohen N, Amar A, Brautbar C (1984) Definition of a new DR2 short associated HLA-D specificity with the ninth histocompatibility workshop reagents. Tissue Antigens 24: 184-186

Dupont B, Hansen JA, Yunis EJ (1976) Human mixed-lymphocyte culture reaction: genetics, specificity, and biological implications. Adv Immunol 23: 107-202

Hardy DA, Bell JI, Long EO, Lindsten T, McDevitt HO (1986) Mapping of the class II region of the human major histocompatibility complex by pulse field gel electrophoresis. Nature 323: 453-455

Honda Y, Doi Y, Juji T, Satake M (1984) Narcolepsy and HLA: positive DR2 as a prerequisite for the development of narcolepsy. Folia Psychiatr Neurol Jpn 38: 360

Jaraquemada D, Okoye R, Ollier W, Awad J, Festenstein H (1984) HLA-D and DR in different populations. In: Albert ED, Baur MP, Mayr WR (eds) Histocompatibility testing 1984. Springer, Berlin Heidelberg New York, pp 472-473

Jaraquemada D, Navarrete C, Ollier W, Awad J, Okoye R, Festenstein H (1986) HLA-D specificity assignments are independent of HLA-DQ, HLA-DR and other class II specificities and define a biologically important segregant series which strongly activates a functionally distinct T cell subset. Hum Immunol 16: 259-270

Juji T, Satake M, Honda Y, Doi Y (1984) HLA antigens in Japanese patients with narcolepsy. Tissue Antigens 24: 316-319

Langdon N, Dam MV, Welsh KI, Vaughan R, Parkes D (1984) Genetic markers in narcolepsy. Lancet ii: 1178-1180

Marcadet A, Gebuhrer L, Betuel H, Seignalet J, Freidel AC, Confavreux C, Billiard M, Dausset J, Cohen D (1985) DNA polymorphism related to HLA-DR2 Dw2 in patients with narcolepsy. Immunogenetics 22: 679-683

Mempel W, Grosse-Wilde H, Baumann P, Netzel B, Steinbauer-Rosenthal I, Scholoz S, Bertrams J, Albert ED (1973b) Population genetics of the MLC response: typing for MLC determinants using homozygous and heterozygous reference cells. Transplant Proc 5: 1529-1534

Ollier W, Doxiadis I, Jaraquemada D, Okoye R, Grosse-Wilde H, Festenstein H (1984) First level of HLA-D "blank" HTC. In: Albert ED, Baur MP, Mayr WR (eds) Histocompatibility testing 1984. Springer, Berlin Heidelberg New York, pp 291-285

Ryder LP, Thomsen M, Platz P, Svejgaard A (1975) Data reduction in LD-typing. In: Kissmeyer-Nielsen F (ed) Histocompatibility testing 1975. Munksgaard, Copenhagen, pp 557-562

Sasazuki T, McMichael A, Payne R, McDevitt HO (1977) HLA-D antigens in the Japanese population. Tissue Antigens 9: 267-272

Sasazuki T, Kaneoka H, Tsuji K, Nose Y, Kashiwagi N, Kaneko T (1980) HLA-D in Japan. In: Terasaki PI (ed) Histocompatibility testing 1980. UCLA Tissue Typing Laboratory, Los Angeles, pp 274-276

Schrek R, Donnelly WJ (1961) Differences between lymphocytes of leukemic and nonleukemic patients with respect to morphologic features, motility, and sensitivity to guinea pig serum. Blood 18: 561-571

Schreuder GMT, Degos L (1984) HLA-DR, DQ and DW relationships. In: Albert ED, Baur MP, Mayr WR (eds) Histocompatibility testing 1984. Springer, Berlin Heidelberg New York, p 243

Yunis EJ, Amos DB (1971) Three closely linked genetic systems relevant to transplantation. Proc Natl Acad Sci USA 68: 3031-3035

Chapter 10

HLA-Linked Complement Markers in Narcolepsy

K. TOKUNAGA, K. MATSUKI, T. JUJI, and Y. HONDA

The complement system is composed of a number of plasma proteins that act as important mediators of host defense and inflammation. Two different pathways, the classical and the alternative pathways, are known to achieve the complement activation. The structural genes for three complement components C2, C4, and factor B, which form the C3-convertases in the two pathways, were found to be situated between the loci for HLA-B and HLA-DR on chromosome 6. These complement genes compose the class III genes of the major histocompatibility complex (MHC). Very tight linkage of the C2, factor B (BF), and two C4 (C4A and C4B) genes as well as 21-hydroxylase genes was confirmed by recombinant DNA techniques (Carroll et al. 1984), as shown in Fig. 1. C2 and BF are homologous in structure and function and presumably arose by gene duplication, while C4 is similar to C3 and C5. The adjacent localization of the HLA genes and the class III complement genes has led researchers to associations between diseases and the complement alleles and their possible contribution for MHC-disease associations (Rittner and Bertrams 1981; Dawkins et al. 1983; Porter 1983).

Up to now few studies have been published concerning the associations between the complement markers and narcolepsy (Matsuki et al. 1985). The purpose of this chapter is to present our current knowledge about the complement polymorphisms in narcolepsy. Certain complement alleles may become useful markers for the characterization of the MHC haplotypes carrying the susceptibility gene for narcolepsy.

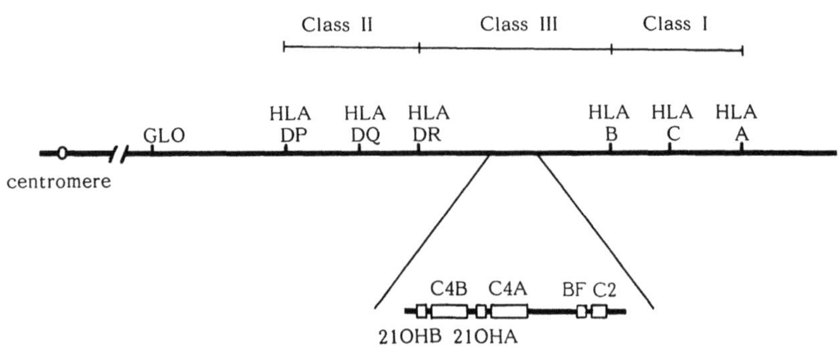

Fig. 1. The MHC class III genes on the short arm of human chromosome 6

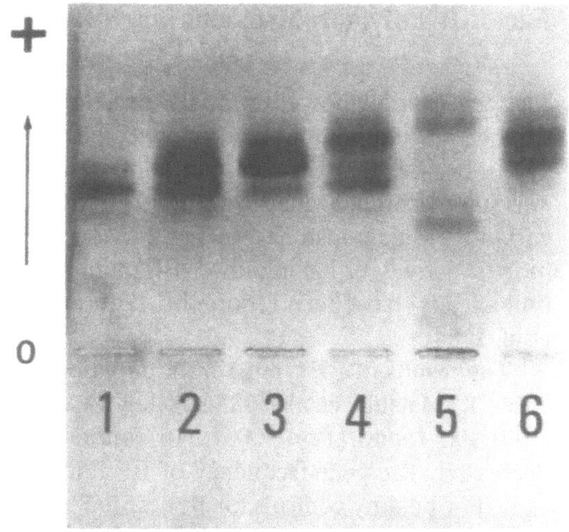

Fig. 2. Factor B phenotypes obtained by agarose gel electrophoresis and immunofixation. 1,BF S; 2,BF FS; 3,BF F; 4,BF F075S(F_TS); 5,BF F1S07(F1S1); 6,BF F075F(F_TF)

Table 1. Phenotype and allele frequencies (%) of BF, C2, C4A, and C4B in Japanese patients with narcolepsy and normal controls

	Narcolepsy		Control		*P* (corrected)	Relative risk
	PF	GF	PF	GF		
	(n=46)		(n=487)[a]			
BF S	80.4	62.0	95.7	80.1	<0.0001	0.2
BF F	56.5	38.0	35.3	19.8	<0.0001	2.4
BF rare	0.0	0.0	0.2	0.1	NS	-
	(n=45)		(n=521)[b]			
C2 C	100.0	87.8	99.6	93.9	NS	-
C2 AT	17.8	8.9	6.5	3.4	<0.025	3.1
C2 B	4.4	2.2	4.4	2.2	NS	1.0
C2 BH	2.2	1.1	1.2	0.6	NS	1.6
	(n=44)		(n=169)			
C4A 3	90.9	68.2	91.1	68.3	NS	1.0
C4A 4	34.1	17.0	25.4	13.6	NS	1.5
C4A 2	9.1	4.5	20.1	10.7	NS	0.4
C4A Q0	9.1	4.5	13.0	6.5	NS	0.7
C4A rare	11.4	5.7	1.8	0.9	NS	7.1
	(n=44)		(n=169)			
C4B 1	77.3	51.1	80.5	58.0	NS	0.8
C4B 2	45.5	26.1	31.9	17.2	NS	1.8
C4B 5	13.6	6.8	17.2	8.9	NS	0.8
C4B Q0	29.5	14.8	30.2	16.0	NS	1.0
C4B rare	2.3	1.1	0.0	0.0	NS	-

PF, frequencies of the positive patients; *GF*, allele frequencies
[a] Data from Tokunaga et al. (1982)
[b] Data from Tokunaga et al. (1981)

Factor B Polymorphism and Narcolepsy

The genetic polymorphism of BF protein is usually detected by agarose gel electrophoresis and immunofixation with specific antiserum to human BF (Alper et al. 1972). Besides the two common allotypes BF S and BF F, a number of rare variants have been described in various populations (Mauff et al. 1978). Five of these variants are demonstrated in Fig. 2. Moreover, particular variants lacking BF hemolytic activity or having lower BF quantity in addition to certain evidence for BF null allele(s) have been reported (Mauff et al. 1980; Raum et al. 1984b; Tokunaga et al. 1984).

The results of BF typing in the Japanese patients with narcolepsy are shown in Table 1 (Matsuki et al. 1985). A highly significant increase of the frequency of BF F was found ($Pc < 0.0001$). In contrast, the BF S frequency was significantly decreased. The gene frequency of BF F in the patients was almost twice as much as that of healthy controls (38.0% vs, 19.8%). The relative risk for BF F-positive individuals for narcolepsy was calculated to be 2.4.

C2 Polymorphism and Narcolepsy

The polymorphism of C2 is usually detected by isoelectric focusing with a specific hemolytic overlay containing antibody-sensitized sheep erythrocytes and C2-deficient (or diluted normal) serum (Alper 1976; Meo et al. 1976). Most individuals possess the common allotype C2 C. A basic variant C2 B is observed with gene frequency of 0.02-0.04 and a few very rare acidic variants have been described in Caucasians. In Japanese, besides the C2 C and C2 B, another acidic variant C2 AT and a few rare basic variants were found, as demonstrated in Fig. 3 (Tokunaga et al. 1981). The product of C2 AT shows a higher hemolytic activity than

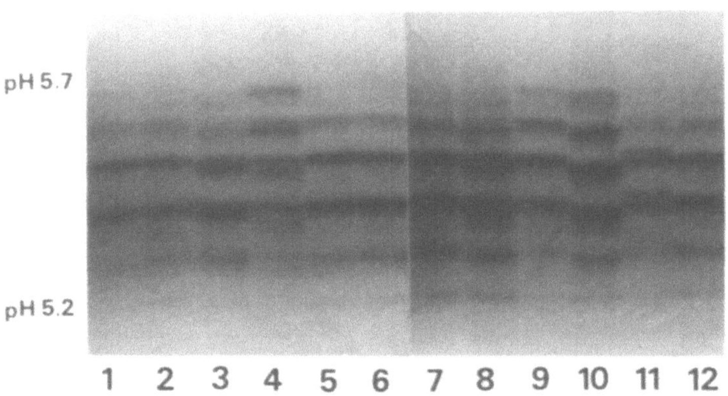

Fig. 3. C2 phenotypes obtained by isoelectric focusing and hemolytic overlay. *1*,C2 C; *2*,C2 C; *3*,C2 A_TC; *4*,C2 B_HC; *5*,C2 C; *6*,C2 C; *7*,C2 C; *8*,C2 A_TC; *9*,C2 C; *10*,C2 A_TB_H; *11*,C2 BC; *12*,C2 C

those of the other alleles. Inherited deficiency of C2 is the most common one of complement components in Caucasians and the gene frequency of the deficient allele (C2 Q0) is assumed to be around 1%. The deficiency state is known to be strongly associated with systemic lupus erythematosus (SLE)-like diseases (Agnello 1978). In contrast, no C2-deficient individuals have been reported in Japanese.

The results of C2 typing in the Japanese patients with narcolepsy are shown in Table 1 (Matsuki et al. 1985). A significant increase of the frequency of C2 AT was found ($Pc < 0.025$). The gene frequency of C2 AT was 8.9% in the patients and 3.4% in healthy controls. The relative risk for C2 AT-positive individuals was 3.1.

C4 Polymorphism and Narcolepsy

After agarose gel electrophoresis with neuraminidase-treated samples, C4A and C4B patterns are detected by immunofixation with specific anti-C4 serum and by a specific C4-dependent hemolytic overlay (Awdeh and Alper 1980; Mauff et al. 1983). C4 shows the highest degree of polymorphism in the HLA-linked complement components, and a large number of different variants have been described for each C4 locus (Mauff et al. 1983). Six C4A and three C4B allotypes occur with frequencies of more than 1% in Caucasians (Awdeh and Alper 1980), while in Japanese three common allotypes exist at each C4 locus, as demonstrated in Fig. 4 (Tokunaga et al. 1985). In addition, there are high frequencies of null alleles, C4A Q0 and C4B Q0, at both C4 loci. On the other hand, some individuals are now known to have duplication of C4A or C4B gene (Bruun-Petersen et al. 1982; Raum et al. 1984a; Rittner et al. 1984). A few variants with antigenical and/or functional abnormalities have also been reported.

The individuals with complete C4 deficiency have been found to suffer from SLE-like diseases (Agnello 1978). Moreover, with the application of the C4 typing, individuals with one, two, or three null alleles were found to be associated with

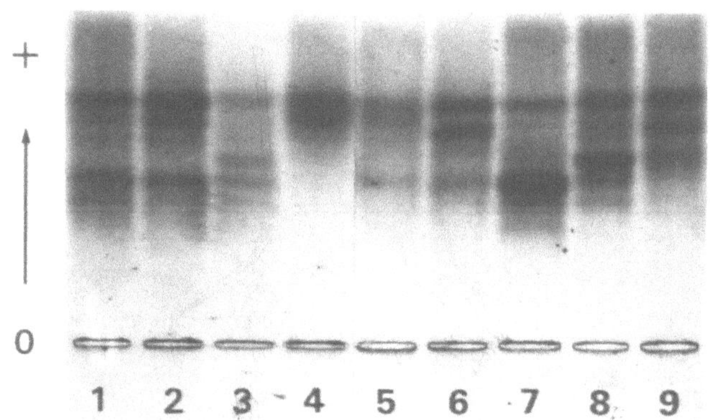

Fig. 4. C4 phenotypes obtained by agarose gel electrophoresis and immunofixation. *1*,C4 A3,3 B1,1; *2*,C4 A3,3 B1,Q0; *3*,C4 A3,Q0 B2,1; *4*,C4 A4,2 BQ0,Q0; *5*,C4 A3,2 B1,Q0; *6*,C4 A3,3 B5,1; *7*,C4 A3,Q0 B1,1; *8*,C4 A4,Q0 B2,2; *9*,C4 A4,3 B5,2

certain autoimmune diseases including SLE (Fielder et al. 1983; Dawkins et al. 1983).

The results of C4A and C4B typing in the Japanese patients with narcolepsy are shown in Table 1 (Matsuki et al. 1985). The increases of the frequencies of C4A rare alleles and C4B 2 and the decrease of C4A 2 were not significant by means of corrected *P* values. However, concerning the estimated frequencies of C4 haplotypes, a significant decrease of C4A 2 B Q0 was found as shown in Table 2. The relative risk for the haplotype was 0.31.

Major Histocompatibility Complex Haplotypes in Narcolepsy

It is well known that HLA-DR2 is 100% positive both in the Japanese and Caucasian patients with narcolepsy (Juji et al. 1984; Langdon et al. 1984; Billiard and Seignalet 1985). As reported by Matsuki et al. (1985), the three most frequent haplotypes in Japanese narcoleptic patients (B35-DR2, B15-DR2, and B51- DR2) are very rare in the healthy population. In contrast, the incidence of the most frequent haplotype in normal Japanese, A24-Bw52-DR2, decreased to one-third in the patients. Analyses on the complement markers support these findings. C4A 2 B Q0, which is associated with the common haplotype A24-Bw52-DR2 (Tokunaga et al. 1985), was also significantly decreased (Table 2). Moreover, from association analyses between the complement and the HLA alleles in narcoleptic patients in addi-

Table 2. Estimated C4 haplotype frequencies (%) in Japanese patients with narcolepsy and normal controls

	Narcolepsy ($n=43$)	Control ($n=169$)	*P*	Relative risk
C4A3 B1	46.3	53.0	NS	0.8
C4A4 B2	15.3	12.0	NS	1.3
C4A3 B2	13.1	3.9	NS	3.7
C4A3 B5	6.1	5.7	NS	1.1
C4A4 B1	5.9	1.5	NS	4.1
C4A2 BQ0	3.6	10.8	<0.005	0.3
C4AQ0 B1	1.1	6.0	NS	0.2
Others	8.6	7.1	NS	1.2

Table 3. DR2-linked HLA/complement haplotypes in Japanese patients with narcolepsy

"High-risk haplotype"					
B35	- C2C	- BFF	- C4A4 B2	- DR2	- DQw1
B15	- C2AT	- BFF	- C4A3 B1	- DR2	- DQw1
B51	- C2C	- BFS	- C4A3 B1	- DR2	- DQw1
"Low-risk haplotype"					
Bw52	- C2C	- BFS	- C4A2 BQ0	- DR2	- DQw1

tion to several multiple-case families, we could infer that certain complement alleles are linked to the high-risk haplotypes of narcolepsy, as summarized in Table 3. BF F and C4A 4 B 2 are associated with the haplotype B35-DR2, while BF F and C2 AT are associated with B15-DR2.

On the other hand, in Caucasians a common haplotype in the normal population, B7-DR2-DQw1, may also be associated with narcolepsy (Langdon et al. 1984; Seignalet and Billiard 1984; Billiard and Seignalet 1985).

Conclusion

Associations between the HLA-linked complement components and narcolepsy were less strong than that between HLA-DR2 and the disease. It is assumed that the association of narcolepsy with DR2 or DQw1 is primary, while the associations with the complement alleles as well as with the HLA-A and -B alleles are secondary. Nevertheless certain complement markers, such as BF F, C2 AT, and C4A 4 B 2 in Japanese, may become useful markers in order to define the high-risk and low-risk haplotypes.

References

Agnello V (1978) Complement deficiency states. Medicine 57: 1-23

Alper CA (1976) Inherited structural polymorphism in human C2. Evidence for genetic linkage between C2 and Bf. J Exp Med 144: 1111-1115

Alper CA, Boenisch T, Watson L (1972) Genetic polymorphism in human glycine-rich beta-glycoprotein. J Exp Med 135: 68-80

Awdeh ZL, Alper CA (1980) Inherited structural polymorphism of the fourth component of human complement. Proc Natl Acad Sci USA 77: 3576-3580

Billiard M, Seignalet J (1985) Extraordinary association between HLA-DR2 and narcolepsy. Lancet I: 226-227

Bruun-Petersen G, Lamm LU, Jacobsen BK, Kristensen T (1982) Genetics of complement C4. Two homoduplication haplotypes C4S C4S and C4F C4F in a family. Hum Genet 61: 36-38

Carroll MC, Campbell RD, Bentley DR, Porter RR (1984) A molecular map of the human major histocompatibility complex class III region linking complement genes C4, C2 and factor B. Nature 307: 237-241

Dawkins RL, Christiansen FT, Kay PH, Garlepp M, McCluskey J, Hollingsworth PN, Zilko PJ (1983) Disease associations with complotypes, supratypes and haplotypes. Immunol Rev 70: 5-22

Fielder AHL, Walport MJ, Batchelor JR, Rynes RI, Black CM, Dodi IA, Hughes GRV (1983) Family study of the major histocompatibility complex in patients with systemic lupus erythematosus: importance of null alleles of C4A and C4B in determining disease susceptibility. Br Med J 286: 425-428

Juji T, Satake M, Honda Y, Doi Y (1984) HLA antigens in Japanese patients with narcolepsy. All the patients were DR2 positive. Tissue Antigens 24: 316-319

Langdon N, Welsh KI, van Dam M, Vaughan RW, Parkes D (1984) Genetic markers in narcolepsy. Lancet II: 1178-1180

Matsuki K, Juji T, Tokunaga K, Naohara T, Satake M, Honda Y (1985) Human histocompatibility leukocyte antigen (HLA) haplotype frequencies estimated from the data on HLA Class I, II, and III antigens in 111 Japanese narcoleptics. J Clin Invest 76: 2078-2083

Mauff G, Hauptmann G, Hitzeroth HW, Gauchel F, Scherz R (1978) The nomenclature of properdin factor B allotypes. Z Immunitatsforsch 154: 115-120

Mauff G, Federmann G, Hauptmann G (1980) A hemolytically inactive gene product of factor B. Immunology 158: 96-100

Mauff G, Alper CA, Awdeh ZL, Batchelor JR, Bertrams J, Bruun-Petersen G, Dawkins RL, Demant P, Edwards J, Grosse-Wilde H, Hauptmann G, Klouda P, Lamm L, Mollenhauer E, Nerl C, Olaisen B, O'Neill G, Rittner C, Roos MH, Skanes V, Teisberg P, Wells L (1983) Statement on the nomenclature of human C4 allotypes. Immunobiology 164: 184-191

Meo T, Atkinson J, Bernoco M, Bernoco D, Ceppellini R (1976) Mapping of the HLA locus controlling C2 structural variants and linkage disequilibrium between alleles C2 and Bw15. Eur J Immunol 6: 916-919

Porter RR (1983) Complement polymorphism, the major histocompatibility complex and associated diseases: a speculation. Mol Biol Med 1: 161-168

Raum D, Awdeh Z, Anderson J, Strong L, Granados J, Teran L, Giblett E, Yunis EJ, Alper CA (1984a) Human C4 haplotypes with duplicated C4A or C4B. Am J Hum Genet 36: 72-79

Raum D, Surgenor T, Awdeh ZL, Marcus D, Blumenthal M, Yunis EJ, Alper CA (1984b) An unusual "morphologic" variant of BF S. Am J Hum Genet 36: 346-351

Rittner C, Bertrams J (1981) On the significance of C2, C4, and factor B polymorphisms in disease. Hum Genet 56: 235-247

Rittner C, Giles CM, Roos MH, Demant P, Mollenhauer E (1984) Genetics of human C4 polymorphism: detection and segregation of rare and duplicated haplotypes. Immunogenetics 19: 321-333

Seignalet J, Billiard M (1984) Possible association between HLA-B7 and narcolepsy. Tissue Antigens 23: 188-189

Tokunaga K, Araki C, Juji T, Omoto K (1981) Genetic polymorphism of the complement C2 in Japanese. Hum Genet 58: 213-216

Tokunaga K, Araki C, Juji T, Omoto K (1982) Polymorphism of properdin factor B in Japanese: description of a rare variant and data of association with HLA and C2. Hum Genet 60: 42-45

Tokunaga K, Omoto K, Yukiyama Y, Sakurai M, Saji H, Maruya E (1984) Further study on a BF silent allele. Hum Genet 67: 449-451

Tokunaga K, Omoto K, Akaza T, Akiyama N, Amemiya H, Naito S, Sasazuki T, Satoh H, Juji T (1985) Haplotype study on C4 polymorphism in Japanese. Associations with MHC alleles, complotypes and HLA-complement haplotypes. Immunogenetics 22: 359-365

Chapter 11

DNA Typing in Narcolepsy

H. Inoko

Introduction

Human chromosome 6 contains a set of genes, known as the major histocompatibility complex, that encode polymorphic cell surface glycoproteins composed of two noncovalently associated 33000- to 35 000-dalton α (heavy) and 26000- to 29000-dalton β (light) chains. Alleles at these loci determine the ability to confer the immune response and thus control the susceptibility to a wide variety of human diseases (Dausset and Svejgaard 1975; Ryder et al. 1979; Terasaki 1980; Benacerraf 1981; Korman et al. 1984; Bodmer 1984). Serological as well as cellular reagents have allowed the identification of three sets of molecular entities that display a similar function and tissue distribution to HLA-D products. These antigens are named DR, DQ (DC), and DP (SB) and the latter mainly carries the polymorphic determinants (Owenbach et al. 1983; Cohen et al. 1984), although the α chain is also polymorphic with respect to the DQ antigen (Trowsdale et al. 1983; Tosi et al. 1984). Each chain of all class II antigens consists of four domains, an amino terminal domain ($\alpha1$ or $\beta1$ domains), a membrane proximal domain ($\alpha2$ or $\beta2$ domains), a transmembrane region, and an intracytoplasmic domain (Kaufman and Strominger 1983; Korman et al. 1985).

We and others have isolated and characterized a large number of cDNA and genomic clones for class II antigens including the newly identified antigen heavy chain, DOα (DZα) (Inoko et al. 1985a; Inoko et al. 1985b; Korman et al. 1985). The genomic cloning data reveal a surprising large number of genes, including at least six α chain genes and at least eight β chain genes (see Fig. 8). One DRα chain and three DRβ chain (DRβ1, DRβ2, DRβ3) genes, two DQα chain (DQα, DXα) and two DQβ chain (DQβ, DXβ) genes, two DPα chain (DPα1 and DPβ1) and two DPβ chain (DPβ1 and DPβ2) genes, one DOα chain gene, and at least one DOβ chain gene were found. These numbers are in accord with those obtained from genomic hybridization studies using HLA-homozygous cell lines. These cloned DNA probes should allow understanding at the molecular level of the HLA gene organization, its polymorphism, and HLA-disease association.

In this paper, I present some studies on restriction enzyme polymorphisms using class II cDNA probes (DNA typing) and the application of such typing to definition of polymorphism at the genomic level to differentiate between narcoleptic patients and healthy individuals with DR2 homo- or heterozygotes. Marked differences were observed between narcoleptic patients and normal controls when DQβ cDNA was used as a probe (Inoko et al. 1986). Thus, HLA-DQβ chain DNA restriction fragments can differentiate between healthy and narcoleptic individuals with HLA-DR2. These restriction fragment polymorphisms were found to be due to polymorphism within the HLA-DQβ gene, especially around the β1 exon, second intron, and β2 exon, not within the DXβ gene by analysis of overlapping genomic clones derived from the HLA-DR2-Dw2 haplotype, providing a promising clue for isolation of the gene controlling susceptibility to narcolepsy.

Southern Hybridization Analysis of DNA Polymorphisms in the HLA-D Region

In an attempt to establish standard Southern blot patterns for different DR specificities with the HLA class II antigen α and β chain probes, genomic DNAs from 28 EB-transformed HLA-homozygous B-lymphoblastoid cell lines with Dw1-Dw19 specificity (Table 1) were digested with four different restriction endonucleases (*Eco*RI, *Hin*dIII, *Pst*I, and *Bam*HI) and with the DRβ (pDRβ101),

Table 1. EB-transformed HLA homozygous lymphoblastoid cell lines

Cell lines	9th International Workshop number or source	HLA type	
		DR	Dw
Sa	local	1	1
CI	9W0201	2	2
PGF	Festenstein (London)	2	2
Ys12	local	2	2
TOK	9w1202	2	12
72-4	Reinsmoen (Minneapolis)	2	MN2
Nancy	Reinsmoen (Minneapolis)	2	MN2
Kathy	Reinsmoen (Minneapolis)	2	MN2
Bacilio	9W1801	2	DB9
Remigio	9W1903	2	DB9
JAH	9W2403	4	4
AL10	9W1001	4	10
PEA	9W1302	4	13
Ls40	9W1403	4	14
YT59	local	4	15
Wa	Wakisaka (Sapporo)	4	15
HVB	9W0504	5	5
GECK	9W0903	6	9
WDV	9W0605	6	18
SLE	9W0608	6	19
KT11	9W0610	6	19
HOR	local	6	19
SH	Katagiri (Asahikawa)	6.2	New
BOR	9W0701	7	7
WE5	9W0705	7	7+71
BTB	9W0801	8	8
HID	local	9	DB5
ISK	Aizawa (Sapporo)	9	New

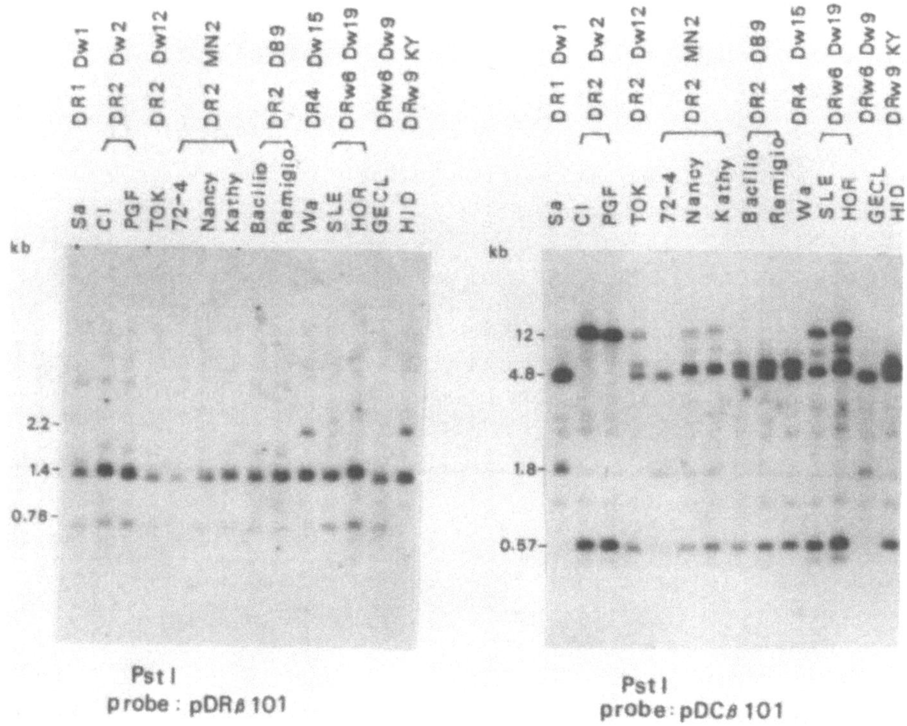

Fig. 1. Autoradiogram of blot hybridization analysis of HLA homozygous B-cell lines with the DRβ cDNA (pDRβ101) and DQβ cDNA (pDCβ101) as probes after *Pst*I digestion. DNAs were isolated from EB-transformed HLA-homozygous B-lymphoblastoid cell lines by solubilizing at 50 °C for 16 h in 50 m*M* Tris HCl (pH 8.0), 20 m*M* ethylenediaminetetraacetate (EDTA), 100 m*M* NaCl, 1% sodium dodecyl sulfate (SDS), and 150 γ/ml proteinase K. Protein was removed from the DNA by 400 m*M* Tris-saturated phenol, and the DNA aqueous phase was incubated with RNase A (80 γ/ml) and RNase T_1 (30 units/ml) at 37 °C. The DNA was recovered by ethanol precipitation. Samples of *Eco*RI-cleaved genomic DNA (7.5 μg) were subjected to electrophoresis on 0.7% agarose and transferred to nitrocellulose paper (BA85, S&S) with 20 × SSC (3 *M* NaCl, 0.3 *M* sodium citrate) (Southern 1975; Thomas 1980). The size marker was a mixture of *HindIII* and (*Eco*RI + *Hind*III)-digested λDNA. After transfer, the filters were prehybridized (0.9 *M* NaCl, 90 m*M* Tris HCl pH 7.4,6 m*M* EDTA, 0.5% SDS, 5 × Denhardt's solution, and 100 γ/ml heated, denatured salmon sperm DNA) at 65 °C for 4 h. A radioactively labeled cDNA insert from the almost full-length DQβ cDNA clone, pDCβ101 (Inoko et al. 1985 b), and λDNA were added to a concentration of 1×10^6 cpm/ml and 1×10^4 cpm/ml in the hybridization mixture (0.9 *M* NaCl, 90 m*M* Tris HCl, pH 7.4, 6 m*M* EDTA, 0.5% SDS, 10% dextran sulfate, 5 × Denhardt's solution, and 100 γ/ml heated, denatured salmon sperm DNA), respectively, and incubated with the filters at 65 °C for 16 h. The filters were washed in 3 × SSC, 0.1% SDS for 5 min at room temperature, in 2 × SSC, 0.1% SDS for 5 min at room temperature, in 1 × SSC, 0.1% SDS for 20 min at 68 °C, and in 0.2 × SSC, 0.1% SDS for 20 min at 68 °C. The filters were then exposed to Kodak XRP-5 film with an intensifying screen at −70 °C

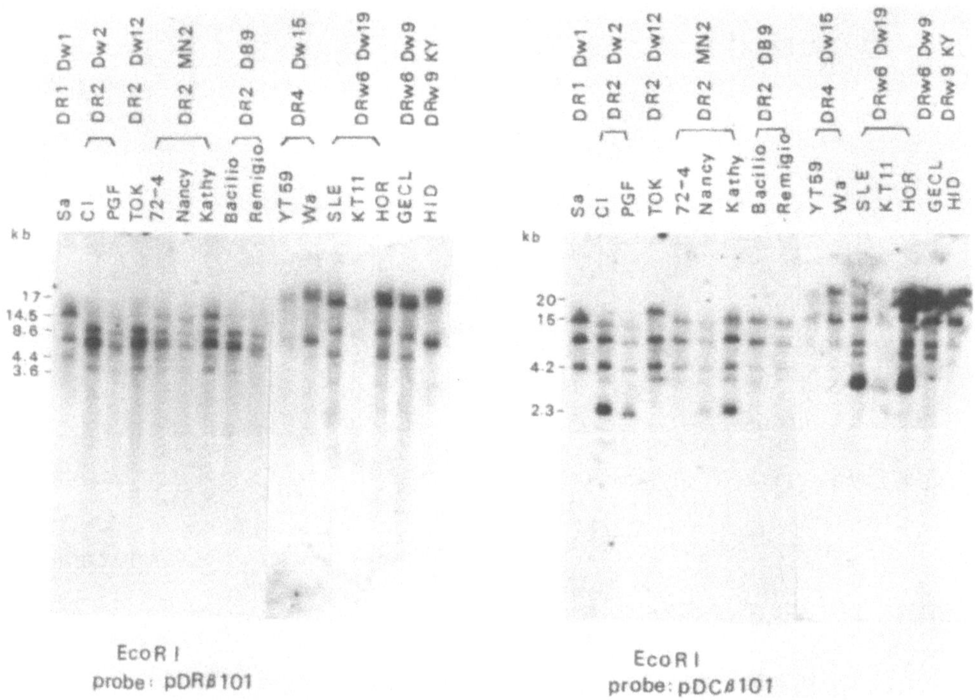

Fig. 2. Autoradiogram of blot hybridization analysis HLA homozygous B cell lines with the DRβ cDNA and the DQβ cDNA as probes after *Eco*RI digestion. See the legend to Fig. 1 for details

DQα(pDCα107), DQβ(pDCβ101), and DPβ(pDAβ5) cDNA probes (Inoko et al. 1985a, Inoko et al. 1986). Figures 1 and 2 shows the polymorphic restriction fragments of some DNA samples hybridizing DRβ and DQβ cDNA probes after *Pst*I and *Eco*RI digestion, respectively. Multiple hybridizing fragments were encountered in DNA from all HLA-homozygous B-lymphoblastoid cell lines with both the DR and DQβ cDNA probes and the patterns of bands were distinct between DR or DQ types for each enzyme. The DQα cDNA probe could also detect polymorphic fragments specific for HLA-DR or -DQ specificities. On the other hand, the DPβ cDNA probe could primarily discriminate between HLA-DP specificities.

Hybridization with the DRβ cDNA probe generally gave identical patterns with DNA from different Dw specificities with an identical DR type [for example, four Dw subtypes of DR2 (Dw2, Dw12, MN2, DB9) or two Dw subtypes of DR6 (Dw9, Dw19). See Figs. 1, 2], although restriction fragment polymorphism was easily detected in different DR types as described above. In contrst, the DQβ cDNA could easily distinguish not only DR specificities, but also different Dw specificities (Figs. 1, 2).

The distribution of all of these fragments detected with the DRβ and DQβ cDNA probes in 27 HLA-homozygous B-lymphoblastoid cell lines were studied in relation to the DR and DQ specificities by cluster analysis. Figure 3 illustrates the

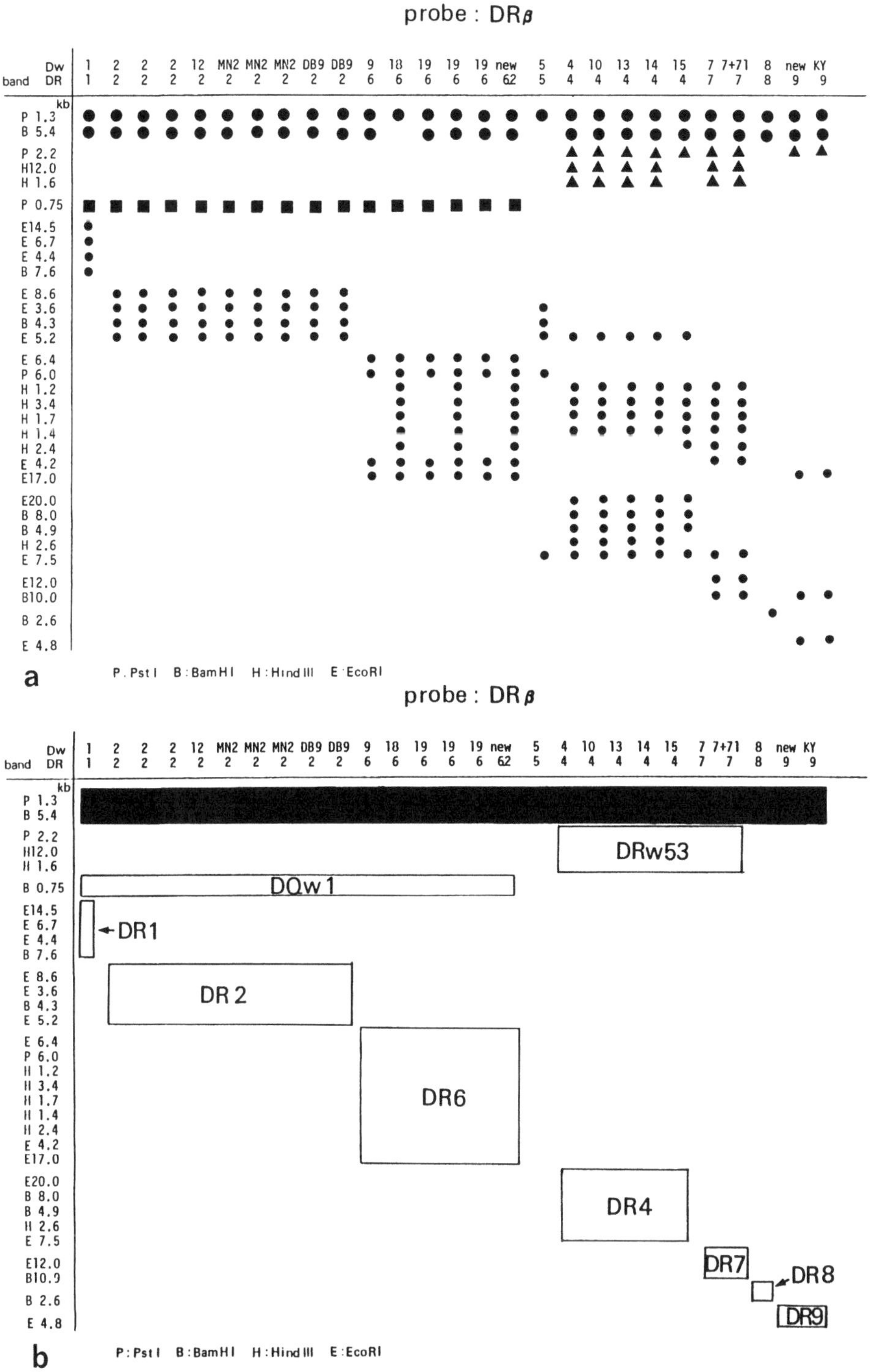

Fig. 3. **a** Distribution of the fragments hybridizing to the DRβ cDNA probe in 27 HLA homozygous B-cell lines in relation to the DR types. **b** Schematic representation of **A**, showing the various clusters. Data of (DR4, Dw15) are derived from only Wa. ● all DR specificities; ▲ depicts DRw53; ■ depicts DQw1; • depicts the single DR serotype

distribution of each fragment hybridizing to the DRβ cDNA probe in each haplotype, and the allelic behavior of the clusters of fragments or some single fragments can be seen. At the top of Fig. 3 (large black circles), two fragments (*Pst*I, 1.3 kb, and *Bam*HI, 5.4 kb) cover all of the haplotypes. The following three fragments (*Pst*I, 2.2 kb, *Hin*dIII, 12.0 kb, and *Hin*dIII, 1.6 kb) (black triangles) correlate with DR4 and DR7, i.e., DRw53. Next, one fragment (*Pst*I, 0.75 kb) (black squares) is present in the DR1, DR2, and DR6 haplotypes which belong to the DQw1 family. The other fragments (small black circles) strongly correlate with the single DR serotype, forming the DR-type-specific clusters. Four fragments (*Eco*RI, 14.5 kb, *Eco*RI, 6.7 kb, *Eco*RI, 4.4 kb, *Bam*HI, 7.6 kb) coincide with the DR1 haplotype. The following four (*Eco*RI, 8.6 kb, *Eco*RI, 3.6 kb, *Bam*HI, 4.3 kb, *Eco*RI, 5.2 kb) and nine (*Eco*RI, 6.4 kb, *Pst*I, 6.0 kb, *Hin*dIII, 1.2kb, *Hin*dIII, 3.4 kb, *Hin*dIII, 1.7 kb, *Hin*dIII, 1.4 kb, *Hin*dIII, 2.4 kb, *Eco*RI, 4.2 kb, *Eco*RI, 17.0 kb) fragments determine the DR2 and DR6 haplotype, respectively, although some of them are also detected in other DR haplotypes. The DR4 and DR7b haplotypes are specified by five fragments (*Eco*RI, 20.0 kb, *Bam*HI, 8.0 kb, *Bam*HI, 4.9 kb, *Hin*dIII, 2.6 kb, *Eco*RI, 7.5 kb) and two fragments (*Eco*RI, 12.0 kb, *Bam*HI, 10.0 kb), respectively. The last two (*Bam*HI, 2.6 kb, and *Eco*RI, 4.8 kb) fragments define the DR8 and DR9 haplotype, respectively. These results suggest that the DRβ cDNA probe permits definite HLA-D region genotyping at the DNA level.

It became clear that genomic hybridization with class II antigen β chain probes provides valuable information regarding the definition and typing of new class II antigen loci and alleles as a complementary method of conventional tissue typing and studies of new markers for diseases associated with HLA. So, we decided to apply this DNA typing technique to narcoleptic patients to understand the molecular mechanism that underlies HLA-DR2 susceptibility to narcolepsy.

DNA Typing in Narcolepsy

A remarkably high level of association between HLA-DR2, -DQw1, and narcolepsy was first reported by Honda et al. (1984). All 111 narcoleptic patients tested were found to be DR2-positive ($\chi^2 = 141$, $P < 10^{-29}$) (Juji et al. 1984, Matsuki et al. 1985). This high level of association was also observed for all the 37 Caucasoid patients studied by Langdon et al. (1984). The DQβ cDNA probe was used to define polymorphisms at the genomic level in order to differentiate between narcoleptic patients and healthy individuals with DR2 homozygotes or heterozygotes. Marked differences were found between narcoleptic patients and normal healthy individuals. All the narcoleptic patients shared DQβ *Eco*RI 2.4-kb and *Pst*I 12-kb fragments, which were detected in healthy controls only at decreased frequencies (37.9% and 82.9%, respectively). Furthermore, all of the patients except one possessed DQβ *Bam*HI 2.9-kb fragments, which were observed in healthy controls at a decreased frequency of 55.1%. In contrast, the narcoleptic patients showed a decreased frequency of an *Eco*RI 18-kb fragment (34.8%) which was present in all the healthy controls. On the other hand, the DRβ cDNA has so far been unable to detect any significant difference(s).

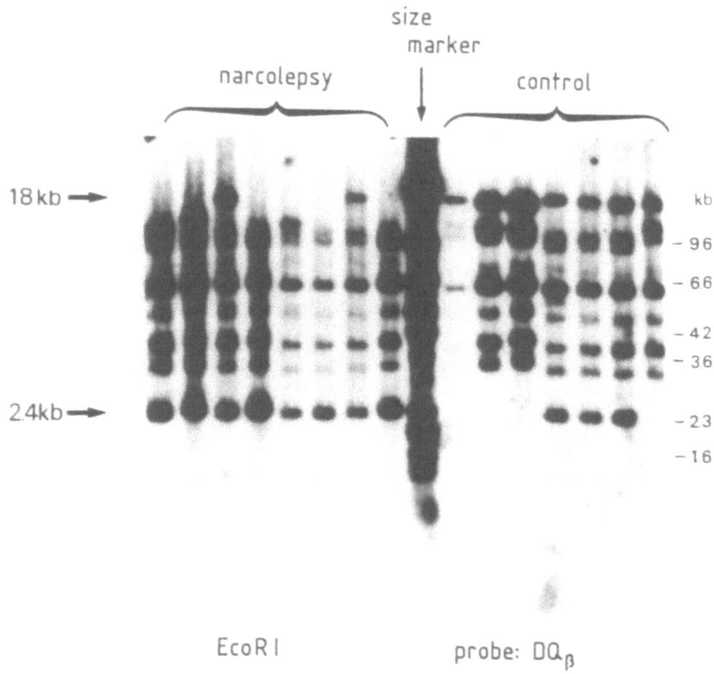

Fig. 4. Autoradiogram of blot hybridization analysis of eight narcoleptic patients (DR2/- = DR2/DR2 or DR2/DR2 blank) and seven healthy controls (DR2/-) with DQβ cDNA (pDCβ101) after *Eco*RI digestion. See the legend to Fig. 1 for details. *Arrows* indicate the positions of 2.4-kb and 18-kb bands

DNA was isolated from the peripheral lymphocytes of 46 narcoleptic patients who were typed as being either HLA-DR2/($n=24$, DR2/DR2 or DR2/DR blank) or DR2/DRx ($n=22$, DR/DR alleles other than DR2: DR1, $n=1$; DR4, $n=8$; DR5, $n=4$; DR6, $n=2$; DR8, $n=3$; DR9, $n=4$). Twenty-nine HLA-DR2 healthy individuals (the number was increased to 35 individuals for *Pst*I digestion) were selected, being either HLA-DR2/-($n=15$) or DR2/DRx ($n=14$: DR4, $n=4$; DR5, $n=3$; DR6, $n=2$; DR8, $n=3$; DR9, $n=3$). The DNA samples (7.5 µg) were digested with the restriction endonucleases *Eco*RI, *Bam*HI, and *Pst*I. After electrophoresis and transfer, the restriction fragments were probed with the DQβ cDNA insert, which was isolated from the almost full-length DQβ cDNA clone, pDCβ101 (Inoko et al. 1985b), by digestion with *Pst*I (see legend to Fig. 1 for details).

The DQβ cDNA probe detected six to ten *Eco*RI, seven to ten *Pst*I, and six to eight *Bam*HI fragments. Significant differences in hybridization band patterns between patients and controls were as follows. The *Eco*RI 2.4-kb fragment was found in all 46 narcoleptic patients, but it was absent in 18 out of 29 healthy controls (Figs. 4, 5). In contrast, *Eco*RI sequences of 18 kb were present in all 29 healthy individuals, but this fragment was detected in only 16 out of 46 narcoleptic patients (Figs. 4, 5). The *Bam*HI 2.9-kb fragment was found in all 45 narcoleptic patients except one (Fig. 6). The frequency of this fragment was, however,

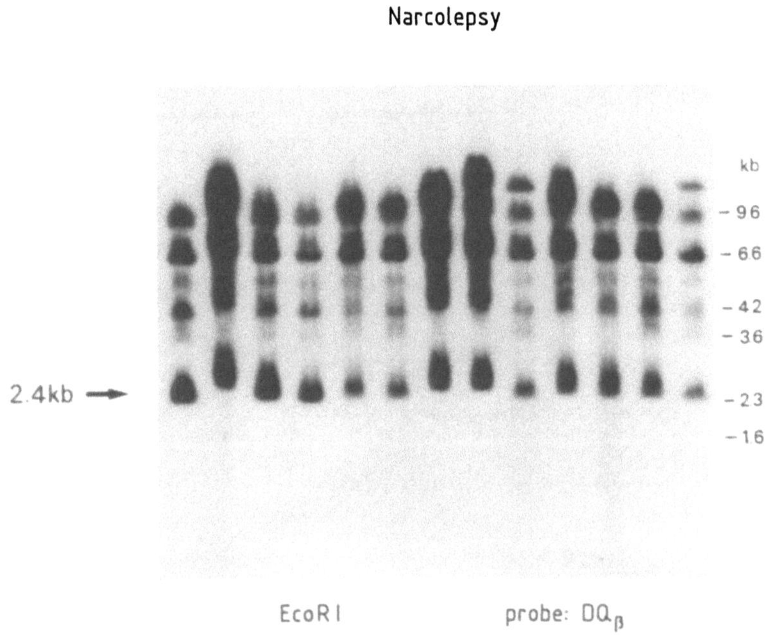

Fig. 5. Autoradiogram of blot hybridization analysis of 13 narcoleptic patients (DR2/- or DR2/DRx) with DQβ cDNA (pDCβ101) after *Eco*RI digestion. See the legend to Fig. 1 for details. An *arrow* indicates the position of the 2.4-kb band

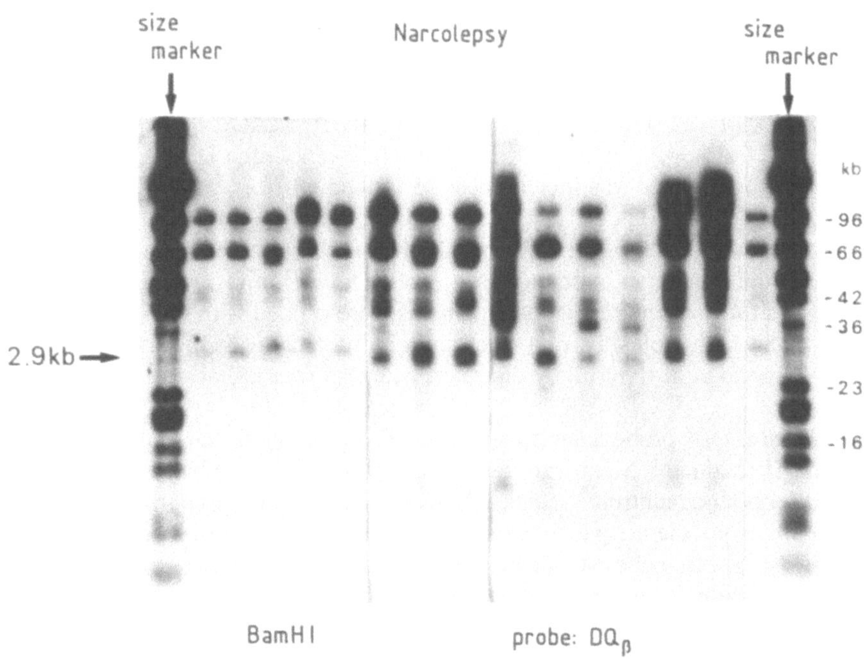

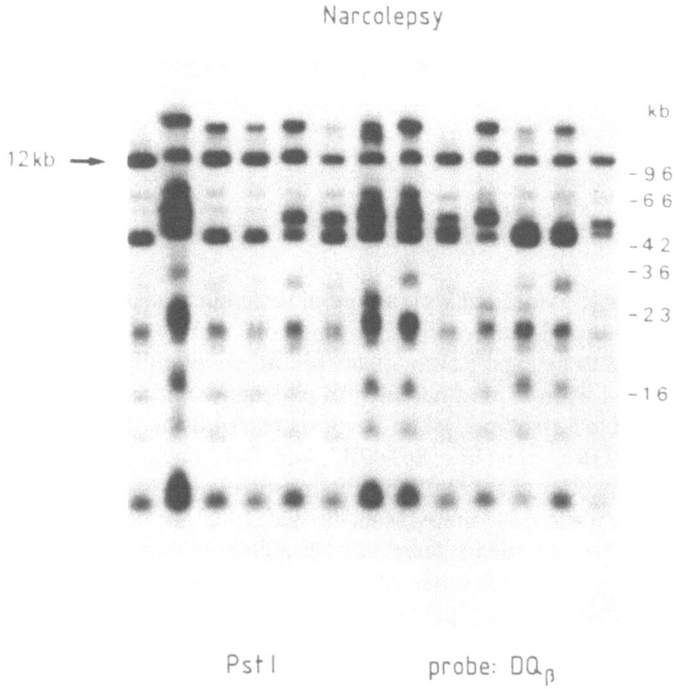

Fig. 7. Autoradiogram of blot hybridization analysis of 13 narcoleptic patients (DR2/- or DR2/DRx) with the DQβ cDNA after *Pst*I digestion. See the legend to Fig. 1 for details. An *arrow* indicates the position of the 12-kb band

clearly decreased in healthy individuals (16 out of 29 controls). Furthermore, *Pst*I sequences of 12 kb were present in all 46 patients, but were only present at a decreased frequency in healthy individuals (29 out of 35 controls) (Fig. 7). These marked differences were observed between narcoleptic patients and healthy controls with DR2/DRx as well as with DR2/DR- (Figs. 4–7), indicating susceptibility to the disease does not correlate with the DR2 homo- or heterozygous genotype.

On the other hand, the DRβ cDNA probe gave almost similar hybridization patterns between patients and healthy controls, not detecting significant differences when *Eco*RI, *Bam*HI, and *Pst*I were used for digestion (data not shown). This result may only reflect the fact that the HLA-D subregion around the DRβ gene is less polymorphic than that around the DQβ gene.

Southern hybridization analysis demonstrated that, compared with healthy controls, all the narcoleptic patients examined had the DQβ *Eco*RI 2.4-kb (χ^2 = 37.6) and *Pst*I 12-kb (χ^2 = 8.5) sequences (Table 2). The *Bam*HI 2.9-kb sequence

Fig. 6. Autoradiogram of blot hybridization analysis of 15 narcoleptic patients (DR2/-) with the DQβ cDNA (pDCβ101) after *Bam*HI digestion. See the legend to Fig. 1 for details. An *arrow* indicates the position of the 2.9-kb band

Table 2. Restriction fragment frequency in narcolepsy

	Narcolepsy ($n=46$)	Control ($n=29$)	χ^2	*RR*
DQ *Eco*RI 2.4 kb	46 (100%)	11 (37.9%)	37.6	>73.6
DQ *Pst*I 12 kb	46 (100%)	24 (82.7%)	8.5	>9.4
DQ *Bam*HI 2.9 kb	45 (97.8%)	16 (55.1%)	21.3	36.6
DQ *Eco*RI 18 kb	16 (34.8%)	29 (100%)	31.5	>58.0

was also associated with all the narcoleptic patients except one ($\chi^2=21.3$). Unexpectedly, all the healthy controls had the DQβ *Eco*RI 18-kb fragment which was found to be significantly decreased in narcoleptic patients ($\chi^2=31.5$). These clear results showed that narcoleptic patients commonly share a relatively rare DR2-positive haplotype, which is consistent with the findings that the rare haplotypes (B35-DR2, B15-DR2, B51-DR2, and DR2-Dw2) increased in their frequencies in narcoleptics compared with the most frequent haplotype, B52-DR2-Dw12, found in the normal Japanese (Matsuki et al. 1985). In fact, hybridization band pattern of narcoleptic patients detected by the DQβ cDNA are quite similar to those of the DR2, Dw2 homozygous cell line, CI and PGF (see Figs. 1, 2).

Location of Restriction Fragments Specific for Narcolepsy Within the DQβ Chain Gene

Seventeen genomic clones representing a length of about 95 kb DNA derived from the DR2, Dw2, DQw1 haplotype of healthy individuals (PGF and Man) were isolated by successive screening of the human phage and cosmid gene libraries (Fig. 8). The DQ subregion consists of two pairs of α and β genes, which include the genes (DQα, DQβ) for the DQ antigen (Kornman et al. 1985). The other α–β pair has been named DXα and DXβ (Okada et al. 1985). The DXα and DXβ genes have strong homology to the DQα and DQβ, respectively. There is no evidence that the DX region is capable of expressing an HLA class II-like heterodimer so far although the sequence data indicate no defect in the gene structure of DXα and DXβ. Restriction enzyme mapping studies demonstrated that all of these restriction fragments specific for narcolepsy are located within the expressible DQβ gene in spite of the fact that nucleotide homology between the DQβ and DXβ gene is more than 90% and so the DQβ cDNA can efficiently detect not only the DQβ gene, but also the DXβ gene when used as a probe in Southern hybridization experiments (Fig. 9). It must be noted that polymorphic sites possibly related to susceptibility to narcolepsy are mapped around exon 2 (representing the β1 domain), intron 2, and exon 3 (representing the β2 domain) of the DQβ gene.

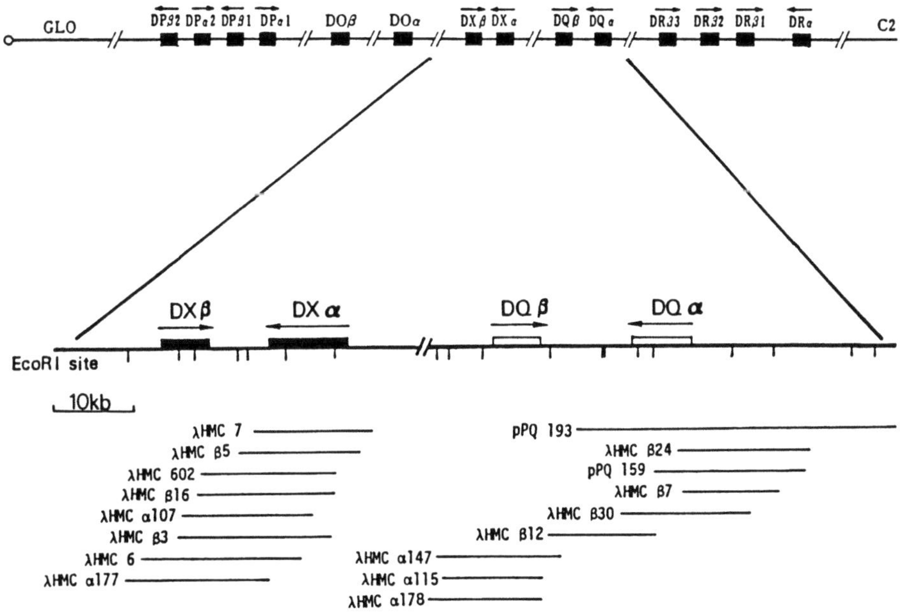

Fig. 8. Schematic map of the HLA-D region and molecular map of the HLA-DQ subregion (DR2, Dw2, DQw1) defined by nine overlapping genomic clones for the DQα and DQβ genes and eight overlapping genomic clones for the DXα and DXβ genes. *Arrows* indicate the direction of transcription of genes. See the text for details. O, centromere of chromosome 6; *GLO*, glyoxalase I; *C2*, component of the complement system

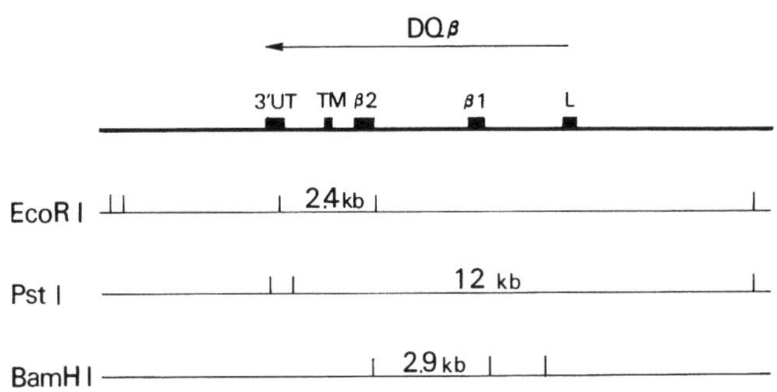

Fig. 9. Location of three restriction fragments specific for narcolepsy within the DQβ gene. The restriction map was constructed according to the data on overlapping genomic clones derived from healthy HLA-DR2, Dw2, DQw1 haplotypes (PGF and Man) (Fig. 7). The location and orientation of exons of the DQβ gene *shown as black boxes* was determined by Southern blot analysis of restriction fragments from the genomic clones with separated 5′ and 3′ end fragments from the DQβ cDNA clone, pDCβ101, used as hybridization probes. *L*, leader sequence; *TM*, transmembrane region; *3′ UT*: *3′*, untranslated region

Conclusions and Speculations

DNA typing techniques of HLA class II antigen based on restriction fragment length polymorphism have been developed in our laboratory and applied to 46 narcoleptic patients. Three restriction fragments specific for narcolepsy (*Eco*RI, 2.4 kb, *Bam*HI, 2.9 kb, and *Pst*I, 12 kb) and one restriction fragment significantly decreased in narcoleptic patients (*Eco*RI, 18 kb) were detected. Analysis of overlapping genomic clones encoding the HLA-DQ subregion of the DR2, Dw2 haplotype mapped these polymorphic sites in the DQβ gene region, especially around the β1 exon, second intron, and β2 exon. These results are of great interest when the following facts are taken into acount. The HLA class II antigens are essential for cellular recognition and cooperation between macrophages or B cells and T cells, determining immune response as restriction molecules. Underlying these phenomena is thought to be the cell-to-cell interaction where T-cell antigen receptor recognizes HLA antigens, especially β1 and β2 domain. Cloning of these narcolepsy-specific fragments and characterization of their function will help to understand not only the molecular mechanism of susceptibility to narcolepsy, but will also clarify the genetic basis and the mode of disease linkage of certain HLA class II antigen specificities.

Acknowledgments. The author acknowledges the efforts of his coworkers and collaborators: Drs. A. Ando, K. Tsuji, S. Nezu, K. Shirakura (Tokai University School of Medicine), K. Matsuki, T. Juji (Tokyo University Hospital), and Y. Honda (Seiwa Hospital, Neuropsychiatric Research Institute). The author wishes to thank Miss A. Ohki for her assistance in preparing this manuscript.

References

Benacerraf B (1981) Role of MHC gene products in immune regulation. Science 212: 1229-1238

Bodmer WF (1984) The HLA system, 1984. In: Histocompatibility testing 1984. Springer, Berlin Heidelberg New York, pp 11-22

Cohen D, Gall IL, Marcadet A, Font MP, Lalovel JM, Dausset J (1984) Clusters of HLA class II restriction fragments describe allelic series. Proc Natl Acad Sci USA 81: 7870-7874

Dausset J, Svejgaard A (1975) HLA and disease. Munksgaard, Copenhagen

Honda, H, Doi Y, Juji T, Satake M (1984) Narcolepsy and HLA: positive DR2 as a prerequisite for the development of narcolepsy. Folia Psychiatr Neurol Jpn 38: 360

Inoko H, Ando A, Kimura M, Tsuji K (1985a) Isolation and characterization of the cDNA clone and genomic clones of a new HLA class II antigen heavy chain DOα. J Immunol 135: 2156-2159

Inoko H, Ando A, Kimura M, Tsuji K (1985b) Isolation and characterization of the cDNA clones and genomic clones of the HLA class II antigens. In: Tsuji K (ed) Present and future development of transplantation. Tokai University Press, Tokyo, pp 188-220

Inoko H, Ando A, Tsuji K, Matsuki K, Juji T, Honda Y (1986) HLA-DQβ chain DNA restriction fragments can differentiate between healthy and narcoleptic individuals with HLA-DR2. Immunogenetics 23: 126-128

Juji T, Satake M, Honda Y, Doi Y (1984) HLA antigens in Japanese patients with narcolepsy. Tissue Antigens 24: 316

Kaufman JF, Strominger JL (1983) The extracellular region of light chains from human and murine MHC class II antigens consists of 2 domains. J Immunol 130: 808-812

Korman JF, Auffray C, Korman AJ, Shackelford DA, Strominger J (1984) The class II molecules of the human and murine major histocompatibility complex. Science 36: 1-13

Korman AJ, Boss JM, Spies T, Sorrentino R, Okada K, Strominger JL (1985) Genetic complexity and expression of human class II histocompatibility antigens. Immunol Rev 85: 45-86

Langdon N, Welsh KI, Dam MV, Vaugham RW, Parkes D (1984) Genetic markers in narcolepsy. Lancet ii: 1178-1180

Matsuki K, Juji T, Tokunaga K, Naohara T, Satake M, Honda Y (1985) Human histocompatibility leukocyte antigen (HLA) haplotype frequencies estimated from the data on HLA class I, II and III antigens in 111 Japanese narcoleptics. J Clin Invest 76: 2078-2083

Okada K, Boss JM, Prentice H, Spies T, Mengler R, Auffray C, Lillie J, Grossberger D, Strominger JL (1985) Gene organization of DC and DX subregions of the human major histocompatibility complex. Proc Natl Acad Sci USA 82: 3410-3414

Owenbach D, Lernmark A, Rask L, Peterson PA, Platz P, Svejgaard A (1983) Detection of HLA-D/DR-related DNA polymorphism in HLA-D homozygous typing cells. Proc Natl Acad Sci USA 80: 3758-3761

Ryder LP, Anderson E, Svejgaard (eds) (1979) HLA and disease registry. Munksgaard, Copenhagen

Southern EM (1975) Detection of specific sequences among DNA fragments separated by gel electrophoresis. J Mol Biol 98: 509-517

Terasaki PI (ed) (1980) Disease studies. In: Histocompatibility testing 1980. UCLA Tissue Typing Laboratory, Los Angeles, pp 638-735

Thomas PS (1980) Hybridization of denatured RNA and small DNA fragments transferred to nitrocellulose. Proc Natl Acad Sci USA

Tosi R, Tanigaki N, Sorrentino R, Centis D, Ferrara GB (1984) Serologically detectable polymorphism of the HLA-DC-subunit. J Immunol 132: 277-281

Trowsdale J, Lee J, Carey J, Grosweld F, Bodmer J, Bodmer W (1983) Sequences related to the HLA-DRα chain on chromosome 6: restriction enzyme polymorphism detected with DCα chain probes. Proc Natl Acad Sci USA 79: 1972-1976

Chapter 12

Immunological Features of Narcolepsy in Japan

K. Matsuki, T. Juji, and Y. Honda

Narcolepsy has traditionally been regarded as a nonimmunological disease. However, the findings of a strong association between narcolepsy and an HLA antigen have led to a new speculation: an altered regulatory system of immune response may underlie the pathogenesis of narcolepsy (Billiard and Seignalet 1985; Matsuki et al. 1985; Langdon et al. 1986).

One possible way to substantiate this speculation is to investigate various immunological parameters in narcoleptic patients. In this chapter, we will summarize our findings.

Lymphocyte Subsets in Narcolepsy

The immune system consists of functionally distinct subsets of lymphocytes. These subsets can be identified by their cell surface differentiation antigens. The quantitative measurements of lymphocyte subpopulations with these cell surface antigens usually provide sensitive and reproducible indices for the immune status in patients.

We have analyzed 31 Japanese patients with narcolepsy and 55 age- and sex-matched controls. The patients were randomly selected with informed consent, all were DR2 positive, and they had no apparent illnesses other than narcolepsy. They were all under medication for narcolepsy. All of them had at least a 5-year history of narcolepsy. Part of this study was previously reported (Matsuki et al. 1985).

Table 1 shows the monoclonal antibodies used in this and succeeding studies and the lymphocyte subsets and/or epitopes recognized by these monoclonal antibodies.

No significant deviation was observed quantitatively for $CD2^+$, $CD3^+$, $CD4^+$, $CD8^+$, $OKIa1^+$, $OKB7^+$, $Leu7^+$, and $Leu11^+$ subpopulations (Table 2). The ratio of CD4:CD8 was in the normal range. On the other hand, three subsets, $OKIa1^+$, $OKM1^+$, and $CD10^+$, showed significant increases.

The $CD3^+$, $CD4^+$, and $CD8^+$ subpopulations and the CD4:CD8 ratio are among the most widely used immunological parameters. The number and percentage of each subset is not affected by the subjects' HLA-DR types (Bertrams et al. 1986). Our data suggest that no major helper/inducer and suppressor/cytotoxic T-cell subsets alterations were present in these patients, at least quantitatively. We

Table 1. Monoclonal antibodies

Monoclonal antibodies	Reactivity
CD2	CD2, all T cells forming an E-rosette
CD3	CD3, mature T cells
CD4	CD4, helper/inducer T cells
CD8	CD8, suppressor/cytotoxic T cells
CD4:CD8	Helper/suppressor ratio
OKIa1	HLA-class II positive cells
OKB7	Mature B cells
Leu7	Large granular lymphocytes
Leu11	CD16, natural killer cells
OKM1	C3b receptor, monocytes
CD10	Activated T cells
Tac	Activated T cells

Table 2. Lymphocyte subpopulations*

Monoclonal antibodies	Narcolepsy		Controls		*P*
	Mean	SD	Mean	SD	
CD2	74.9	6.6	75.0	5.1	
CD3	67.2	9.0	70.6	4.7	
CD4	42.0	9.5	40.8	5.6	
CD8	26.2	7.1	27.8	4.7	
CD4:CD8	1.76	0.74	1.83	0.53	
OKIa1	16.6	5.2	11.9	3.6	<0.000005
OKB7	10.2	3.7	12.9	7.5	
Leu7	22.6	9.1	20.1	7.6	
Leu11	17.1	9.8	17.0	7.0	
OKM1	24.3	10.3	12.5	5.3	<0.0005
CD10	15.6	5.8	7.0	4.1	<0.000005

* Lymphocyte subpopulations were determined by the previously described method (Matsuki et al. 1985)

have no qualitative or functional information on these subsets. However, it should be noted that in many diseases these parameters reflect disease activity and usually have good correlations with functional parameters such as mitogen stimulation indices.

It is difficult to interpret the increase of OKIa1$^+$, OKT10$^+$, OKM1$^+$ subpopulations. The changes of these subpopulations do not necessarily imply the aberrant immune status in narcolepsy. These subsets may differ among subjects with different DR antigens. Besides, the medications prescribed for narcolepsy may have altered the numbers of these subpopulations.

A 1-Year Follow-up Study on Newly Developed Cases

To further investigate the immunological status in narcolepsy, we have also studied various immunological parameters on three newly developed cases. They were not included in the study described above. The laboratory tests were performed serially for 1 year.

Case 1

A 7-year-old girl had been well and had not experienced daytime sleepiness until 5 May 1985, when she suddenly fell asleep at a relative's house in the morning and again in the afternoon. From that day on, she began to fall asleep at least twice during the daytime. Frequent cataplectic attacks developed almost simultaneously. She lost muscle strength when she laughed, while crossing the street, while riding a bicycle, etc. She dreamt dreadful dreams; when she seemed to wake up from the dreams, she found that she was unable to move her hands or entire body. She was hospitalized for 5 weeks without receiving a definite diagnosis. She was referred to our hospital on 16 July 1985. She was 130 cm tall and weighed 30 kg. She had gained 5 kg in 2 months between May and July.

Her HLA typing results were A2, B35, B51, Cw3, DR2, DRw12, DQw1, DQw3. An all-night polysomnography performed during the 3rd night of admission revealed a marked tendency to fall asleep and 6 c/s positive spike trains and sporadic spikes during the non-REM sleep. However, a rapid eye movement (REM) period was not detected within 15 min after the onset of sleep. A multiple sleep latency test (MSLT) performed on the next day showed clear sleep-onset REM periods on all of the four daytime records. The REM latencies were 0 min on all the records. The patient experienced frightening hypnagogic hallucinations during the third and fourth MSLT recordings performed at 2 p.m. and 4 p.m. Her daytime sleepiness was eliminated with the administration of 25 mg pemoline and 40 mg methylphenidate. Clomipramine at bedtime was effective in controlling cataplexy and improving nocturnal sleep.

On August 1, 2 months and 3 weeks after the onset, we performed extensive laboratory examinations. The data were all within the normal range. Her white cell count was 7300, with 44% lymphocytes; erythrocyte sedimentation ratio, 9 mm/h; C-reactive protein, negative; rheumatoid factor, negative; total protein, 7.1 g/100 ml; albumin, 66.1%; γ-globulin, 15.9%; IgG, 1211 mg/100 ml; IgA, 299 mg/100 ml; IgM, 137 mg/100 ml; CH_{50}, 31.7 units/ml; C3, 101 mg/100 ml; C4, 27 mg/100 ml; LE factor, negative; antinuclear antibodies, negative; anti-DNA antibodies <1 unit/ml; immunosuppressive acid protein, 435 mmol/ml.

The lymphocyte subpopulations were as follows: CD3, 61.1%; CD4, 24.8%; CD8, 24.9; CD4:8 ratio, 1.00; CD2, 64.7%; Leu11, 9.2%; OKIa1, 23.3%; OKB7, 20.8%; Leu7, 14.5%; Tac, 2.3%. Stimulation indices with phytohemagglutinin (PHA), concanavalin A (ConA), and pokeweed mitogen (PWM) were 544, 334, and 150, respectively. They were all within the normal range.

Fig. 1 shows the 1-year follow-up results of the cytological markers. None of the markers showed any significant deviations in the course of a year. Mitogen stimulation indices varied widely and were not suitable for the time-course follow-up.

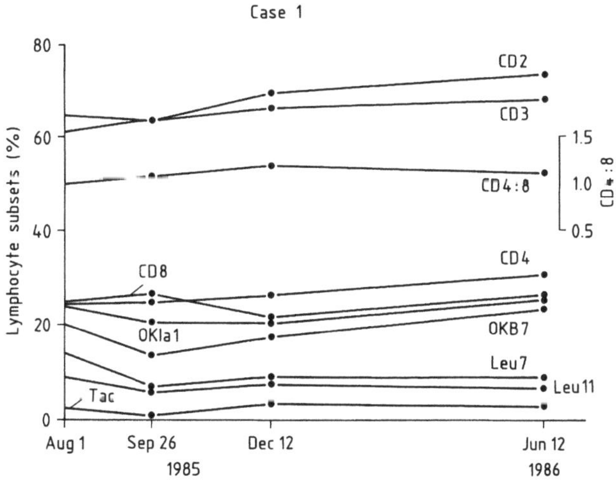

Fig. 1. Changes of lymphocyte subsets in case 1

Case 2

A 10-year-old girl had been well until the end of May 1985. The onset was insidious. She had exercised strenuously for 1 week for an athletic event on May 25. During that week, she often fell asleep when she came home from school. The sleepiness continued even after the athletic event. In June, she began to fall asleep at home almost every evening for about 2 h. After the sleep, she felt good and could stay awake until she went to bed. In early June, she experienced sudden weakness in various muscles of her body, especially when she laughed. She dreamt a lot, but the dreams were usually pleasant. She did not experience sleep paralysis. She came to our hospital on June 25. She was 142 cm tall and weighed 35 kg. No significant weight gain was observed.

Her HLA typing results were A24, Bw61, Cw3, DR2, DR4, DQw1, DQw3. An all-night polysomnography performed during the 8th night of her admission showed a marked tendency to fall asleep (sleep latency = 3 min) and a REM period at 3 min after the onset of sleep. MSLT on the next day revealed sleep-onset REM periods on all the four daytime recordings (see Chap. 2, Fig. 14). Administration of 25 mg pemoline and 10 mg methylphenidate in the morning and after lunch eliminated daytime sleepiness during school hours; after school, she used to nap for ½ h and could then stay awake without medicine. Her cataplexy disappeared with the administration of 10 mg clomipramine and 12.5 mg chlorpromazine.

The results of the serological examination on 1 August, about 2½ months after the onset, were all within the normal range except for a positive rheumatoid factor. Her white-cell count was 6700, with 23% lymphocytes; erythrocyte sedimentation ratio, 4 mm/h; C-reactive protein, negative; rheumatoid factor, 1+; sensitized sheep cell agglutination (SSCA) for rheumatoid factor activity, negative; total protein, 7.3 g/100 ml; albumin, 67.3%; γ-globulin, 15.6%; IgG, 1106 mg/100 ml; IgA,

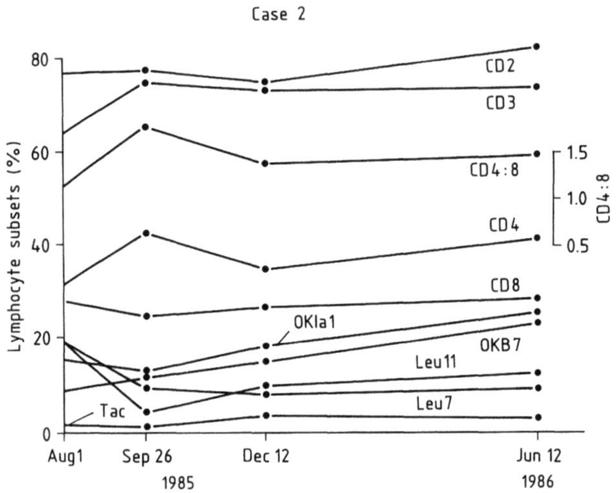

Fig. 2. Changes of lymphocyte subsets in case 2

229 mg/100 ml; IgM, 146 mg/100 ml; CH_{50}, 39.3 units/ml; C3, 91 mg/100 ml; C4, 16 mg/100 ml; LE factor, negative; antinuclear antibodies, negative; immunosuppressive acid protein, 300 mmol/ml.

The lymphocyte subsets were as follows: CD3, 63.9%; CD4, 32.0%; CD8, 28.4%; CD4:8 ratio, 1.13; CD2, 76.2%; Leu11, 18.2%; OKIa1, 15.3%; OKB7, 8.8%; Leu7, 19.4%; Tac, 1.1%. Stimulation indices with PHA, Con A, and PWM were also normal: 257, 188, and 58, respectively.

The results of the serial cytological tests are shown in Fig. 2. The various lymphocyte subpopulations showed no significant deviations. The rheumatoid factor was positive until the end of September; in December it was negative. SSCA was negative throughout the course of the study.

Case 3

A 12-year-old boy had been well until September 1984, when he joined a soccer club. He started falling asleep, usually for a while after school, before he went to the soccer practice. In October, he found himself unable to play well because of frequent attacks of muscle weakness during the soccer matches. In December, both his sleepiness and attacks of muscle weakness became aggravated. He had difficulty watching television comedies, for his head sagged when he laughed at funny scenes and dialogues. When walking his knees buckled suddenly; he reported feeling as if his body were sinking a little into the ground. On 18 December, he was admitted to hospital; after 1 month of hospitalization, his condition remained undiagnosed. On 20 March 1985, he was transferred to another hospital. In April, he was measured as 1 cm taller and 3 kg heavier than in September 1984. He also complained of disturbed sleep at night. He came to our hospital on 9 May 1985.

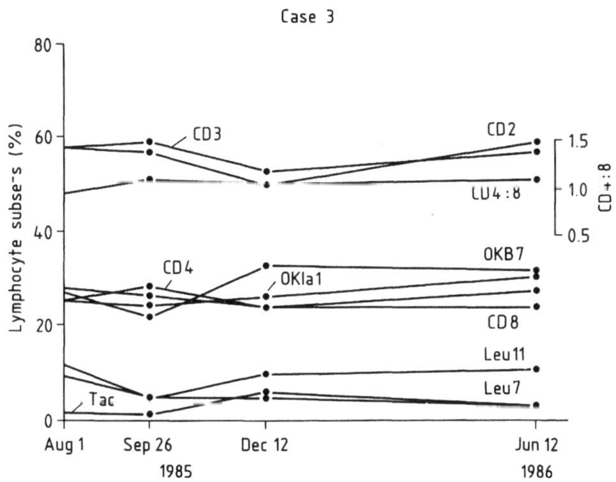

Fig. 3. Changes of lymphocyte subsets in case 3

His HLA typing results were A24, A26, B35, Cw3, DR2, DRw8, DQw1, DQw3. A polysomnography performed on one afternoon showed a marked tendency to fall asleep and a REM period at 5 min after the onset of sleep. Daytime sleepiness was decreased with the administration of 100 mg pemoline and 30 mg methylphenidate. Attacks of cataplexy were reduced and nocturnal sleep was improved with the administrations of 100 mg clomipramine, 12.5 mg chlorpromazine, 50 mg phenobarbital, and 5 mg diazepam.

The laboratory tests performed on 1 August were generally normal. The lymphocyte subpopulations were CD3, 58.0%; CD4, 25.8%; CD8, 28.2%; CD4:8 ratio, 0.91; CD2, 58.1%; Leu11, 9.4%; OKIa1, 26.2%; OKB7, 27.1%; Leu7, 11.1%; Tac, 1.5%. Stimulation indices with PHA, Con A, and PWM were 90, 46, and 91, respectively. No significant deviations of lymphocyte subsets were observed in the time-course follow-up (Fig. 3).

Narcolepsy is Not an Autoimmune Disease

Our study failed to demonstrate immunological abnormalities in the newly developed narcoleptics with extensive laboratory tests. This finding suggests that narcolepsy is not an autoimmune disease in the usual sense.

Cases 1 and 2 were examined within 3 months from the onset of the disease The normal erythrocyte sedimentation ratio and negative C-reactive protein suggest the absence of an acute inflammatory process shortly after the onset of the disease. Inflammatory reactions are among the most common laboratory findings in autoimmune disorders.

The complement levels were also normal in these cases. Altered complement levels are also common in autoimmune disorders. Immunoglobulin concentrations proved normal, too.

The lymphocyte subpopulations of these three newly developed cases were all within the normal range and did not show significant deviations during the 1-year follow-up. In line with the previous study, this suggests the absence of major quantitative changes of lymphocyte subpopulations from the very early stages through the developed stages in narcolepsy.

Two neurological disorders are well known to be associated with autoimmune mechanisms: multiple sclerosis and myasthenia gravis. In cases of multiple sclerosis, the pathology is usually confined to the nervous system. However, it tends to show more or less general inflammatory reactions during the active stages; we often encounter altered lymphocyte subsets not only in the nervous system and cerebrospinal fluid but also in the general circulation. Myasthenia gravis, which involves only neuromuscular junctions, also shows abnormal lymphocyte subsets in the general circulation. These cases of narcolepsy displayed none of these abnormalities.

The possibility is not excluded that some unknown immune mechanism(s) participate(s) in the development of narcolepsy: an aberrant immune reaction absolutely restricted within the nervous system that regulates sleep and arousal mechanisms; a possible regulatory function of the HLA molecules in normal sleep; specific autoantibodies to sleep substances or receptors that cannot be detected with current technologies; a possible influence of the HLA antigens in the production of interleukins, prostaglandins, or other substances that participate in both sleep and immune processes, etc. However, there is no evidence at present substantiating or refuting these possibilities.

"Sleep Gene" Hypothesis

Absence of immunological abnormalities favors another hypothesis for the development of narcolepsy. This hypothesis may be termed the "sleep gene" hypothesis. This hypothesis postulates that a gene encodes an essential protein for normal sleep. This gene may be the HLA gene itself, or other genes located in very close proximity to the HLA genes.

The normal function of this hypothetical gene may be lost or altered in the narcoleptic DR2/Dw2 haplotype. Kilduff et al. (1986) showed an increased number of the M2 muscarinic cholinergic receptors in the brain stem of narcoleptic dogs. If this putative gene encodes an enzyme for neurotransmitter synthesis or a protein essential for the transmitter release, mutation of this gene will most likely lead to an impaired release of the neurotransmitters and a compensative increase of the receptors. Otherwise, this gene may directly regulate the production of the receptors in the brain stem.

If this gene is located very close to the DR2 gene where crossovers seldom, if ever, occur, then narcolepsy and HLA-DR2 will almost always be found together (Matsuki et al. 1985).

According to this hypothesis, immunological abnormalities are not necessarily present in cases of narcolepsy. Absence of abnormal immunological profiles favors this hypothesis. However, direct evidence supporting this hypothesis is yet to be obtained.

References

Bertrams J, Luboldt W, Dannehl K, Baur MP (1986) Homogeneity of HLA-DQ, DR phenotypes in lymphocyte subsets of normal individuals. Hum Immunol 15: 330-335

Billiard M, Seignalet J (1985) Extraordinary association between HLA-DR2 and narcolepsy. Lancet i: 226-227

Kilduff TS, Bowersox SS, Kaitin KI, Baker TL, Ciaranello RD, Dement WC (1986) Muscarinic cholinergic receptors and the canine model of narcolepsy. Sleep 9: 102-106

Langdon N, Lock C, Welsh K, Vergani D, Dorow R, Wachtel H, Palenschat D, Parkes JD (1986) Immune factors in narcolepsy. Sleep 9: 143-148

Matsuki K, Honda Y, Naohara T, Satake M, Someya T, Harada S, Juji T (1985) Lymphocyte subsets in HLA-DR2-positive narcoleptic patients. Folia Psychiatr Neurol Jpn 39: 499-506

Chapter 13

Immune Factors in Narcolepsy in the United Kingdom

J. D. Parkes, K. Welsh, N. Langdon, and C. Lock

Introduction

In this and the following chapter, we discuss the importance of genetic and environmental factors in the development of narcolepsy. Narcolepsy, with a near-100% HLA DR2/DQ relationship (Honda et al. 1984; Langdon et al. 1984; Billiard and Seignalet 1985), is an ideal neurological disorder in which to consider the genetic basis of disease, despite marked heterogeneity in clinical expression. The tight HLA linkage may suggest that environmental factors are less important than inherited factors, although this is not necessarily the case. In contrast to the tight HLA and genetic linkage in narcolepsy, Parkinson's disease is at the opposite pole, and concordance rates for Parkinson's disease in twin studies are the lowest of any neurological disorder investigated by this method (Ward et al. 1984). Unfortunately, insufficient twins with narcolepsy have been described as yet to help elucidate either genetic or environmental components in the disease, despite one intriguing report of multiple sclerosis and narcolepsy-cataplexy in one of a monozygotic twin pair (Schrader et al. 1980). Other twin studies have been reported by Imlah (1961) and Mitchell and Cummins (1965). For proper assessment of genetic and environmental factors in narcolepsy, it is necessary to consider the known familial associations and clinical presentation, as well as data at the laboratory and molecular level.

Definitions of the Narcoleptic Syndrome

Narcolepsy is defined here as the clinical association of narcolepsy with cataplexy (Guilleminault et al. 1976). Narcolepsy implies excessive and abnormal persistent daytime drowsiness, with sleep under unusual circumstances. These include in particular monotony, which is rarely if ever a habitual trigger of daytime sleep in nonnarcoleptics. Cataplexy is best defined as brief or prolonged (1 s to several minutes) episodes of loss of muscle tone, with partial or complete paralysis involving in particular postural muscles. In contrast to the precipitation of narcolepsy by monotony, the usual trigger of cataplexy is a sudden increase in arousal, with laughter, surprise, or other stimuli. Electrophysiological criteria, if positive, with a short sleep latency on multiple sleep latency test, and REM sleep onset, help to confirm the clinical diagnosis (Rechtshaffen et al. 1963; Richardson et al. 1978; Billiard et al. 1983), although the finding of a normal sleep latency and non-rapid eye movement sleep onset does not exclude the diagnosis if strongly indicated on clinical grounds (Mosko et al. 1984). The addition to these clinical and electrophysiological diagnostic criteria of HLA, DR2-positive status may improve the definition of narcolepsy.

Narcolepsy and HLA Linkage

The strongest histocompatibility (MHC)-disease linkage so far discovered is that between narcolepsy and HLA DR2. With only three exceptions, all the 76 narcoleptics (70 of 71 Caucasoid and 4 of 5 Negroid) so far investigated by us have proved to be DR2 positive, compared with 21.5% of 200 controls. Narcolepsy occurs in the United Kingdom with an estimated frequency of 0.05%. If narcolepsy cannot occur without the DR2 gene, some 30000 of the approximate 12 million population of the United Kingdom expected to be DR2 positive will have narcolepsy (0.25%).

Theories of Narcolepsy

There have been many different theories as to the cause of narcolepsy:

1. The earliest of these, the *psychiatric* hypothesis, has been totally disproved by the discovery of the familial basis of narcolepsy and, on careful analysis, the absence of any convincing feature of known psychiatric illness in narcoleptics.
2. This theory was displaced by the *metabolic* hypothesis, the idea that narcolepsy, cataplexy, hypnogogic hallucinations, and sleep paralysis had a metabolic and perhaps gene-determined basis, due to an inborn neurotransmitter, enzymic, or receptor defect, resulting in a *physiological* disturbance of normal sleep-wake and sleep cycle mechanisms. In support of this theory have been the occasional findings of low amine neurotransmitter metabolite concentration in the CSF of humans with narcolepsy, and changes in dopamine metabolism and neurotransmitter receptor systems in the brains of narcoleptic dogs (Kilduff et al. 1986). Observations of low aspartate and glutamate concentration in the CSF of narcoleptics (Parkes et al. 1974) remain unconfirmed and have not been associated causally with the disease.
3. Linked to the metabolic theory is the idea that narcolepsy may be due to excess of some naturally occurring sleep-promoting substance, hypnotoxin or 'REM' juice within the blood, CSF, or brain (Pieron 1913). At least 20 such compounds have been proposed this century, including Pappenheimer's factor S (Pappenheimer et al. 1967), delta-sleep-inducing peptide (DSIP; Schoenenberger and von Graf 1985), and sleep-promoting factors, obtained from the brain stem of sleep-deprived rats. A physiological role has not been proved for any of these substances; neither has a sleep-promoting compound been demonstrated in narcolepsy.
4. Linked to the metabolic or sleep-juice theory of narcolepsy is the concept that any metabolic or receptor defect may reside in DR2, with perhaps the DR2

gene itself, or with a cell surface configuration controlled by the DR2 genetic region expressed in the brain as well as the lymphocyte, forming a constituent part of neuronal or receptor mechanisms in the sleep-wake system.
5. An *infective* hypothesis, studied (but rejected) by Adie (1926), suggests that some if not most cases of narcolepsy are due to acquired disease. Translated into a modern idiom, do foreign organisms have DR2 determinants which cross-react with the host, or alternatively provoke the expression of DR antigens in the brain (Wong et al. 1984)? The problem here is to separate examples of so-called "secondary" narcolepsy, i.e., narcolepsy due to a definite structural abnormality of the brain (Bonduelle and Degos 1976), from "idiopathic" or true narcolepsy, in which no structural lesion has yet been demonstrated.
6. The *immune* hypothesis of narcolepsy (Parkes et al. 1986; Langdon et al. 1986) derives from the HLA-disease association. There is striking evidence for a role of the HLA complex in immunobiology. This comes partly from the finding of disease associations with specific HLA antigens. Positive HLA DR2 associations have been reported in multiple sclerosis (Welsh 1984, for review); older onset (over 40) myasthenia gravis (Compston et al. 1980); antiglomerular basement membrane disease (Rees et al. 1978); dermatitis herpetiformis, certain Guillain-Barré syndrome variants, and specific allergies, for example to ragweed pollen (Marsh et al. 1982). In contrast, rheumatoid arthritis and juvenile type 1 diabetes mellitus, especially the latter, have a lower or zero incidence of a subtype of HLA-DR2.

The immune hypothesis of narcolepsy states: *Narcolepsy is an immune-mediated disease, occurring in susceptible (DR2-positive) subjects.* To satisfy this hypothesis, several criteria need to be met. These include

(1) the presence of a specific antigen;
(2) specific cellular or humoral immunity, directed to the specific antigen;
(3) possible association of narcolepsy with other immune disorders;
(4) passive transfer of narcolepsy between subjects may occur, using suitable experimental techniques;
(5) antecedents of narcolepsy may include known precipitants of immune disorders; and
(6) immunosuppression may improve narcolepsy.

Evidence for the Genetic Basis of Narcolepsy

Does the Immune Theory Fit the Known Facts About the Inheritance of Narcolepsy?

A genetic basis for narcolepsy has been recognized for over a century (Westphal 1877), but there are still no wholly satisfactory family studies available. This is due to the critical factors of incomplete and inaccurate case ascertainment. Large population surveys are biased by incomplete case ascertainment, as well as by the method of search, and small surveys are imprecise, with large sampling errors.

Most of the available genetic studies have relied for the diagnosis of narcolepsy on history alone, sometimes reported secondhand, and unaided by electrophysiological or HLA typing studies. These difficulties probably account for the different results reported in genetic studies. In particular, attempts at genetic modeling in narcolepsy are doomed to failure until more accurate clinical data are available.

The first report of familial narcolepsy came from Westphal (1877), who described a mother and a son who both had sleep paralysis and narcolepsy. Krabbe and Magnussen (1942) described a family of 12 sibs, 4 of whom had narcolepsy. In a review of the literature they found 54 narcoleptics in 19 families, with a distribution suggestive of a single dominant mode of inheritance, among a total of 200-300 people with excessive sleep. However, the diagnosis of narcolepsy was unconvincing in many of these cases. Yoss and Daly (1960) initially found a hereditary occurrence of narcolepsy in 40 of 400 of their cases, but on close questioning a much higher familial occurrence was revealed, and up to 30% of subjects with the narcoleptic syndrome had an affected relative. Other estimates of the number of affected first-degree relatives of index cases of narcolepsy vary from 12% (Sours 1963) to 52% (Kessler et al. 1974). The study of Baraitser and Parkes (1978) was based on personal interview of all the probands, all of the children, 50% of the parents, and 66% of the siblings. This revealed that 52% of the probands of 50 subjects with narcolepsy had an affected first-degree relative; 42% of the sibs of these probands with an affected parent were similarly affected; 33% of the parents of two affected sibs, and 41% of the children, had narcolepsy, cataplexy, or both.

As judged by this study, it is likely that, in the United Kingdom families investigated, narcolepsy is transmitted by a single gene mechanism with a Mendelian autosomal dominant pattern of inheritance. If this is correct, these findings imply that the pathogenesis of narcolepsy, no matter how complex, is related to an abnormality in a single protein molecule. It is not at present possible to identify the protein directly concerned.

Many of the observed features of narcolepsy in this and other studies are in keeping with the idea of autosomal dominant inheritance. The features of such inheritance include (Goldstein and Brown 1983):

(1) Each affected individual has an affected parent.
(2) An affected individual will bear, on average, an equal proportion of affected and nonaffected children.
(3) Normal children of an affected individual will have only normal offspring.
(4) Males and females are affected in equal proportions.
(5) Each sex is equally liable to transmit the condition to male and female offspring, with male-male transmission occurring.
(6) Vertical transmission of the condition occurs through successive generations.

One major objection to the autosomal dominant theory of narcolepsy is the lack of an affected parent in the majority of cases, although narcolepsy may arise by new mutation. If susceptibility to narcolepsy does arise in cases without parental involvement by new mutation, parental age may be higher in newly arising cases than in those with an involved parent (since the expected mutation rate in germ cells increases with age). Present data, although scanty, do not support this view.

Table 1. Types of narcolepsy

	Familial[a] (n=35)	Nonfamilial (n=78)
DR2 status	All positive except two subjects	All positive
RFLP-DR2 status[b] (restriction enzyme *Bgl*$_{II}$ DQ$_\beta$: probe-band at 3 kb)	Similar HLA-DQ + DQα restriction fragments in familial and nonfamilial cases (also in individual DR2-negative subjects)	
Onset		
Age (mean range)	21.5 (7-48) years	23 (3-70) years
Sudden or slow	Sudden onset in 14%	Sudden onset in 15%
Previous infection?	History of infection in 10%	History of infection in 8%
Recovery	Nil	Single instance
Blood/CSF abnormalities		
Antibodies in blood?	Not found	Not found
T-cell abnormality?	Not demonstrated	Not demonstrated
α-1-Trypsin phenotype	Association unremarkable	Association unremarkable
Immunoglobulin Allotype	Association unremarkable	Association unremarkable
CSF abnormality	Occasinal increased cell count, minor increase in protein	Minor abnormalities in about 20% of cases
"Sleep factors" present in blood/CSF?	Not detected	Not detected
Benzodiazepine receptor-binding activity in CSF	Not excessive	Not excessive

[a] Familial: definite narcolepsy, cataplexy, or both present in first-degree relative (parent, sib, or child)
[b] DR2 RFLP status: similar RFLP present in DR2-positive subjects with multiple sclerosis

"Familial" and "Nonfamilial" Narcolepsy

Between one-tenth and one-half of all narcoleptics have an affected first-degree relative. Are familial cases in any way different in clinical presentation from nonfamilial cases? (Any clinical distinction need not imply a genetic distinction, although environmental factors may be different in the two groups. Immune factors, if relevant to the disease, might possibly be expected to play a larger part in so-called "nonfamilial" than in "familial" cases). In our experience, the clinical presentation, disease prodromata, mode of onset (slow or sudden), age of onset, severity of illness, and distribution of the four cardinal symptoms of narcolepsy, cataplexy, sleep paralysis, and hypnagogic hallucinations are closely similar in "familial" and in "nonfamilial" cases (Table 1).

Clinical Evidence for an Immune Basis for Narcolepsy

There is a marked heterogeneity in the incidence of narcolepsy, with wide differences in age of onset, disease severity, frequency of the associated factors of cataplexy, sleep paralysis, and hypnagogic hallucinations; variable expression in different members of the same family; and in females occasional menstrual relationship. The causes of disease heterogeneity are not known.

Onset of Narcolepsy

The onset of narcolepsy has been recorded between the ages of 3 and 70 years, sometimes at the menarche, but late puberty is the usual time. The onset of narcolepsy is either gradual (over 1-2 years in 85% of our patients) or sudden (over a few days in the remainder).

In most cases there is no definite antecedent to narcolepsy, or at best the report is anecdotal. In the initial patient described by Gélineau (1880), narcolepsy started after a brawl, while Wilson (1928) described cases after head injury, encephalitis, and influenza. Other typical cases may follow systemic infection or, rarely, exposure to toxins. Vein (1966) and Roth (1980) described the development of "narcolepsy" after typhoid, pneumonia, mumps, scarlet fever, malaria, and various neurotropic infections, as well as nephritis, Sydenham's chorea, infectious hepatitis, and sinusitis. Some of these examples are not cases of true narcolepsy.

In our experience, 3 of 36 patients with the sudden onset of narcolepsy gave a definite history of previous respiratory infection, as compared with 11 of 177 patients with a gradual onset. Other described prodromata were the menarche (four patients), pregnancy (six), nonrespiratory infection (seven), electric shock (one), psychiatric illness (three), and glandular fever (one).

Once established, minor fluctuations in the severity of narcolepsy are usual, but long or complete remissions are rare (see Ohta et al. 1979).

Neonatal Narcolepsy

Neonatal narcolepsy (i.e., narcolepsy in the offspring of narcoleptic mothers) has not been recorded, but it would be difficult if not impossible to detect in newborn infants with a very different sleep pattern from that of adults.

Precipitate Narcolepsy

Although very unusual, the onset of narcolepsy-cataplexy over 24 h is sometimes recorded.

> A 44-year-old housewife, previously in good health and with no family history of narcolepsy, had her first attack of cataplexy while playing with her 5-year-old daughter on holiday. Several further attacks of cataplexy, and also narcolepsy, occurred the same day, and the condition has now been established for 20 years, with a short sleep latency and REM sleep onset. The subject is DR2 positive.

Remission of Narcolepsy

A complete remission has been witnessed by us in only a single patient. This DR2-positive subject, with nonfamilial narcolepsy, developed severe narcolepsy and cataplexy at the age of 24, and had a complete symptomatic remission of both conditions from the age of 40.

Disease Associations with Narcolepsy

"Secondary Narcolepsy" (Bonduelle and Dégos 1976)

Narcolepsy has often been considered to be secondary to encephalitis, head injury, brain tumor, or other pathological process. However, the evidence that "secondary" narcolepsy ever occurs is inadequate. In most instances with this diagnosis, the sleep disturbance is atypical, cataplexy is absent, evidence of REM sleep onset is lacking, and, unlike the idiopathic disease, recovery usually occurs.

Most cases of secondary narcolepsy after *head injury* bear no relation to the idiopathic disease; Bonduelle and Degos (1976) in a review of many patients with "symptomatic narcolepsy" could find only a single example of this type they considered to be genuine and, even here, the sleep disturbance did not commence until 5 years after head injury.

Narcolepsy, cataplexy, and sleep-onset REM activity have occasionally been described with *infiltrating tumors* of the pons. In a patient with unilateral cataplexy and systemic lupus reported by Lascelles et al. (1976), cataplexy was assumed to be due to direct pontine vascular involvement, but no postmortem findings were available, and an immunological mechanism may have accounted for narcolepsy-cataplexy in this case.

The frequency of narcolepsy-cataplexy following *encephalitis lethargica* has been grossly overstressed. The condition was a rarity. We have never seen an example, although postencephalitic parkinsonism is still not uncommon. However, there are isolated case reports of unequivocal narcolepsy-cataplexy developing within 1 year of an acute febrile encephalitic illness, with midbrain involvement, behavioral disturbance, and/or parkinsonian features (Symmonds 1926). The situation here is complicated by the possibility that narcolepsy was not due to encephalitis lethargica, but occurred as an aftermath to the simultaneous widespread pandemic of influenza.

Pathological Changes in the Narcoleptic Syndrome

No definite pathological change has ever been associated with idiopathic narcolepsy-cataplexy. However, only one definitive report, that of Erlich and Itabashi (1985), has appeared to date. In contrast, there are many reports of periventricular and periaqueductal cellular infiltration attributed to encephalitis lethargica or polioencephalitis in children and adults with "narcolepsy" (Pohl 1966; Castaigne and Escourelle 1967).

Neuroradiology not infrequently reveals minor abnormalities in subjects with idiopathic narcolepsy. CT head scans in ten of the King's College Hospital series have been normal, but others have reported abnormalities, mainly a dilated third ventricle or abnormally shaped ventricle in between 5% and 70% of all narcoleptics (Roth 1980).

Diseases Associated with the Narcoleptic Syndrome

Narcolepsy has been associated with a wide variety of other diseases (Table 2). These relationships are usually considered to be fortuitous; or the diagnosis of narcolepsy to be incorrect, in reality the result of sleep apnea. However, both of these premises may sometimes be incorrect.

1. There are a few isolated examples of apparent narcolepsy in association with *blood dyscrasias,* lymphoma, polycythemia, or systemic lupus erythematosus. Narcolepsy is not a usual manifestation of any of these disorders, and was not listed as a symptom in more than 500 patients with primary polycythemia investigated by Blood (1950). In some instances, polycythemia is undoubtedly associated with sleep apnea.

A 29-year-old physiotherapist with no family history of sleep disorder developed a malignant stage 4 lymphoma with ovarian and axillary gland involvement in 1976. She was treated with thiotepa, methotrexate, and whole head irradiation, with no subsequent sign of lymphoma recurrence, but the subsequent year developed persistent severe narcolepsy, cataplexy, automatic behavior and hyp-

Table 2. Association between "narcolepsy" and other diseases

Disease associated with narcolepsy	Notes
Possible immune mechanisms	
Polycythemia	Occasional association with narcolepsy, but very uncommon in all instances
Lymphoma	
Systemic lupus erythematosus	
Disseminated sclerosis	
Pernicious anemia	
Probable sleep apnea, not narcolepsy	
Acromegaly	Probably always sleep apnea
Myotonic dystrophy	
Dysautonomias	
Ocular disorders	
Extrinsic muscle paralysis	?Embryonic defect
Cataract	
Glaucoma	
Metabolic disorders	
Diabetes mellitus	Not true narcolepsy. DR2+ve rare in type 1 diabetes mellitus
Thyroid disease	
Miscellaneous	
Essential tremor	(Single patient only)
Parkinsonism	(Two patients)

nogogic hallucinations with a short sleep latency and REM sleep onset. The connection between lymphoma and narcolepsy in this patient is speculative.

2. The likely explanation for the not infrequent association between sleep disorders, acromegaly, and myotonic dystrophy (Carroll et al. 1977) is that so-called narcolepsy is the result of *sleep apnea*. However, the sleep disturbance of myotonia is sometimes unusually severe, or may antedate muscle weakness, and a central sleep disturbance related to narcolepsy may occur in myotonia.
3. *Oculomotor paralysis,* which is sometimes familial, is found in between 0.25% and 0.5% of all narcoleptics (see Roth 1980; Parkes 1985). Other ocular abnormalities, in particular cataracts, are occasionally present. The brain stem of these patients has not been examined, but a possible nuclear agenesis, also with involvement of pontine "burst" cells, which generate saccadic eye movements and some aspects of sleep, may be present. These areas are derived from a common embryonic source, the cell bands of Essick, maldevelopment of which may possibly explain these examples.
4. Narcolepsy is associated with *multiple sclerosis,* although this is uncommon (reviews by Bonduelle and Degos 1976; Parkes 1985). There have been at least 16 case reports in which narcolepsy-cataplexy has preceded, accompanied, or followed by up to 1 decade the establishment of probable or definite multiple sclerosis. Postmortem examination has shown midbrain plaques in one such case. We have observed one such patient in whom narcolepsy-cataplexy preceded the onset of multiple sclerosis by 14 years.

> A 49-year-old Caucasian housewife with no family history of any neurological illness developed severe narcolepsy, frequent sleep paralysis, cataplexy, and hypnogogic hallucinations following hysterectomy and ovarian cyst puncture at the age of 29. She had a short sleep latency and REM sleep onset. Apart from narcolepsy, she remained well until the age of 43, when she developed total incontinence with an internuclear ophthalmoplegia, ocular dysmetria, and saccadic pursuit eye movements, followed by a spastic paraplegia, frequent episodes of visual blurring, optic atrophy, prolonged latency of visual evoked responses, and gait ataxia. The CT scan showed no definite abnormality apart from mild enlargement of the superior cerebellar cistern, but the NMR scan revealed multiple paraventricular lesions. Serum autoantibody studies were negative. The cerebrospinal fluid had a protein content of 50 mg/ml with no white cells present.

In this case it was considered that narcolepsy was associated with, but not caused by, multiple sclerosis. Restriction fragment length polymorphism studies have shown that 97% of subjects with multiple sclerosis who are DR2 positive have the same DR2 subtype as occurs in narcolepsy (Marcadet et al. 1985; Table 1).
5. The symptoms of narcolepsy have a superficial resemblance to those of *myasthenia gravis,* although we know no examples of disease concurrence. Both are long-term disorders with fluctuating levels of disability, influenced by the degree of rest and activity. In both conditions symptoms are worst in the evening, and just as rest improves motor fatigue in myasthenia, a short sleep period will improve subsequent alertness in narcolepsy. Pathophysiological mechanisms may be com-

parable in the two conditions, with reduction in the safety factor of neuromuscular or synaptic transmission.

Experimental Studies

An Antigen in Narcolepsy?

The biochemical lesion in narcolepsy is likely to be in the tegmentum of the pons, an area of the reticular formation important for the generation of REM sleep and control of sleep atonia (review by Sakai 1984). At least 20 different neurotransmitters occur within a small area of the brain stem. Although biogenic amine theories of sleep control have concentrated on serotonin and the catecholamines, and a possible defect in these has been sought for in narcolepsy, nonmonoamine mechanisms may be equally or more important. A genetically determined or acquired protein receptor defect in this area may be present in narcolepsy. The recent finding of proliferation of muscarinic cholinergic receptors in the brain stem of dogs with narcolepsy suggests, however, a fundamental problem in neurotransmitter release rather than receptor function in these animals (Kilduff et al. 1986).

Circulating Antibodies in Narcolepsy?

Lymphocytosis and a slight increase in protein occur in about one-fourth of all patients with narcolepsy, although many of these are atypical examples or have been considered to have "secondary" narcolepsy. Rennert (1956) and Janzen et al. (1969) found hyperalbuminosis, increase in protein content of up to 75 mg% and/or lymphocytosis (11-19 WBC/cm) in 25% of their cases, and Roth (1980) made similar observations in 8 of 32 subjects. In 17 narcoleptics we reported in 1974, CSF cell count and protein concentration were all normal (Parkes et al. 1974), although subsequent studies have revealed minor CSF abnormalities, including in one instance the presence of oligoclonal bands, in a minority of narcoleptics (Parkes et al. 1986).

Many of the diseases and features associated with P_i and G_m systems (alpha-1-antitrypsin phenotype and the immunoglobulin heavy chain allotype, localized on chromosome 14) are also associated with HLA antigens. Several diseases have been reported to be associated with the alpha-1-antitrypsin heterozygotes MZ or MS, or with G_m allotypes. In particular, multiple sclerosis and myasthenia (usually with thymoma) are associated with G_m allotypes, while Honda et al (1986) have associated narcolepsy in Japanese subjects with the antitrypsin phenotype (present in 54% of narcoleptics, 20% of controls). In the present subjects, no association between narcolepsy and P_i or G_m systems was shown.

Cell-Mediated Immunity in Narcolepsy?

From our results (Briggs et al. 1987), and those of Honda and his colleagues (1986), the T-cell subsets and complement studies of narcoleptics show no significant changes, although all cases investigated in the United Kingdom had been established for several years.

Treatment of Narcolepsy

The immunotherapy of narcolepsy has not been investigated. Hazards of such treatment outweigh any potential theoretical benefit.

We have investigated the effect of plasmapheresis in one severely disabled subject with severe narcolepsy and status cataplecticus, resistant to drugs, and with the precedent of the successful use of plasmapheresis in Goodpasture's syndrome before the final antigen recognition was made.

> This 57-year-old Caucasian housewife had the HLA type A2/3; B7/44; C5/7; DR2. There was no family history of any sleep disorder or cataplexy. Narcolepsy commenced in Nigeria at the age of 20, with frequent sleep in inappropriate surroundings, restless night sleep, with frequent nocturnal arousals, sleep paralysis, pre-sleep dreams, and severe cataplexy from the age of 30 resulting in four separate fractures of the ankles and severe head injury. Dexamphetamine (60 mg daily), mazindol (12 mg), clomipramine (150 mg), and fluoxetine (100 mg) caused at best only partial symptom control, or tolerance, weight gain, and indigestion. Polysomnogram studies showed REM sleep onset with short sleep latency, without sleep apnea. CT scan was normal. The development of diabetes mellitus at the age of 47, and osteoarthrosis at the age of 54, did not greatly alter the severity of narcolepsy or cataplexy. The CSF Ig G concentration was raised, and CSF oligoclonal bands were present.

Plasmapheresis was done during an episode of severe drug-unresponsive status cataplecticus. Plasmapheresis (2 liters over 4 h) was achieved on three subsequent days without complication (equipment from Haemonetics). Subjective assessment by the patient of the frequency and severity of narcolepsy-cataplexy, and the overall degree of motor control at hourly intervals before, during, and for the week after plasmapheresis remained unchanged. There was no alteration in the number of sleep attacks, degree of wakefulness, frequency of pre-sleep dreams, or the number and duration of attacks of powerlessness and tonelessness. Near-continuous partial cataplexy with facial flickering, involuntary eye divergence, and inability to sit erect, with laughter-evoked collapse, persisted throughout.

Conclusion

At present there is no convincing evidence for an immune basis of narcolepsy. No specific antigen has been determined, no unequivocal evidence of immune abnormality found, and there is no clear relationship of narcolepsy with other immune-mediated diseases. The mysterious occasional relationship between narcolepsy and multiple sclerosis probably depends on a common genetic rather than environmental factor in the two diseases. However, the occasional cerebrospinal fluid abnormality in narcolepsy remains unexplained. As was the case with type 1 (juvenile onset) diabetes mellitus (Gorsuch et al. 1981; Srikanta et al. 1985), evidence of immune disorder in narcolepsy may require a long search, as well as the study of patients with the recent onset of symptoms.

References

Adie WJ (1926) Idiopathic narcolepsy: a disease sui generis: with remarks on the mechanisms of sleep. Brain 49: 257-306

Baraitser M, Parkes JD (1978) Genetic study of narcoleptic syndrome. J Med Gent 15: 254-259

Billiard M, Seignalet J (1985) Extraordinary association between HLA-DR2 and narcolepsy. Lancet 1: 226-227

Billiard M, Besset A, Cadilhac J (1983) The clinical and polygraphic development of narcolepsy. In: Guilleminault C, Lugaresi E (eds) Sleep-wake disorders: natural history, epidemiology and long-term evolution. Raven, New York, pp 171-185

Blood AM (1950) Polycythaemia vera. Analysis of 41 cases with special emphasis on neurologic and psychiatric manifestations. Mississippi Doctor 28: 6-12

Bonduelle M, Degos C (1976) Symptomatic narcolepsies: a critical study. In: Guilleminault C, Dement WC, Passouant P (eds) Narcolepsy. Spectrum, New York, pp 313-332

Briggs DC, Lock CB, Welsh KI, Trowsdale J, So A, Parkes JD (1987) Complement in narcolepsy. (in press)

Carroll JE, Zwillich CW, Weil JV (1977) Ventilatory response in myotonic dystrophy. Neurology (Minneap) 27: 1125-1128

Castaigne P, Escourelle R (1967) Etude topographique des lésions anatomiques dans les hypersomnies. Rev Neurol 116: 547-584

Compston DA, Vincent A, Newsom Davis J, Batchelor JR (1980) Clinical, pathological, HLA antigen and immunological evidence for disease heterogeneity in myasthenia gravis. Brain 103: 579-601

Erlich SS, Itabashi HH (1985) Narcolepsy: a neuropathological study. In: Proc 2nd International symposium on narcolepsy, Stanford, July 6-7, 1985

Gelineau JBE (1880) De la narcolepsie. Gaz Hop (Paris) 55: 626-628, 635-637

Goldstein JL, Brown MS (1983) Genetic aspects of disease. In: Petersdorf RG, Adams RD, Braunwald E, Isselbacher KJ, Martin JB, Wilson JD (eds) Harrison's principles of internal medicine, 10th edn. McGraw Hill, New York, pp311-322

Gorsuch AN, Spencer KM, Lister J, McNally JM, Dean BM, Bottazzo GF, Cudworth AG (1981) Evidence for a long prediabetic period in type 1 (insulin-dependent) diabetes mellitus. Lancet ii: 1363-1365

Guilleminault C, Dement WC, Passouant P (eds) (1976) Narcolepsy. Spectrum, New York

Honda Y, Dol Y, Juji T, Satake M (1984) Narcolepsy and HLA. Positive DR2 as a prerequisite for the development of narcolepsy. Proc 6th Jap Soc Biol Psychiatry, Tokyo, March 23-24, 1984, p 6

Honda Y, Juji T, Matsuki K, Naohara T, Satake M, Inoko H, Someya T, Harada S, Dol Y (1986) HLA-DR2 and DW2 in narcolepsy and in other disorders of excessive somnolence without cataplexy. Sleep 9: 133-142

Imlah NW (1961) Narcolepsy in identical twins. J Neurol Neurosurg Psychiatry 24: 158-160
Janzen R, Bushart W, Wender G (1969) Hirnbiolektrische Studien und klinische Betrachtungen bei Narkolepsiekranken. In: Jovanovič UJ (ed) Der Schlaf. Barth, Munich, pp 207-221
Kessler S, Guilleminault C, Dement W (1974) A family study of 50 REM narcoleptics. Acta Neurol Scand 50: 503-512
Kilduff TS, Bowersox SS, Kaitin KI, Baker TL, Ciaranello RD, Dement WC (1986) Muscarinic cholinergic receptors and the canine model of narcolepsy. Sleep 9: 102-106
Krabbe F, Magnussen G (1942) Familial narcolepsy. Acta Psychiatr Neurol 17: 149-173
Langdon N, Welsh K, van Dam M, Vaughan RM, Parkes JD (1984) Genetic markers in narcolepsy. Lancet ii: 1178-1180
Langdon N, Lock C, Welsh K, Vergani D, Dorow R, Wachtel H, Palenschat D, Parkes JD (1986) Immune factors in narcolepsy. Sleep 9: 143-148
Lascelles RG, Mohr PD, Peart I (1976) Unilateral cataplexy associated with systemic lupus erythematosus. J Neurol Neurosurg Psychiatry 39: 1023-1026
Marcadet A, Massart C, Semona G et al. (1985) Association of class II HLA-DQ beta restriction fragments with multiple sclerosis. Immunogenetics 22: 93-96
Marsh DG, Hsu SH, Roebber M et al (1982) HLA-DW2: a genetic marker for human immune response to short ragweed pollen allergen Ra5.1. Response resulting primarily from natural antigenic exposure. J Exp Med 155: 1439-1451
Mitchell SA, Cummins LE (1965) Idiopathic narcolepsy in one of monozygotic twins Paper presented at the Association for the Psychophysiological Study of Sleep, Washington DC
Mosko SS, Shampain DS, Sassin JF (1984) Nocturnal REM latency and sleep disturbance in narcolepsy. Sleep 7: 115-125
Ohta T, Honda Y, Kameyama T, Kurita H, Takahashi Y (1979) A long-term prognosis of narcolepsy. Sleep Res 8: 206
Pappenheimer JR, Miller TB, Goodrich CA (1967) Sleep-promoting effects of cerebrospinal fluid from sleep-deprived goats. Proc Natl Acad Sci 58: 513-517
Parkes JD (1985) Sleep and its disorders. Saunders, Eastbourne
Parkes JD, Fenton GW, Struthers G, Curzon G, Kantamaneni BD, Buxton BH, Record C (1974) Narcolepsy and cataplexy. Clinical features, treatment and cerebrospinal fluid findings. Q J Med 43: 525-536
Parkes JD, Lock C, Langdon N (1982) Narcolepsy and immunity. Br Med J 292: 359-360
Pieron H (1913) Le problème physiologique du sommeil. Masson, Paris
Pohl O (1966) Ein Beitrag zur Pathologie der symptomatischen Narkolepsie. Dtsch Z Nervenheilkd 189: 211-217
Rechtschaffen A, Wolpert EA, Dement WC, Mitchell SA, Fisher C (1963) Nocturnal sleep of narcoleptics. Electroencephalogr Clin Neurophysiol 15: 599-609
Rees AJ, Peters DKP, Compston DAS, Batchelor JR (1978) Strong association between HLA-DR2 and antibody mediated Goodpasture's syndrome. Lancet i: 966-969
Rennert H (1956) Die Narkolepsie. Mschr Psychiatr Neurol 132: 155-172
Richardson G, Carskadon M, Flagg W, van der Hoed J, Dement W, Mitler M (1978) Excessive daytime sleepiness in man: multiple sleep latency measurement in narcoleptic and control subjects. Electroencephalogr Clin Neurophysiol 45: 621-627
Roth B (1980) Narcolepsy and hypersomnia. Karger, Basle
Sakai K (1984) Central mechanisms of paradoxical sleep. In: Borbely A, Valatx JL (eds) Sleep mechanisms. Springer, Berlin Heidelberg New York, pp 3-18
Schoenberger GA, von Graf M (1985) Effects of DSIP and DSIP-P on different biorhythmic parameters. In: Wauquier A et al. (eds) Sleep: neurotransmitters and neuromodulators. Raven, New York, pp 265-277
Schrader H, Gotlibsen OB, Skomedal GN (1980) Multiple sclerosis and narcolepsy-cataplexy in a monozygotic twin. Neurology (NY) 30: 105-108
Sours JA (1963) Narcolepsy and other disturbances in the sleep-waking rhythm: a study of 115 cases with review of the literature. J Nerv Ment Dis 137: 527-542
Srikanta S, Ganda OmP, Rabizadeh A, Soeldner JS, Eisenbarth GS (1985) First-degree relatives of patients with Type 1 diabetes mellitus: islet cell antibodies and abnormal insulin secretion. New Engl J Med 313: 461-464
Symmonds CP (1926) Narcolepsy as a symptom of encephalitis lethargica. Lancet ii: 1214-1215

Vein AM (1966) Syndrome of hypersomnia (narcolepsy and other forms of pathological sleepiness). Izd Meditsina, Moskva, p 236

Ward CD, Duvoisin RC, Ince SE, Nutt JD, Eldridge R, Calne DB, Dambrosia J (1984) Parkinson's disease in twins. In: Hassler RG, Christ RF (eds) Parkinson-specific motor and mental disorders. Raven, New York, pp 341-344

Welsh KI (1984) Genetic markers in neurological diseases. In: Behan P, Spreafico F (eds) Neuroimmunology. Raven, New York, pp 469-473

Westphal C (1877) Eigentümliche, mit Einschlafen verbundene Anfälle. Arch Psychiatr Nervenkr 7: 631-635

Wilson SAK (1928) The narcolepsies. Brain 51: 62-109

Wong GHW, Bartlett PF, Clark-Lewis I, Battye F, Schrader JW (1984) Inducible expression of H-2 and 1a antigens on brain cells. Nature 310: 688-691

Yoss RE, Daly DD (1960) Hereditary aspects of narcolepsy. Trans Am Neurol Assoc 85: 239-240

Chapter 14

Disorders of Excessive Daytime Sleepiness Without Cataplexy, and Their Relationship with HLA in Japan

S. HARADA, K. MATSUKI, Y. HONDA, and T. SOMEYA

Since ancient times, astute philosophers, scientists, and clinicians have observed and investigated disorders of sleep. Due to these efforts, some of these disorders have now emerged as clearly defined clinical entities: narcolepsy, sleep-apnea syndrome, and restless legs syndrome, to name a few. However, a number of sleep disorders remain obscure, undefined, and unclassified.

This is especially true for disorders of excessive sleepiness (DOES) without cataplexy. Controversies continue even today over the concept, terminology, definition, and diagnostic criteria for these sleep disorders. In this chapter, we will deal with this controversial area and present our findings on the HLA antigens.

Essential Hypersomnia

We have used the term *essential hypersomnia* to denote disorders of excessive daytime sleepiness of unknown etiologies. Essential hypersomnia is defined by the following criteria:

(a) excessive daytime sleepiness which occurs almost every day over a period of at least 6 months;
(b) absence of cataplexy;
(c) not due to other known disorders associated with daytime somnolence, such as sleep-apnea syndrome.

This definition encompasses a diverse group of unknown etiologies, including idiopathic hypersomnia, aborted forms of narcolepsy, and other disorders which are diverse and therefore difficult to categorize (Table 1).

Idiopathic Hypersomnia

Roth (1961, 1976, 1980) first used the term of *idiopathic hypersomnia* to denote disorders which share the following specific characteristics of sleepiness: nonimperative sleepiness and lengthy daytime sleep episodes. Because sleepiness in idiopathic hypersomnia is not as overwhelming as in narcolepsy, the patients can usually resist falling asleep with conscious efforts. Daytime sleep episodes are usually

Table 1. Four possible subtypes of essential hypersomnia

	I	II	III	IV
Mean duration of daytime sleep	>1 h	<1 h	<1 h	≷1 h
Intensity of sleepiness	Controllable	Overwhelming uncontrollable	Mild and controllable	Controllable
Restorative naps	-	+	+	−/+
Effects of CNS stimulants	-	++	++	+
Nocturnal sleep	Deep prolonged	Disrupted	Normal	Impaired
Personality	Often neurotic	Narcoleptoid	Often neurotic	Neurotic/ nonneurotic

Type I, idiopathic hypersomnia
Type II, aborted forms of narcolepsy
Type III, mild hypersomnia with neurotic attitudes
Type IV, possibly related with underlying mild sleep-related respiratory impairments
It should be noted that only a small fraction of the patients with essential hypersomnia can be subcategorized

longer than in cases of narcolepsy, lasting from one to several hours. Some patients show only daytime sleepiness (monosymptomatic form), while other patients experience prolonged and deep nocturnal sleep and difficulty in waking up known as sleep drunkenness (polysymptomatic form).

The Association of Sleep Disorders Centers (ASDC) and the Association for the Psychophysiological Study of Sleep (APSS) (1979) adopted Roth's concept and coined the term *idiopathic CNS hypersomnolence* to describe the above conditions. The nature of sleepiness in this category is essentially the same as described by Roth: lengthy daytime sleep and nonimperative sleepiness. However, they added several clinical characteristics to expand the description: deepening of nocturnal sleep; resistance to CNS stimulants; associated symptoms such as headaches, migraines, and nausea; nonrestorative nature of daytime naps; and lack of abnormal REM sleep manifestations. The following three case studies of idiopathic hypersomnia have been documented by the authors.

Case 1

A 47-year-old housewife complained of excessive daytime sleepiness which had persisted for 7 years. Before the diagnosis of her illness, she had complained of difficulty in waking up in the morning and used to take a nap daily after lunch. At the age of 41, she felt that her legs fatigued easily. She went to an orthopedist and was diagnosed as having spondylolysis. She believed that her sleepiness worsened after receiving this diagnosis. Since then, she has experienced relentless daytime sleepiness. She usually awoke at 5:30 a.m. She got out of bed only with great effort, and did not feel fully alert. She usually napped for 3 h in the morning and 1 h following lunch. Although her naps were lengthy, they were nonrestorative: she still felt drowsy and unrefreshed after naps. She very often stayed in bed, feeling tired and worn-out. She also complained of dull headaches, a sense of impaired alertness, and difficulty in concentration. She usually went to bed around 11 p.m. and slept for 7 h. Nocturnal sleep was deep and without disruptions. She tended to snore but not very loudly. She did not experience cataplexy, sleep paralysis, hypnagogic hallucinations, or epileptic seizures. There was no family history of excessive daytime sleepiness. She often worried about her sleepiness; she thought herself to be punctual, unsociable, and overconcerned with trivial details.

She was 146 cm tall and weighed 53 kg. Daytime polysomnographic examinations revealed left central and parietal positive spikes in a drowsy state, generalized slowing and appearance of slow bursts on hyperventilation, and a marked tendency to fall asleep. Sleep-onset micro-REM episodes were observed twice on Multiple Sleep Latency Test (MSLT). Apneic episodes during sleep were not observed. CNS stimulants and antiepileptic drugs had no effects on her sleepiness. On the other hand, cyclandelate, a vascular dilator, had a limited effect on her sleepiness; that is, her sleepiness slightly declined for ½ year while taking this medication. Her HLA types were A24, A31, B51, Bw61, C blank, DRw11, DRw9, DQw3.

This case meshes well with the descriptions of polysymptomatic idiopathic hypersomnia (Roth 1980) and idiopathic CNS hypersomnolence in the ASDC-APSS classification (1979), except for MSLT findings.

Although the ASDC-APSS classification defines idiopathic CNS hypersomnolence as a syndrome without abnormal manifestations of REM sleep, we have encountered further cases in which characteristic sleepiness of idiopathic hypersomnia and abnormal REM manifestations coexist, such as the following two cases.

Case 2

A 28-year-old male office worker complained of prolonged daytime sleepiness. His sleepiness started at 22 years of age. While in university, he often dozed off during classroom lectures. After graduation he started working for a company and claimed to be sleepy all day long. He sometimes dozed off while talking with his customers or during important meetings. He usually woke up around 7 a.m. but with great effort. He said that his drowsiness persisted all day long. He sometimes took a nap in the afternoon, which usually lasted more than 1 h. He did not report feeling refreshed after the naps. He went to bed around 11 p.m. and usually slept for 7–8 h without awakening. He snored and complained of dull headaches, impaired alertness, malaise, and epigastralgia. He had no experience of cataplexy, sleep paralysis, hypnagogic hallucinations, or nocturnal myoclonus. He was reported as hard working and syntonic, although he had a tendency to be overconcerned with trivial details. He reported that his deceased grandfather also had excessive sleepiness and often fell asleep in the daytime.

He was 173 cm tall and weighed 63 kg. A polysomnographic examination showed a marked tendency to fall asleep and a REM period starting 10 min after the onset of sleep and lasting for 5 min. Apneic episodes during sleep were not observed. Administration of pemoline was effective against his sleepiness. His HLA types were A24, Aw33, A13, B44, C blank, DR7, DRw13, DQw1, DQw2.

The ADSC-APSS classification (1979) defined narcolepsy as a syndrome consisting of excessive daytime sleepiness and abnormal manifestations of REM sleep. Since he showed a sleep-onset REM period, this case might well be classified as narcolepsy within the parameters of this definition. However, the nature of his daytime sleep lapses and sleepiness was different from that of narcolepsy and more similar to that of idiopathic CNS hypersomnolence in that naps were lengthy yet unrefreshing, nocturnal sleep was deep and without disruption, and, sleepiness persisted all day long.

According to our diagnostic criteria, he is not a true narcoleptic because of the absence of cataplexy. According to Roth's classification, this case is categorized as polysymptomatic idiopathic hypersomnia. Should he be diagnosed as a narcoleptic, this would be a case of DR2-negative narcolepsy.

Case 3

An 18-year-old male student complained of anxiety and intense sleepiness. Symptoms of sleepiness began at the age of 17. He claimed to be sleepy all day and often lapsed into sleep during the dull lectures. Although he once fell asleep at an entrance examination for a university, he could usually voluntarily resist sleepiness and therefore avoid falling asleep. He tended to nap three or four times a day, and the sleep durations were usually more than 1 h, sometimes lasting up to 3 h. He did not snore, nor did he report feeling refreshed after long diurnal sleep. He usually slept well at night for about 7 h without disruptions. His sleepiness seemed to intensify when under psychological stress, such as when he was preparing for university entrance examinations or when he broke up with his girlfriend. Sleep paralysis and hypnagogic hallucinations also developed at the age of 17. In one reported dream, he met a faceless lady who tried to choke him to death. During this dream, he was not able to move his arms at all. He had no experience of cataplexy, nor a family history of sleepiness. He feared that other people often stared and avoided him because of his "ugly" face (*taijin-kyofu*) (Honda 1983). He was described as nervous, introverted, tense, and a hypochondriac.

He was 159 cm tall and weighed 52 kg. A polysomnogram revealed a tendency to fall asleep, but no sleep-onset REM periods were noted. CNS stimulants were ineffective in alleviating his daily sleepiness. His HLA types were A2, A24, Bw52, Bw56, Cw1, Cw4, DR2, DQw1.

The nature of his sleepiness is similar to that of polysymptomatic idiopathic hypersomnia and idiopathic CNS hypersomnolence: prolonged and nonrestorative diurnal sleep, deep and undisrupted nocturnal sleep, ineffective response to CNS stimulants, etc.

Thus, according to Roth's classification, this case would be categorized as polysymptomatic idiopathic hypersomnia. On the contrary, he experienced frequent episodes of hypnagogic hallucinations and sleep paralysis. This distinguishes his sleep disorder from idiopathic CNS hypersomnolence as defined by the ASDC-APSS classification. In terms of the ASDC-APSS classification, this case would be diagnosed as narcolepsy due to the presence of hypnagogic hallucinations and sleep paralysis. Yet, on the other hand, his personality traits differed markedly from those of narcoleptics.

From these case studies, we are led to consider that the essential features of idiopathic hypersomnia are

(a) the characteristic sleepiness which is less overwhelming than that in narcolepsy;
(b) nonrestorative and lengthy (usually more than 1 h) daytime sleep; and
(c) unresponsiveness to CNS stimulants (type I in Table 1).

Abnormal REM manifestations except for cataplexy may or may not accompany idiopathic hypersomnia. To date, we have HLA-typed six cases which met our definition of idiopathic hypersomnia; three were DR2 negative and three were DR2 positive.

Aborted Forms of Narcolepsy

At times, we encounter patients with sleepiness similar to that of narcolepsy. In such patients, the sleep attacks are overwhelming and imperative as in narcolepsy; the daytime sleep episodes are brief, usually lasting less than 1 h; the naps are most often refreshing; nocturnal sleep is often disrupted; and CNS stimulants show marked effect to sleepiness (type II in Table 1). The patients may experience hypnagogic hallucinations and sleep paralysis; however, they do not experience cataplexy throughout long-term clinical follow-ups.

Case 4

A 34-year-old male office worker came to our hospital because of his excessive sleepiness. He had developed duodenal ulcer at the age of 25. He reported that he was not sleeping well at night and that he often fell asleep during the daytime at work. By the age of 29, he started to experience general muscle weakness. For example, when he was lying on a sofa, watching television, or relaxing in the bathtub, he tended to become very drowsy and then found himself unable to move or utter a word for about 2 or 3 min. He got up at 7 a.m. but with great difficulty. He often took naps around 8 a.m. on the commuter to his office; around noon after lunch; and around 6 p.m. on the train returning home. The naps were usually less than 30 min long and left him feeling refreshed. He usually went to bed at 11 p.m. and dreamt a lot and sometimes woke up several times at night. He was reported to be punctual, patient, passive, enduring, and generally good natured. He had no family history of somnolence.

He was 175 cm tall and weighed 92 kg. A polysomnogram revealed a marked tendency to fall asleep and a REM period at 3 min after sleep onset. Methylphenidate and imipramine were markedly effective in controlling his sleepiness and improving nocturnal sleep, respectively. He has been followed up for 17 years. Even under these prescribed medications, he often experienced sleep paralysis, hypnagogic hallucinations, and attacks of muscle weakness, e.g., he dropped a glass after drinking a small amount of alcohol; his knees tended to buckle when he stood up quickly; he could not speak up even though he wanted to; he could not move his body or arms in the bathtub. He once fell asleep while reading a book, and he found he could not move his arms after he had woken up. As far as he could recollect, all of these attacks of muscle weakness occured only when he was sleepy. He never experienced muscle weakness triggered by laughter or any other kinds of emotion. His HLA types were A2, A31, B35, B51, Cw1, Cw3, DR2, DRw11, DQw1, DQw3.

In this case, the question is whether the frequent attacks of muscle weakness were cataplexy or not. Some of the attacks may have been due to excessive sleepiness itself. He may have fallen asleep for an unnoticeable brief period, during which he may have dropped things in his hand. The attacks that occurred when this patient was drowsy seem to be attacks of sleep paralysis. Since sleep paralysis and cataplexy are both manifestations of dissociated REM sleep, they may sometimes look similar. However, they are essentially different in regard to their triggers. Cataplexy is triggered by strong emotions, mostly of a pleasant and exciting nature, whereas sleep paralysis can occur without apparent emotional triggers. Sleep paralysis may be accompanied with hypnagogic hallucinations, which is usually associated with unpleasant emotions, such as fear, sadness, terror, and weirdness. In addition, cataplexy occurs when a patient is fully alert, while sleep paralysis occurs in a transitional state between sleep and wakefulness. Since he had no experience of muscle weakness apparently triggered by emotion, we do not consider his muscle weakness as cataplexy and would not diagnose his condition as narcolepsy.

Case 5

A 20-year-old male student came to our hospital because of prolonged daytime sleepiness. The onset was insidious. He dozed off twice in the daytime at school at the age of 12. At the age of 13, he began to fall asleep more frequently, one to three times at school almost every day. The duration of such sleep lapses was between 20 and 30 min. After sleeping, he felt somewhat refreshed. By 14, he started experiencing sudden and short attacks of knee weakness once or twice a week. For example, his knees would buckle for a moment when he stood up from a sitting position, and he reported feeling as if he were sinking a little into the floor. During these attacks, he was fully alert and did not experience dizziness or vertigo. He had no other attacks of muscle weakness or attacks preceded by emotional states. At the age of 14, he began to have frightening dreams at the onset of nocturnal sleep. He tried to move his arms but could not. He woke up several times every night. During senior high school, although the attacks of knee buckling subsided and eventually ceased, his sleepiness seemed to increase: he slept for 30-40 min three to four times every day. Sometimes the sleepiness was so intense that he could not voluntarily resist falling asleep. He did not snore. He was described as mild mannered, passive, introverted, easygoing, and quiet. He had no family history of excessive daytime sleepiness.

He was 165 cm tall and weighed 71 kg. Two separate polysomnographic sessions revealed tendencies to fall asleep; however, sleep-onset REM periods were not detected in either session. Methylphenidate was effective in controlling his sleepiness. His HLA types were A2, A11, Bw31, Cw1, Cw7, DR2, DR4, DQw1. He has been followed up for 12 years on the prescription of methylphenidate. Throughout the follow-up course, cataplexy has been absent.

This case showed excessive daytime somnolence, hypnagogic hallucinations, sleep paralysis, sleep attacks, and disturbed nocturnal sleep. According to both the ASDC-APSS and Roth's classification, he would without question be diagnosed as having narcolepsy. Although he had attacks of knee weakness, these attacks do not satisfy our criterion for cataplexy, for emotional triggers were absent in these attacks.

Possible cases of aborted forms of narcolepsy are also found in families with a narcoleptic relative(s). The patients may share a HLA-DR2 haplotype with the relative(s).

Case 6

A 16-year-old female student self-referred to our hospital because of excessive daytime sleepiness. She underwent an appendectomy at the age of 13. After the operation, she had a high fever which lasted for about 1 month. She believed that her sleepiness developed as a result. By the age of 14, she could not concentrate on studying because of intensive sleepiness which occurred almost daily. Her appetite increased with sleepiness. Her mother usually woke her up at 7 a.m. She was reluctant to get up and used abusive language, which she later claimed that she did not remember. She was sleepy throughout the day and often dozed off during classes. When she came home from school, she usually slept for about ½ h. She usually went to bed about 9 p.m. She dreamed a lot, though her dreams were usually pleasant. She often woke up at midnight, and stayed awake for 1-2 h, watching video movies and raiding the refrigerator. She had no experience of hypnagogic hallucinations, sleep paralysis, or cataplexy. She did not snore. She was described as soft spoken, subdued, mild, and gentle. One of her relatives had narcolepsy and shared a DR2-positive HLA haplotype (A26-Cw3-B35-DR2-DQw1) with her. Family study confirmed that she had this haplotype and an A2-Cx46-Bw46-DRw8-DQw1 haplotype.

She was 149 cm tall and weighed 57 kg. She reported that she gained weight after the onset of sleepiness. A polysomnogram revealed a tendency to fall asleep but no sleep-onset REM periods. Pemoline was very effective in decreasing her sleepiness. She lost 10 kg in 2 months after the start of treatment. She has been followed up for 3 years; cataplexy has been absent throughout the course.

Her bouts of sleepiness are difficult to classify. According to Roth's classification, she is categorized as having monosymptomatic narcolepsy, for she experienced excessive sleepiness and recurrent short sleep lapses during the daytime but did not have any signs or symptoms of abnormal REM sleep. According to our criteria and the ASDC-APSS classification, she is not narcoleptic, although there is still a chance that she may develop cataplexy in the future. The best description for this case in the ASDC-APSS classification is the "not otherwise specified" category. Since she had the same HLA-DR2 haplotype as that of a narcoleptic relative, she is most likely to have an aborted or latent form of narcolepsy.

Other Forms of Essential Hypersomnia

The aforementioned two subclasses of essential hypersomnia, i.e., idiopathic hypersomnia and aborted forms of narcolepsy, occupy only small fractions of the total body of essential hypersomnia. Most cases are difficult to subclassify or categorize. Two such cases are presented here.

The first case (case 7) looks similar to aborted forms of narcolepsy. The diurnal sleep episodes were short and refreshing, and CNS stimulants were effective. However, her sleepiness was not as imperative and irresistible as in genuine narcolepsy or aborted forms of narcolepsy (type III in Table 1). She was also DR2 negative.

Case 7

A 55-year-old housewife came to our hospital because of excessive sleepiness. Her sleepiness began around the age of 14. She remembers often dozing off in classrooms. She got married at the age of 20. She often fell asleep while talking with a friend, sitting relaxed, or watching television. She had frightening hallucinations at sleep onset; she usually reported that somebody tried to attack her, and that she could not move or shout for help. By the age of 54, after her husband had died of heart failure, she had to take care of her mother-in-law handicapped with senile dementia. Her sleepiness seemed to increase after her husband's death. She usually woke up at 5 a.m., feeling refreshed, but became sleepy around 10 a.m. She sometimes lapsed into sleep in the afternoon. The sleep was usually 30 min long and refreshing. Her sleepiness increased in the evening; she usually slept from 8 p.m. to 10 p.m., then woke up again. She went to bed again around midnight and fell asleep easily. The nocturnal sleep was deep and without disruptions. She did not dream or snore. She also had various somatic complaints, such as headaches, general malaise, hiccups, and dull pains in her shoulders. She was described as nervous, irritable, neurotic, a hypochondriac, and anxious about her sleepiness. She tended to be overconcerned about trivial details. She had no family history of sleepiness.

She sometimes felt weakness in her whole body when she was sitting in a relaxed position. She did not have attacks; the onset of weakness was neither sudden nor clear cut. She felt as if she had lost all her energy, and she found it very difficult to move for several minutes. She had reported no experiences of muscle weakness triggered by emotional situations.

She was 153 cm tall and weighed 45 kg. A polysomnogram revealed a marked tendency to fall asleep, but sleep-onset REM periods were not observed. Pemoline was prescribed and was effective. Her HLA types were A24, A31, Bw62, B39, Cw1, Cw7, DR4, DRw11, DQw3.

Her sleepiness is difficult to classify. Since she had hypnagogic hallucinations and sleep paralysis, she could be classified as a narcoleptic according to the ASDC-APSS classification. According to Roth's classification, she could also be diagnosed as having polysymptomatic narcolepsy.

At times, she experienced general muscle weakness. However, her weakness was different from cataplexy: she did not experience sudden attacks, and muscle weakness was not triggered by emotions. Her muscle weakness may be due to sleep paralysis or cerebrovascular insufficiency. It may also only be a product of her neurotic concern regarding her physical conditions, or it may be a mere subjective malaise. Her attitude toward sleepiness was characterized by overconcern and irritation. The total clinical description was completely different from that of narcolepsy. However, should she be diagnosed as narcoleptic, she would become another case of DR2-negative narcolepsy.

The next case falls into another subcategory (type IV in Table 1). The patients in this subcategory feel daytime sleepiness which is not as intense as in genuine narcolepsy. The sleep episodes are usually short, but sometimes may last over 1 h, and are generally unrefreshing. CNS stimulants are moderately effective. The patients may have impaired night-time sleep; they may snore and have limited sleep-induced respiratory impairments which do not meet the criteria for the sleep-apnea syndrome.

Case 8

A 56-year-old male business executive was referred to our hospital because of his sleepiness. He had long been a short sleeper. He had usually slept 5-6 h a night and had not felt any daytime sleepiness until the age of 54, when his daytime sleepiness started. He usually woke up about 7 a.m. but often became sleepy after 10 a.m. He dozed off during inactive moments at work, such as during monotonous business meetings; on the train; while reading a book, etc. The duration of sleep ranged from a few seconds to 30 min. He still felt sleepy after naps. He never experienced attacks of intense sleepiness, and he could control his sleepiness with voluntary efforts. He usually went to bed at 2 a.m. and woke up two or three times during the night. He snored. He did not feel better even if he slept longer at night. He had no experience of cataplexy, sleep paralysis, or hypnagogic hallucinations. He was described as being punctual, compulsive, energetic, and good natured. He reported that his father had always complained of daytime sleepiness, too.

He was 168 cm tall and weighed 70 kg. A daytime polysomnogram did not show sleep-apneic episodes. Prescribed pemoline was effective in controlling his sleepiness. His HLA types were A11, A24, Bw52, Bw61, Cw3, DR2, DQw1.

There is no suitable category for this case in the ASDC-APSS classification. His colleagues and his family unanimously noted his sleepiness, suggesting that his sleepiness was not simply subjective. It is apparent that he is not narcoleptic according to our criteria or the ASDC-APSS classification. He does not appear to have idiopathic CNS hypersomnia either, since his naps were generally short, and the CNS stimulant was quite effective. According to Roth's classification, this case could be categorized as monosymptomatic narcolepsy.

Abnormal Manifestations of REM Sleep

In cases 1-3, the nature of sleepiness was similar to that of idiopathic hypersomnia and idiopathic CNS hypersomnolence: diurnal naps were lengthy and nonrestorative; nocturnal sleep was deep and without disruptions; and CNS stimulants were not effective. However, these cases apparently experienced REM sleep-related abnormalities: sleep-onset REM periods in cases 1 and 2, hypnagogic hallucinations and sleep paralysis in case 3. These findings show that patients with characteristic sleepiness of idiopathic hypersomnia can have "auxiliary symptoms of narcolepsy", with the exception of cataplexy. This further indicates that sleep paralysis, hypnagogic hallucinations, and sleep-onset REM periods are *not* the pathognomonic features; we can neither make a diagnosis of narcolepsy nor exclude a diagnosis of other disorders such as idiopathic CNS hypersomnolence on the basis of these three features.

This, in turn, shows that the definition of narcolepsy provided by the ASDC-APSS classification is indeed insufficient to discriminate narcolepsy from other somnolent disorders. Except for cases involving cataplexy, the REM-related signs and symptoms can be found in various etiologies other than narcolepsy. If the description of narcolepsy is expanded to include the coexistence of these REM-related symptoms other than cataplexy, then narcolepsy will encompass heterogeneous and diverse pathologies. They are different in the nature of sleepiness, duration of daytime naps, continuity and depth of nocturnal sleep, efficacies of drugs, personality traits, and so on. Such a definition is of little, if any, help for investigating sleep disorders, much less for the study involving the association with HLA.

Muscle Weakness in Essential Hypersomnia

The correct diagnosis of cataplexy is the cornerstone in differentiating narcolepsy from other disorders of excessive somnolence. In cases 4 and 5, both patients experienced attacks of knee weakness when they stood up quickly. These attacks may have the same pathophysiology as that of cataplexy, although they are not apparently triggered by emotions. Most of the muscle weakness in case 4 seemed to be due to sleep paralysis. Some of the attacks of muscle weakness in case 4 may have been due to microsleeps; the patient may have fallen asleep for unnoticeable periods, and during those short sleeps the patient may have dropped articles the patient was holding. The muscle weakness in case 7 may be merely a subjective and/or a hypochondriac symptom.

If these attacks are considered as cataplexy, the patients will be misdiagnosed as narcoleptics. This misdiagnosis will likely lead to a false "discovery" of DR2-negative narcoleptics. The possibility is strong that this may be the case for some of the currently reported non-DR2 narcoleptics. Previous publications on non-DR2 narcolepsy have been generally ambiguous in regard to the presence of cataplexy. Most reports do not describe the nature of the attacks of muscle weakness, nor do they clarify whether the attacks were triggered by emotionally charged situations.

Attitudes Toward Sleepiness

Patients develop certain attitudes toward sleepiness during the course of their disorders. Although these attitudes are influenced by prior personalities, they seem to correlate with the intensity of sleepiness. At the very early onset, most patients seem anxious and worried about their excessive daytime sleepiness. When the sleepiness becomes so overwhelming and persistent as in narcolepsy, most patients find it very difficult to continue fighting off bouts of sleepiness. Because of uncontrollable sleepiness, the patients may feel ashamed in social situations, which may indeed lead to partial social withdrawal and development of shame, anxiety, or feelings of inferiority. The patients often try to suppress awareness of somnolence and to function as normally as possible despite their sleepiness. Although they are very often concerned and anxious about somnolence, they gradually develop acclimation to and acceptance of their sleepiness. At later stages, they may appear as if they were unaware of their obvious sleepiness and may even deny it to themselves and others. In spite of internal conflicts, the patients often appear gentle, subdued, mild, laid-back, easygoing, not very punctual, and good natured (narcoleptoid personality).

In contrast, when the sleepiness is not as strong as in narcolepsy, the patients may keep on fighting against sleepiness. They may never develop acclimation to or acceptance of their sleepiness. They may always be anxious about their sleepiness, trying to overcome it, and be overconcerned with their sense of fatigue, tiredness, headaches, and other so-called neurasthenic symptoms. They usually look nervous, act neurotically, and may even become hypochondriacs. It is not rare that subjective complaints of sleepiness seem to surpass real or "objective" sleepiness.

Among our observations, most patients with possible aborted forms of narcolepsy acclimate to sleepiness at earlier stages. The patients with idiopathic hypersomnia tend to assume neurotic and neurasthenic attitudes. The patients with other forms of essential hypersomnia may take either neurotic or nonneurotic attitudes toward their sleepiness (Table 1).

Table 2. HLA antigen frequencies in essential hypersomnia

Ag	Patients (n=41)	Controls (n=310)	Ag	Patients (n=41)	Controls (n=310)
A1	1 (2.4%)	3 (1.0%)	B7	1 (2.4%)	35 (11.3%)
A2	22 (53.7%)	127 (41.0%)	B13	2 (4.9%)	11 (3.5%)
A3	0 (0.0%)	5 (1.6%)	B27	0 (0.0%)	1 (0.3%)
A11	5 (12.2%)	56 (18.1%)	B35	6 (14.6%)	55 (17.7%)
A24	25 (61.0%)	185 (59.7%)	B37	0 (0.0%)	3 (1.0%)
A26	8 (19.5%)	65 (21.0%)	B39	2 (4.9%)	23 (7.4%)
A31	6 (14.6%)	50 (16.1%)	B44	7 (17.1%)	39 (12.6%)
Aw33	7 (17.1%)	50 (16.1%)	Bw46	4 (9.8%)	26 (8.4%)
			Bw48	5 (12.2%)	14 (4.5%)*
Cw1	13 (31.7%)	85 (27.4%)	B51	8 (19.5%)	53 (17.1%)
Cw3	16 (39.0%)	142 (45.8%)	Bw52	10 (24.4%)	72 (23.2%)
Cw4	1 (2.4%)	33 (10.6%)	Bw54	7 (17.1%)	45 (14.5%)
Cw5	0 (0.0%)	3 (1.0%)	Bw55	2 (4.9%)	21 (6.8%)
Cw7	8 (19.5%)	60 (19.4%)	Bw56	1 (2.4%)	3 (1.0%)
			Bw59	1 (2.4%)	13 (4.2%)
Bw4	24 (58.5%)	170 (54.8%)	Bw60	3 (7.3%)	41 (13.2%)
Bw6	34 (82.9%)	274 (88.4%)	Bw61	8 (19.5%)	56 (18.1%)
			Bw62	7 (17.1%)	65 (21.0%)
			Bw67	2 (4.9%)	5 (1.6%)
DR1	0 (0.0%)	45 (14.5%)*	DRw52	26 (63.4%)	178 (57.4%)
DR2	23 (56.1%)	104 (33.5%)**	DRw53	20 (48.8%)	189 (61.0%)
DR4	14 (34.1%)	125 (40.3%)			
DRw8	11 (26.8%)	84 (27.1%)	DQw1	29 (70.7%)	213 (68.7%)
DRw9	5 (12.2%)	85 (27.4%)*	DQw3	20 (48.8%)	157 (50.6%)
DRw10	0 (0.0%)	2 (0.6%)			
DRw11	5 (12.2%)	20 (6.5%)			
DRw12	6 (14.6%)	41 (13.2%)			
DRw13	7 (17.1%)	51 (16.5%)			
DRw14	1 (2.4%)	8 (2.6%)			

* $P<0.05$, $Pc>0.05$; ** $P<0.005$, $Pc>0.05$; Ag: antigen

HLA Antigen Frequencies in Essential Hypersomnia

HLA antigen frequencies in 41 patients with essential hypersomnia were examined (Table 2). Parts of this study were reported elsewhere (Honda et al. 1986). The HLA antigens did not show any significant deviations when compared with normals. The frequency of DR2 was 57.5% in essential hypersomnia.

Clinical features of the DR2-positive and DR2-negative patients with essential hypersomnia are presented in Table 3. The two groups were indistinguishable in regard to several clinical features: ages at onset, frequencies of sleep paralysis, hypnagogic hallucinations, disturbed night sleep, sleep-onset REM periods, possible precipitating exogenous factors, and family histories of excessive daytime sleepiness. It should be noted that all the patients that had a relative with narcolepsy were DR2 positive. This suggests that the DR2-positive group included the patients with aborted or latent forms of narcolepsy.

Table 3. Clinical features of DR2-positive and -negative essential hypersomnia

		DR2+ (*n*=23)	DR2− (*n*=18)
Age at onset (years) mean ± SD		22.3 ± 13.4	24.7 ± 14.9
Sleep paralysis		10 (43%)	8 (44%)
Hypnagogic hallucinations		8 (35%)	7 (39%)
Disturbed Nocturnal sleep		10 (43%)	10 (56%)
Sleep onset REM periods		5 (22%)	2 (11%)
Exogenous factors[a]	++	1 (4%)	1 (6%)
	+	6 (26%)	5 (28%)
	−	16 (70%)	12 (67%)
Family history of excessive daytime sleepiness[b]	++	7 (30%)	4 (22%)
	+	2 (9%)	2 (11%)
	−	14 (61%)	12 (67%)
Family history of narcolepsy		4 (17%)	0 (0%)

[a] ++, exogenous stressors found within 3 months prior to the onset of the disorders; +, exogenous factors found more than 3 months before the onset; −, no exogenous factors

[b] ++, excessive daytime sleepiness in the first-degree relatives; +, excessive daytime sleepiness in other relatives; −, no excessive daytime sleepiness in relatives

Of the 23 DR2-positive patients, 8 (35%) had Bw52. This frequency is lower than that of normal DR2-positive subjects (about 60%), but higher than that of narcoleptics (6.8%). The Bw52-DR2/Dw12 haplotypes have no association with narcolepsy (see Chap. 3). This indicates that DR2-positive patients with essential hypersomnia may not always have a DR2/Dw2-linked narcolepsy susceptibility gene. In fact, cases 3 and 8, which were DR2 and Bw52 positive, showed sleepiness and personality traits different from those of genuine narcoleptics.

Various Disorders with Excessive Daytime Somnolence and HLA Antigens

In addition to essential hypersomnia, we have HLA-typed the patients with various disorders with excessive daytime somnolence (Table 4). Parts of this study were reported by Honda et al. (1986). The patients consist of 11 with sleep-apnea DOES syndrome, 7 with periodic somnolence including a case of Kleine-Levin syndrome, 6 with disorders of the sleep-wake schedule, 2 with sleep paralysis, 2 with mental retardation, a pair of identical twins with myotonic dystrophy, 2 due to poor sleep hygiene, and 3 with psychoreactive transient somnolence.

Table 4. DR2 in various disorders of excessive daytime somnolence

Disorders	DR2+ (*n*)	DR2− (*n*)	Total (*n*)
Sleep apnea DOES syndrome	3	8	11
Periodic hypersomnia	1	6	7
Irregular sleep/wake schedule	0	6	6
Myotonic dystrophy	0	2	2
Mental retardation	1	1	2
Sleep paralysis	1	1	2
Poor sleep hygiene	0	2	2
Psychoreactive, transient	1	2	3
Total	7	28	35

No disorders showed complete associations with DR2. This suggests that the DR2-linked narcolepsy-susceptibility gene is not required for the manifestation of these disorders. The pathogenesis of these disorders is thus most likely different from that of narcolepsy.

References

Association of Sleep Disorders Centers and the Association for the Psychophysiological Study of Sleep (1979) Diagnostic classification of sleep and arousal disorders. Sleep 2: 5-121

Honda Y, Juji T, Matsuki K, Naohara T, Satake M, Inoko H, Someya T, Harada S, Doi Y (1986) HLA-DR2 and Dw2 in narcolepsy and in other disorders of excessive somnolence without cataplexy. Sleep 9: 133-142

Honda Y (1983) DSM-III in Japan. In: Spitzer RL, Williams JBW, Skodol AE (eds) International perspectives on DSM-III. American Psychiatric Press, Washington DC, pp 185-201

Roth B (1961) Narkolepsie und Hypersomnie. Veb Verlag Folk und Gesundheit, Berlin

Roth B (1976) Narcolepsy. In: Guilleminault C, Dement WC, Passouant P (eds) Narcolepsy. Spectrum, New York, pp 333-349

Roth B (1980) Narcolepsy and hypersomnia. Karger, Basel

Chapter 15

HLA in Disorders of Excessive Daytime Sleepiness Without Cataplexy in Canada

J. MONTPLAISIR and G. POIRIER

Introduction

Diseases presenting a genetic basis often exhibit characteristic features. They tend to be concentrated in families in which the prevalence of the illness is higher than in the general population. Studies of families with more than one case of idiopathic hypersomnia argue in favor of a genetic basis for this affection (Roth et al. 1972; Guilleminault and Faull 1982).

Narcolepsy and nonnarcoleptic idiopathic hypersomnia share clinical, polygraphic, and pharmacological features. As for narcoleptics, idiopathic hypersomniacs complain of EDS, have short sleep latency during the MSLT, and also report improvement of EDS with the use of stimulants such as amphetamine and methylphenidate. In addition, low concentration of free dopamine was found in the cerebrospinal fluid of both narcoleptics and idiopathic CNS hypersomniac patients (Montplaisir et al. 1982). However, narcolepsy has specific features, such as the symptom of cataplexy and the presence of sleep-onset REM periods; part of its physiopathology has also been elucidated (Godbout and Montplaisir 1986) while little is known about idiopathic hypersomniacs.

There is a heterogeneous group of patients corresponding to several diagnoses of the Diagnostic Classification of Sleep and Arousals Disorders (Association of Sleep Disorder Centers 1979), namely idiopathic CNS hypersomnolence, and subjective hypersomnia without objective findings. After the discovery of a genetic marker for narcolepsy, one question arises: are these forms of hypersomnia different clinical presentations of the same illness, incomplete forms of narcolepsy, or completely different entities? The strategy used in the present study was to separate a group of idiopathic hypersomniacs into three subgroups based on results of polygraphic recordings and then to compare the results of HLA determination obtained in these subgroups with those of narcoleptics and normal controls.

Methods

Patient Selection

Thirty unrelated Caucasoid patients with a clinical complaint of excessive daytime sleepiness (EDS) and/or sleep attacks without cataplexy were selected. In all cases the diagnosis was made blind with regard to the HLA typing. Patients with sleep apneas and periodic movements in sleep, documented by two all-night polygraphic recordings, were excluded from the study, as were patients with evidence of psychiatric disorders or drugs and alcohol abuse. Patients were divided into three groups according to the results of their polysomnographic investigation. The first group (*n*, 6; mean age, 37.3 years) was patients with severe EDS and sleep attacks without cataplexy. During the MSLT, they showed short sleep latencies (mean, 4.7 min) and the presence of at least one sleep-onset REM period (SOREMP). Consequently, they were called REM hypersomniacs. The second group (*n*, 18; mean age, 39.2 years) was composed of patients presenting the same clinical picture but without SOREMP during the MSLT. Polygraphic sleep recording also revealed short latencies (mean, 6.1 min). The third group was composed of patients (*n*, 6; mean age, 34.7 years) referred to the sleep clinic for a complaint of severe EDS interferring with their social, professional, and personal activities but who presented long sleep latencies (mean, 12.9 min) and no SOREMP during the MSLT. Despite their complaint of hypersomnia, no objective evidence of EDS was thus found during the laboratory investigation of these patients.

HLA Typings

Antigens of loci A, B, and C were detected by the standard microlymphotoxicity technique (Terasaki and McClelland 1964). HLA-DR antigens were detected using the same technique after B-cell enrichment performed by rosetting of T-cells with red blood cells treated with neuraminidase. Fifty-four antigens were typed. Typings were made blind with regard to the patient's diagnosis. National Reference laboratory plates (Red Cross, Toronto) were used for all typings. HLA frequencies were compared for each subgroup of hypersomniacs with those of 158 unrelated Caucasoid control subjects, using the Yate's corrected chi square analysis with one degree of freedom. All of them had already been typed for their HLA-A, B, and C, and 150 of them for their HLA-DR antigens during a previous genetic study conducted by the Canadian Red Cross. Comparison with results obtained in 48 narcoleptics (see Chap. 6) will be considered in the discussion.

Results

Tables 1 and 2 present HLA frequencies of hypersomniacs and controls. All six REM hypersomniacs were HLA-DR2 positive compared with 22.00% for controls. In addition, HLA-Cw2 frequency was elevated in all experimental groups. This increased frequency of HLA-Cw2 was not significant for REM and subjective hypersomniacs, most likely due to the small number of patients included in these subgroups. The frequency of HLA-DR5, an antigen known to be linked to Cw2 in Caucasoids, was also found to be increased in objective hypersomniac patients. No significant difference was found in subjective hypersomniacs for any HLA antigen studied.

Table 1. HLA-A, B, and C frequencies (%) in hypersomniac and control subjects

Antigen	REM H	OBJ H	SUBJ H	CONTR
A1	33.33	11.11	33.33	23.42
A2	50.00	55.55	33.33	52.53
A3	0.00	16.66	33.33	25.32
A11	16.66	5.55	16.66	13.92
A23	0.00	5.55	16.66	3.16
A24	50.00	33.33	0.00	17.72
A25	16.66	5.55	16.66	3.16
A26	0.00	5.55	0.00	2.53
A28	16.66	5.55	0.00	8.23
A29	0.00	22.22	16.66	12.66
A30+31	0.00	11.11	0.00	10.13
B7	16.66	5.55	0.00	19.62
B8	33.33	5.55	16.66	18.99
B13	0.00	5.55	0.00	5.70
B14	0.00	0.00	0.00	13.29
B15	0.00	5.55	16.66	8.86
B16	0.00	22.22	0.00	10.13
B17	0.00	16.66	0.00	6.96
B18	33.33	0.00	16.66	10.76
B21	0.00	5.55	0.00	6.33
Bw22	0.00	5.55	0.00	7.59
B27	16.66	22.22	16.66	10.13
B35	16.66	11.11	0.00	16.46
B37	0.00	0.00	0.00	1.27
B40	0.00	16.66	0.00	6.96
B44	33.33	38.88	33.33	28.48
B45	0.00	0.00	0.00	0.63
B49	0.00	5.55	0.00	3.80
Bw50	0.00	0.00	0.00	2.53
B51	16.66	5.55	33.33	15.19
Bw52	0.00	0.00	0.00	1.27
Bw53	16.66	0.00	0.00	1.27
Bw55	0.00	0.00	0.00	3.16
Bw56	0.00	5.55	0.00	1.27
Bw60	0.00	0.00	0.00	5.70
Bw63	0.00	0.00	0.00	0.63
Cw2	33.33	22.22[a]	33.33	5.70
Cw3	0.00	22.22	0.00	13.29
Cw4	0.00	27.77	16.66	22.15
Cw6	0.00	11.11	0.00	8.86

[a] $P < 0.05$

P value calculated with Yate's corrected chi square, comparing each experimental group with controls

REM H, REM hypersomniacs ($n = 6$); OBJ H, objective hypersomniacs ($n = 18$); SUBJ H, subjective hypersomniacs ($n = 6$); CONTR, controls ($n = 158$)

Table 2. HLA-DR frequencies (%) in hypersomniac and control subjects

Antigen	REM H	OBJ H	SUBJ H	CONTR
DR1	50.00	38.88	33.33	25.33
DR2	100.00[a]	16.66	16.66	22.00
DR3	33.33	16.66	33.33	33.33
DR4	16.66	27.77	50.00	27.33
DR5	0.00	38.88[b]	33.33	14.67
DRw6	0.00	0.00[b]	0.00	23.33
DR7	0.00	44.44	16.66	22.67
DRw8	0.00	0.00	0.00	2.67
DRw9	0.00	0.00	0.00	4.00
DRw10	0.00	0.00	0.00	0.67

[a] $P<0.0005$
[b] $P<0.05$
P value calculated with Yate's corrected chi square, comparing each experimental group with controls
REM H, REM hypersomniacs ($n=6$); OBJ H, objective hypersomniacs ($n=18$); SUBJ H, subjective hypersomniacs ($n=6$); CONTR, controls ($n=150$)

Discussion

Only three (16.66%) objective hypersomniacs were HLA-DR2 positive, while all narcoleptic patients studied by us carried this antigen (see Chap. 6). These results demonstrate that narcolepsy and idiopathic CNS hypersomnia are two different entities.

Of interest is the elevated frequency of HLA-DR5 in non-REM hypersomniacs (with and without objective polygraphic findings). In a recent study of 19 patients with endogenous depression, the frequency of HLA-DR5 was also found to be significantly elevated (52.63%) compared with controls (14.67%) (unpublished personal data). This result raises the possibility of similarities between non-REM hypersomnia and affective disorders, a hypothesis that would be concordant with clinical observations made in several cases of non-REM hypersomnia.

All REM hypersomniacs carried the HLA-DR2 antigen. Narcolepsy and REM hypersomnia thus share immunogenetic and polygraphic characteristics, suggesting that REM hypersomnia is probably an envolving narcolepsy. This conclusion is consonant with the clinical observation that cataplexy frequently develops in narcoleptics several years after the onset on EDS. It should be stressed that one of these patients is still cataplexy free 18 years after the onset of EDS.

The increased frequency of HLA-Cw2 in all experimental groups suggests a possible link between the presence of this antigen and the complaint of hypersomnia. The frequency of this antigen was also found to be elevated in our narcoleptic patients (see Chap. 6), which represent another subgroup of hypersomniacs, but was not reported to be increased in patients with sleep apnea syndrome (Honda et al. 1986; Mitler et al. 1986).

Hypersomniacs without objective polygraphic findings showed no significant difference from normal controls with regard to HLA typing. However, the frequency of HLA-Cw2 was comparable to that other of hypersomnia groups. It is possible that the MSLT is not an appropriate test to demonstrate the presence of EDS in these patients.

These results show that HLA typing used in conjunction with MSLT recording will enable to discriminate between narcolepsy, evolving narcolepsy, and idiopathic hypersomnia.

References

Association of Sleep Disorders Centers (1979) Diagnostic classification of sleep and arousal disorders. Sleep 2: 1-137

Godbout R, Montplaisir J (1986) The effect of zimelidine, a serotonin-reuptake blocker, on cataplexy and daytime sleepiness of narcoleptic patients. Clin Neuropharmacol 9: 46-51

Guilleminault C, Faull KF (1982) Sleepiness in non-narcoleptic non-sleep apneic EDS patients: the idiopathic CNS hypersomnolence. Sleep 5: 175-181

Honda Y, Juji T, Matsuki K, Naohara T, Satake M, Inoko H, Someya T, Harada S, Doi Y (1986) HLA-DR2 and Dw2 in narcolepsy and in other disorders of excessive somnolence without cataplexy. Sleep 9: 133-42

Mitler MM, Shafor R, Sobers M, Hajdukovich RM, Rubin RL (1986) Human leucocyte antigen (HLA) studies in excessive somnolence: narcolepsy versus sleep apnea. In: Chase MH, McGinty DJ, Crane G (eds) Sleep research, vol 15. Brain Information Service, Los Angeles, p 148

Montplaisir J, De Champlain J, Young SN, Missala K, Sourkes TL, Walsh J, Remillard G (1982) Narcolepsy and idiopathic hypersomnia: biogenetic amines and related compounds in CSF. Neurology 32: 1229-1302

Roth B, Nevsimalova S, Rechtschaffen A (1972) Hypersomnia with "sleep drunkenness". Arch Gen Psychiatry 26: 456-462

Terasaki PI, McClelland JD (1964) Microdroplet assay of human serum cytotoxins. Nature 204: 998-1000

Chapter 16

Genetic Markers Other than HLA in Narcolepsy

Part 1: Findings on 16 Genetic Markers

A. ASAKA

Narcolepsy has recently been found to be strongly associated with HLA antigens. All patients with narcolepsy have been shown 100% positive HLA-DR2 relationship in studies from Japan, the United Kingdom, France, Canada, the United States, and the Federal Republic of Germany. These findings suggest that the presence of HLA-DR2 was a sine qua non for the development of narcolepsy, not vice versa; those having HLA-DR2 would not always become narcoleptic. Some triggering factors, therefore, must be necessary for the manifestation of narcolepsy, though it is not clear at present whether these factors may be due to genetic and/or environmental factors. One approach to exploring this phenomenon is to examine the genetic backgrounds of narcoleptic patients. Many studies have been undertaken regarding the association between disease and genetic markers. However, no association study in relation to narcolepsy has appeared to date. This article deals with an association study of genetic markers and the trial of multiple discriminant function analysis using these markers.

Subjects and Methods

The subjects were 118 narcoleptic patients who visited the Sleep Disorders Clinic at Tokyo University Hospital. Sixteen genetic markers were identified after the patients' informed consents. The 16 genetic markers used in this association study were as follows: ABO blood group, MNS, Rh system (rhesus blood group), Km markers, GC (group-specific component), HP (haptoglobin), PI (alpha antitrypsin), ESD (esterase D), GPT (glutamic-pyruvate transaminase), GLO (glyoxylase), PGM1 (phosphoglucomutase-1), TF (transferrin), GOT (glutamic-oxaloacetic transaminase), ACP (acid phosphatase), ADA (adenosine deaminase), and PGD (phosphogluconate dehydrogenase). In the study of multiple discriminant analysis, 117 subjects were used, and in place of GOT, the GM marker was added. The total number of genetic markers used was again 16.

First, an association study was performed. The obtained frequencies were compared with the expected ones calculated from the frequencies among general populations. Second, a trial of discriminant function analysis was made between the patient group and the control model group, using these 16 genetic markers. The narcolepsy group consisted of 117 patients whose 16 genetic markers were completely ascertained. For the multiple discriminant function analysis 51 independent variables were constructed from the 16 genetic markers and were given the value 1 or 0 according to the presence or absence of the phenotype, alleles, or haplotypes of these 16 genetic markers. The control model population consisted of 100 subjects who were selected according to the reported frequencies among general populations. If the randomly generated value (P: $0 < P < 1$) was equal to or greater than the actual reported frequency (p), that is $P \geqslant p$, the value 1 was given to the subject, and if $P < p$ then 0 was assigned to the subject. This procedure was conducted under the limitation that the difference of the frequency between the two groups was not higher than 0.01.

Results

Association Study

Results of the association study are shown in Table 1. Significant associations were seen in GC, HP, PI, ESD, and GOT. In GC, rare variants such as 1F-TK', 2-F, 2-J, 2-N, and 1S-I were included in the phenotype of "others", so the frequency of rare variants increased. Also on GOT, the frequency of rare variant types 2-1 or 3-1 was elevated. In HP, a high frequency of individuals with phenotype 1 was seen and in PI the occurence of phenotype M1-M3 or M2-M2 increased. As for ESD, the frequency of phenotype 1 decreased, whereas that of phenotype 2-1 or 2 increased. Even with the MNS marker, if the number of phenotype MNS was independently counted, the observed number of 2.0 patients was significantly higher than the expected number of 0.1 patients (chi-square = 36.1). Accordingly, the total chi-square (= 40.92) indicated a high significance (d.f., 6; $P < 0.005$). It is remarkable that a comparatively high frequency of the MNS phenotype was seen in narcoleptics, whereas the frequency is low in the general population.

Multiple Discriminant Function Analysis

The 51 variables used are shown in Table 2. The results of discrimination are shown in Fig. 1 and Table 3. The percentage of correct diagnosis was 99.1% (116/117) for narcolepsy patients, and 94.0% (94/100) for the normal groups. The combined percentage of correct diagnosis was 96.8%. The large contributing factors of discrimination as seen in standardized coefficients were: v5 (M of MNSs), v14 (B of ACP), v17 (2 of ESD), v18 (1 of ESD), v32 (1 of ADA), v33 (agz of GM), v37 (b of KM), v50 (M2 of PI), and so on. They included some variables related to

Table 1. Genetic markers in patients with narcolepsy

1. ABO (9q34, C)

Phenotype	Observed	Expected	χ^2
A	46	44.5	0.05
B	24	26.1	0.17
O	36	36.7	0.01
AB	12	10.7	0.16
Total	118	118.0	0.39
df=3	$P>0.90$		

2. MNS (4q28 q31, C)

Phenotype	Observed	Expected	χ^2
Ms	31	28.9	0.15
Ns	22	25.4	0.46
MNs	56	51.0	0.49
MSs	2	4.5	1.39
MNSs	5	5.9	0.14
MNS Others	2	2.3	0.04
Total	118	118.0	2.66
df=5	$P>0.75$		

3. RH (1p36.2-p34, C)

Phenotype	Observed	Expected	χ^2
CCDee	60	51.8	1.30
CcDEe	36	44.3	1.56
CcDee	9	7.8	0.18
ccDEE	7	10.0	0.90
ccDEe	4	2.9	0.42
CcDEE	1		
ccDee	1	1.2	0.53
Others	0		
Total	118	118.0	4.89
df=5	$P>0.25$		

4. IGK (Km markers, 2p12, C)

Phenotype	Observed	Expected	χ^2
b/b	54	57.4	0.20
b/1	55	49.8	0.54
1/1	9	10.8	0.30
Total	118	118.0	1.04
df=2	$P>0.50$		

5. GC (4q12-q13, C)

Phenotype	Observed	Expected	χ^2
1F	26	25.6	0.01
1F-1S	22	28.5	1.48
2-1F	27	28.3	0.06
2-1S	19	15.7	0.69
2	7	7.8	0.08
1S	5	7.9	1.06
Others	12	4.2	14.49
Total	118	118.0	17.87
df=6	$P<0.01$		

6. HP (16q22.1, C)

Phenotype	Observed	Expected	χ^2
1	17	8.4	8.80
2-1	38	46.0	1.39
2	63	63.6	0.01
Total	118	118.0	10.20
df=2	$P<0.001$		

7. PI (14q32.1, C)

Phenotype	Observed	Expected	χ^2
M1-M1	57	64.6	0.89
M1-M2	33	36.7	0.37
M1-M3	14	8.7	3.23
M2-M2	10	5.2	4.43
M2-M3	4	2.5	0.90
Total	118	117.7	9.83
df=4	$P<0.05$		

8. ESD (13q14.1, C)

Phenotype	Observed	Expected	χ^2
1	37	51.1	3.89
2-1	62	53.1	1.49
2	19	13.8	1.96
Total	118	118.0	7.34
df=2	$P<0.05$		

9. GPT (16p, I)

Phenotype	Observed	Expected	χ^2
1	38	43.0	0.58
2-1	60	56.5	0.22
2	20	18.5	0.12
Total	118	118.0	0.92
df=2	$P>0.50$		

Table 1 (continued)

10. GLO1 (6p21.3-p21.1, C)

Phenotype	Observed	Expected	χ^2
1	0	0.3	0.30
2-1	10	11.9	0.30
2	108	105.8	0.05
Total	118	118.0	0.65
df=2		$P > 0.50$	

11. PGM1 (1p22.1, C)

Phenotype	Observed	Expected	χ^2
a1-a1	61	54.0	0.91
a1-a2	21	26.7	1.22
a1-a3	15	14.5	0.02
a1-a4	9	8.9	0.001
a2-a2	2	3.3	0.51
a2-a3	3	3.5	0.07
a3-a3	3	1.0	4.00
a3-a4	2	1.2	0.53
Others	2	4.9	1.72
Total	118	118.0	8.96
df=8		$P > 0.25$	

12. TF (3q21-q26.1, C)

Phenotype	Observed	Expected	χ^2
C1	67	65.9	0.02
C1-C2	42	42.4	0.004
C2	9	6.8	0.21
D	0	1.9	1.90
Total	117	117.0	2.13
df=3		$P > 0.5$	

13. GOT1 (10q25.3, C)

Phenotype	Observed	Expected	χ^2
1	113	116.1	0.08
2-1 4	5	1.9	5.06
3-1 1			
Total	118	118.0	5.14
df=1		$P < 0.025$	

14. ACP1 (2p25 or 2p23, C)

Phenotype	Observed	Expected	χ^2
B	70	70.5	0.004
B-A	43	41.4	0.06
A	5	6.1	0.20
Total	118	118.0	0.26
df=2		$P > 0.75$	

15. ADA (20q13.2-qter, C)

Phenotype	Observed	Expected	χ^2
1	113	113.1	0.001
2-1	5	4.8	0.008
2	0	0.1	0.10
Total	118	118.0	0.12
df=2		$P > 0.90$	

16. PGD (1p36.2-p36.13, C)

Phenotype	Observed	Expected	χ^2
A	99	100.5	0.02
A-C	18	16.8	0.09
C	1	0.7	0.13
Total	118	118.0	0.23
df=2		$P > 0.75$	

Parentheses indicate map position and status according to Human Gene Mapping 8: Helsinki Conference (1985) (C, confirmed; I, inconsistent)
Expected frequency was calculated from data among general population as follows, which were reported in JIBP (Watanabe et al. 1975)

1. ABO: Tanaka 1959 (Tokyo, n=77623)
2. MNS: Nakajima 1971 (Tokyo, n=912)
3. RH: Nakajima 1971 (Tokyo, n=7310)
4. Km: Matsumoto (n=748)
5. GC: Omoto 1978 (Tokyo, n=305)
6. HP: Ishimoto 1967 (Tokyo, n=300)
7. PI: Ishimoto (n=345)
8. ESD: Omoto 1979 (Tokyo, n=1066)
9. GPT: Ueda 1979 (Tokyo, n=603)
10. GLO1: Hashimoto 1978 (Tokyo, n=414)
11. PGM1: Matsumoto (n=596)
12. TF: Matsumoto (n=450)
13. GOT: Yamasawa 1972 (Tokyo, n=543)
14. ACP: Omoto 1969 (Tokyo, n=231)
15. ADA: Yamasawa 1970 (Tokyo, n=360)
16. PGD: Ishimoto 1970 (Tokyo, n=201)

Table 2. Variables used (V1 to V51)

V1	ABO	A	V19	PGM1	a1	V37	Km	b
V2		B	V20		a2	V38		1
V3		AB	V21		a3	V39	GC	1F
V4		O	V22		a4	V40		1S
V5	MNS	M	V23		7	V41		2
V6		N	V24		χ	V42		J
V7		S	V25	GPT	2	V43		V
V8		s	V26		1	V44	HP	2
V9	RH	C	V27	PGD	A	V45		1
V10		D	V28		C	V46	TF	C1
V11		E	V29	GLO	2	V47		C2
V12		c	V30		1	V48		D
V13		e	V31	ADA	2	V49	PI	M1
V14	ACP	B	V32		1	V50		M2
V15		A	V33	Gm	agz	V51		M3
V16		X	V34		axgz			
V17	ESD	2	V35		ab^3stz			
V18		1	V36		afb^1b^3n			

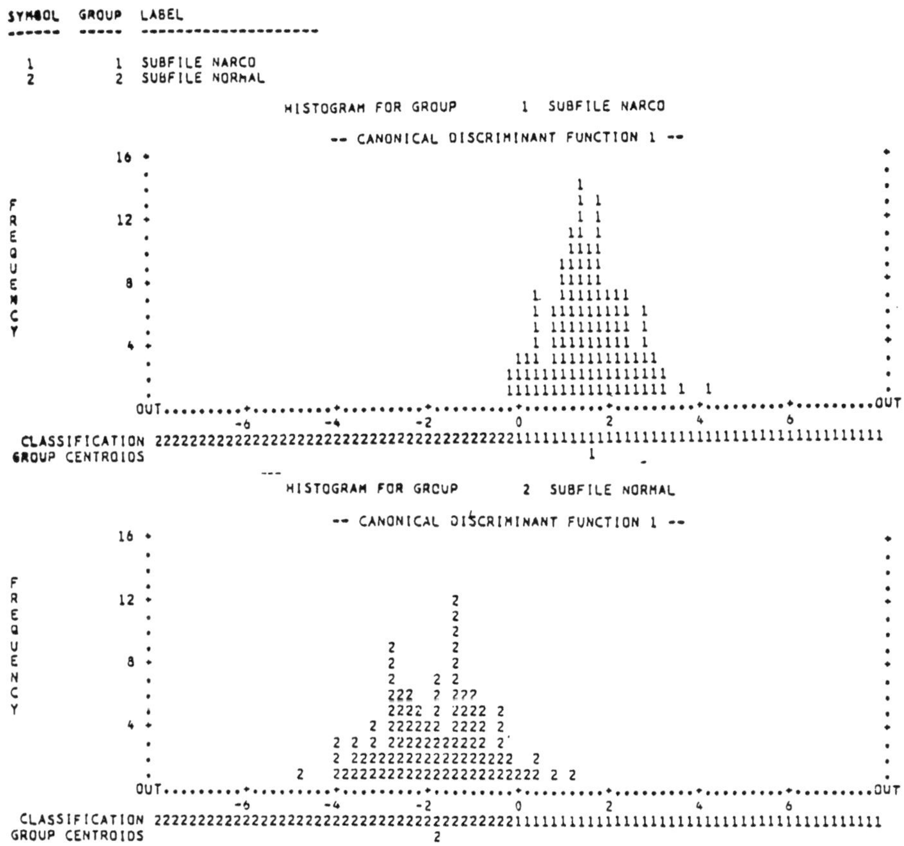

Fig. 1. Histogram of discrimination. *1* indicates narcolepsy group (NARCO) and *2* normal model group (NORMAL)

Table 3. Classification results between narcolepsy group (NARCO) and normal model group (NORMAL) (1), standardized (2), and unstandardized (3) discriminant function coefficients

(1) Classification results:

Actual group	No. of cases	Predicted group membership 1	2
Group 1 Subfile NARCO	117	116 99.1%	1 0.9%
Group 2 Subfile NORMAL	100	6 6.0%	94 94.0%

Percent age of "grouped" cases correctly classified, 96.77%

	(2)		(3)
V1	0.00031	V1	0.1702629D-01
V2	0.02649	V2	0.6453526D-01
V3	0.05103	V3	0.1682869
V4	−0.13454	V4	−0.2867288
V5	0.32749	V5	0.7342288
V6	0.18566	V6	0.3904795
V7	0.10095	V7	0.4096445
V8	−0.07541	V8	−0.4009590
V9	0.14909	V9	0.3812540
V10	0.17926	V10	0.9668482
V11	0.02774	V11	0.5817436D-01
V12	0.11837	V12	0.2421983
V13	0.25579	V13	0.7137600
V14	0.31708	V14	0.9924452
V15	0.14077	V15	0.3048894
V17	0.41734	V17	0.8863923
V18	0.31197	V18	0.7386243
V19	0.25497	V19	0.6637339
V20	0.16179	V20	0.4048737
V21	0.14386	V21	0.4024013
V22	0.14051	V22	0.5370907
V23	−0.16122	V23	−1.688566
V24	0.08755	V24	1.289193
V25	0.22290	V25	0.4654962
V26	0.25864	V26	0.5968631
V27	0.25471	V27	1.363632
V28	0.27663	V28	0.8565437
V29	−0.09109	V29	−0.6128644
V30	0.00409	V30	0.1607217D-01
V31	−0.01176	V31	−0.7143322D-01
V32	0.33292	V32	2.861600
V33	0.31892	V33	0.6766651
V34	0.19486	V34	0.4475247
V35	0.29378	V35	0.6273039
V36	0.11249	V36	0.3341009
V37	0.37994	V37	1.022297
V38	0.21114	V38	0.4374927
V39	−0.01248	V39	−0.2537698D-01
V40	0.08800	V40	0.1879095
V41	−0.01862	V41	−0.3935588D-01
V42	−0.00539	V42	−0.1652307D-01
V43	0.06353	V43	0.4739153

Table 3 (continued)

V44	0.12169	V44	0.3049289
V45	0.24967	V45	0.5266607
V46	0.19950	V46	0.4272673
V47	0.25955	V47	0.7434683
V48	−0.04346	V48	−0.6404236
V49	0.21194	V49	0.5574716
V50	0.33973	V40	0.7467018
V51	0.06644	V51	0.2132352
		(constant)	−13.06171

genetic markers which were significant in the association study such as GC, HP, and MNS. This indicates that the finding of the multivariate analysis is to some extent in accordance with the results obtained by the association study.

Discussion

The usual association studies between 16 genetic markers and narcolepsy indicated the possibility that some predisposing genetic backgrounds are necessary for the development of the disease. For example, those who have rare variants may have increased susceptibility to the disease and go over the threshold according to the threshold theory of the multifactorial inheritance model, which will be discussed later. A trial of multiple discriminant analysis also suggested the presence of several genetic backgrounds which played an important role as genetically predisposing factors to narcolepsy. We started the association study between narcolepsy and these genetic markers in 1980, followed by the study of HLA-A, -B, -C (Juji et al. 1981), and finally the HLA-DR series, in which a strong association between DR2 and the disease was dramatically found (Honda et al. 1984). It was clearly suggested that there exists a gene susceptible to narcolepsy which is closely linked to DR2. It does not mean, however, that those who have positive DR2 always become narcoleptic, but it only indicates that the DR2-positive condition is a prerequisite for the development of the disease. Therefore, some triggering factors must be required, and this assumption was supported, for example, by studies of narcoleptic twins. Five pairs of monozygotic twins with narcolepsy have been reported including ours as is shown in Table 4. They were all discordant or incompletely concordant for narcolepsy. The possible contributing factors seen in the patients were minor biological problems such as neonatal asphyxia, asthma, and dexterity as well as psychological factors such as emotional stress and excessive social demand.

Narcolepsy has generally been classified etiologically into two types: idiopathic and symptomatic. Among 185 Japanese narcoleptic patients, there were at least 11 cases of unquestionable symptomatic narcolepsy (Honda et al. 1986, see also Chap. 3). These symptomatic or major exogenous factors are loss of consciousness, heavy bleeding, or encephalitis which immediately preceded the onset of

Table 4. Reported MZ twins with narcolepsy

Authors	Concordance	Possible contributors
Imlah (1961)	Incompletely concordant	Extrovert personality and poor manual dexterity
Mitchell, Cummins (1965)	Discordant	
Takahashi (in Kessler 1975)	Completely discordant	Neonatal asphyxia and asthma
Mamelak, Caruso, Stewart (1979)	Incompletely concordant	Emotional stress and environmental demands
Asaka, Honda, Takahashi (1986)	Completely discordant	Environmental stress and poor manual dexterity

narcolepsy. It is noteworthy that all of these symptomatic narcoleptics also expressed positive DR2.

As for the mode of inheritance, both a single dominant gene model (Krabbe and Magnussen 1942; Daly and Yoss 1959) and a multifactorial inheritance model (Bruhova and Roth 1972; Kessler et al. 1974) have been proposed. We have analyzed 232 families with a narcolepsy proband and proposed a two-threshold multifactorial model (Honda et al. 1983). These findings, which indicate that the manifestation of the disease can be explained by either a single gene model or a multifactorial inheritance model, appear contradictory. However, if the segregation ratio of the probands' children (4.76%) and the frequency among the general population (0.16%), which were obtained from our family study, are taken into consideration, and if we apply the formula reported by Krüger (1973), both models can coexist under certain specific conditions. That is, the mode of inheritance of narcolepsy fits both a single dominant model with low penetrance and a multifactorial inheritance model with high heritability.

Summary

The finding that all narcoleptic patients had 100% positive DR2 indicates a sine qua non, but not vice versa, condition for the development of narcolepsy. It is suggested that some predisposing factors or other genetic backgrounds are needed, and that some minor or major exogenous factors, biological as well as psychological, are also required as triggering factors for the manifestation of the disease. The mode of inheritance of narcolepsy fits both a single gene model and a multifactorial inheritance model.

References

Asaka A, Honda Y, Takahashi Y (1986) Two pairs of monozygotic twins completely discordant for narcolepsy. Proc 7th International congress of human genetics
Bruhova S, Roth B (1972) Heredofamilial aspects of narcolepsy and hypersomnia. Arch Suisse Neurol Neurochir Psychiatr 11: 45-54
Daly D, Yoss RA (1959) Family with narcolepsy. Proc Staff Mayo Clinic 34: 313-320
Honda Y, Asaka A, Tanimura M, Furusho T (1983) A genetic study of narcolepsy and excessive daytime sleepiness in 308 families with a narcolepsy or hypersomnia proband. In: Guilleminault C, Lugaresi E (eds) Sleep/wake disorders: natural history, epidemiology, and long-term evolution. Raven, New York
Honda Y, Doi Y, Juji T, Satake M (1984) Narcolepsy and HLA: positive DR2 as a prerequisite for the development of narcolepsy. Folia Psychiatr Neurol Jpn 38: 360
Honda Y, Asaka A, Harada S, Juji T, Matsuki K (1986) Exogenous factors triggering the manifestation of narcolepsy. Proc 31st Japanese soceity of human genetics
Human Gene Mapping 8: Helsinki Conference (1985). Cytogenet Cell Genet 40: 1-4
Imlah NW (1961) Narcolepsy in identical twins. J Neurol Neurosurg Psychiatry 2 4: 158-160
Juji T, Maeda H, Honda Y et al. (1981) An analysis of I region associated human B lymphocyte antigens other than HLA-DR locus, and HLA typings in narcolepsy and SLE. In: Watanabe I (ed) Annual report of Research Commitee on Host Factors of Intractable Diseases. Ministry of Health and Welfare, Tokyo
Kessler S, Guilleminault C, Dement WC (1974) A family study of 50 REM narcoleptics. Acta Neurol Scand 50: 503-512
Kessler S (1975) Genetic factors in narcolepsy. Adv Sleep Res 3: 285-302
Krabbe E, Magnussen G (1942) Familial narcolepsy. Acta Psychiatr Neurol 17: 149-173
Krüger J (1973) Zur Unterscheidung zwischen multifaktoriellem Erbgang mit Schwellenwerteffekt und einfachem diallen Erbgang. Humangenetik 17: 181-252
Mamelak M, Caruso VJ, Stewart K (1979) Narcolepsy: a family study. Biol Psychiatry 14: 821-834
Mitchell S and Cummins L (1965) Idiopathic narcolepsy in one of monozygotic twins. Proc APSS meeting, Washington DC
Watanabe S, Kondo S, Matsunaga E (eds) (1975) Anthropological and genetic studies on the Japanese, (JIBP Synthesis 2). University of Tokyo Press, Tokyo

Part 2: Red Blood Cell Antigens in Narcolepsy

K. MATSUKI, M. UCHIKAWA, T. JUJI, and Y. HONDA

The strong association between narcolepsy and an HLA antigen HLA-DR2 demonstrated that at least one genetic factor contributes to the development of narcoloepsy (Honda et al. 1984; Juji et al. 1984; Matsuki et al. 1985). Although this HLA-DR2-related factor is prerequisite, it is insufficient by itself for the development of narcolepsy (Matsuki et al. 1985; Honda et al. 1986). More often than not, the proband is the only member in the family who has narcolepsy. Other family members, who share the same HLA-DR2 haplotype as the proband, are often

Table 1. Red blood cell antigens in narcolepsy

P1		$P=0.51$	
Antigen	Observed N	Expected N	χ^2
P1+	40	36.75	0.287
P1−	65	68.25	0.155
Total	105	105.00	0.442
Lewis (19pter-p13.2)[a]		$P=0.05$	
Antigen	Observed N	Expected N	χ^2
a+b−	25	23.10	0.156
a−b+	64	71.40	0.767
a−b−	16	10.50	2.881
Total	105	105.00	3.804
Duffy (1q12-q21)		$P=0.83$	
Antigen	Observed N	Expected N[b]	χ^2
a+b−	84	84.53	0.003
a+b+	20	19.32	0.024
a−b+	1	1.15	0.020
Total	105	105.00	0.047
Kidd (2p12)		$P=0.56$	
Antigen	Observed N	Expected N	χ^2
a+b−	23	23.1	0.000
a+b+	50	52.5	0.119
a−b+	32	29.4	0.230
Total	105	105.0	0.349
Diego		$P=0.44$	
Antigen	Observed N	Expected N	χ^2
a+	11	8.82	0.539
a−	94	96.18	0.049
Total	105	105.00	0.588

[a] Chromosomal location
[b] Expected numbers were obtained from the normal frequencies of red cell blood types

completely free from narcoleptic symptoms. Factors other than HLA-DR2 are required for the full manifestation of narcolepsy.

If we find another genetic marker of narcolepsy, the clinical value will be high. At present, in a family of a HLA-DR2-positive narcolepsy proband, we can safely say that a member without DR2 has little, if any, chance of developing narcolepsy. However, we cannot forecast anything about a family member with DR2. The member has a certain possibility of contracting narcolepsy, but what is the possibility? Another marker would be very useful in such a case.

Red blood cell antigens are among the first candidates. They are easy to determine, have a certain level of polymorphism, and, for some of the blood types, the chromosomal locations of the coding genes are already known.

These ideas prompted us to examine red blood cell types of Japanese patients with narcolepsy. The antigens examined in the previous study (see the previous section) were excluded in the present study. All the patients met diagnostic criteria and were HLA-DR2 positive. Blood cell types were determined by the standard methods.

Table 1 shows the frequencies of red blood cell antigens in 105 Japanese patients with narcolepsy. To our disappointment, no antigens showed significant deviation of frequency from the general population in Japan.

More extensive study of genetic markers in narcolepsy is certainly required. Determination of restriction fragment length polymorphism with DNA probes will be a promising next step.

References

Honda Y, Doi Y, Juji T, Satake M (1984) Narcolepsy and HLA: positive DR2 as a prerequisite for the development of narcolepsy. Folia Psychiatr Neurol Jpn 38: 360

Honda Y, Juji T, Matsuki K, Naohara T, Satake M, Inoko H, Someya T, Harada S, Doi Y (1986) HLA-DR2 and Dw2 in narcolepsy and in other disorders of excessive somnolence without cataplexy. Sleep 9: 133-142

Juji T, Satake M, Honda Y, Doi Y (1984) HLA antigens in Japanese patients with narcolepsy. All the patients were DR2 positive. Tissue Antigens 24: 316-319

Matsuki K, Juji T, Tokunaga K, Naohara T, Satake M, Honda Y (1985) HLA haplotype frequencies estimated from the data on HLA class I, II, and III antigens in 111 Japanese narcoleptics. J Clin Invest 76: 2078-2083

Subject Index

Abnormal REM manifestations 174, 175, 176
ABO incompatibility 19
Aborted forms 172
- - of narcolepsy 176, 179
Activated T cells 21
- T lymphocyte 17, 21
Activities 53
Adrenal 21-hydroxylase deficiency 21
Age of onset 46
Akinetic seizure 36
Alloantibodies to HLA 14
Alloantigenic determinant 17
Alloantigen system on human leukocytes 10
Alloantisera 14, 15, 17
Allogenotope 19
Alpha chain 17, 81
- 1, 2, 3 domains 17
Ambiguous narcolepsy 110
American Narcolepsy Association (ANA) 2
ANA, *see* American Narcolepsy Association
Ankylosing spondylitis 20, 21, 58, 108
Anti-DQ antiserum 14
Anti-DR antiserum 14
Apneas 187
APSS, *see* Association for the Psychophysiological Study of Sleep
ASDC, *see* Association of Sleep Disorders Centers
Association 192
- for the Psychophysiological Study of Sleep (APSS) 5, 34, 173, 181
- of Sleep Disorders Centers (ASDC) 5, 34, 173, 181
Astatic seizure 36
Attitudes toward sleepiness 182
Autoimmune disease 73, 155
Automatic behavior 32, 37, 102
Autosomal dominant model with low penetrance 45
AZH 82

Baye's theorem 68-69
Beta chain 17, 81
- 1, 2 domains 17
- 2 microglobulin 16, 17
BF 79, 135
- protein 132
Blastogenic transformation 15
B lymphocyte 17, 90
Bone marrow transplantation 19
Broad specificities 13
Bw35 2
Bw52 2

C2 130, 132, 133, 135
C4 130, 133
Cadaver 19
Cataplectic attacks 111, 115
Cataplexy 3, 4, 5, 26, 38, 58-59, 76, 81, 90, 93, 98, 101, 102, 104, 105, 109, 111-114, 152, 153, 155, 159, 166, 174, 176, 177, 178, 186
- age of oneset 46
- muscle weakness 181-182
- without daytime sleepiness 111
C blank 174
cellular proliferation 15
- recognition 146, 148
Chlorpromazine 153
Class I 11, 115
- - antigen 14, 21, 78, 115
- - MHC 81
- - probe 19
- II 11, 78, 115
- - antigen 14, 21
- - probe 19
- III 115
- - HLA system 21
- - MHC 81
Classical narcolepsy 109, 111
- - without DR2 111
Clomipramine 6, 41, 52, 59, 102, 115, 153
Clomipyramine 115
Cluster analysis 140
CN 108
CNS stimulants 37, 41, 52, 53
Combination of alleles 16
Complement 155-156
- C2 130, 132

Complement C4 130, 133
- factor B 130, 132
- gene 21
Concept of narcolepsy 33
Criteria 59, 114
- narcolepsies 109
Cross-reactive antigen 20
Cyclandelate 174
Cyclosporin-A 19
Cytoplasmic tail 17
Cytotoxic T cell 21
- T-lymphocytes 21

Daytime sleep attacks 113
- sleepiness 111, 113
- somnolence 105
Dendritic cell 17
Dermatitis herpetiformus 86
Desipramine 41
Diagnostic criteria 4, 35-36, 42-43, 58, 59, 172, 181-182, 201
- -, EHS 42-43, 59, 172
- -, narcolepsy 4, 57, 72, 181
Differential diagnosis for narcolepsy 36
Diseases 77
Disorders of excessive daytime sleepiness (DOES) 36, 172
- - the sleep-wake schedule 184
Dissociated REM sleep manifestation 38
Disturbed noctural sleep 31, 36
Dizygotic twins 10
DNA 7, 18, 104, 123, 130
cDNA 19, 43
EcoR1-digested DQ beta DNA 21
Taq-1-digested DQ alpha DNA 21
DNA analysis 82, 91
cDNA clone 18
DNA, genomic 18
cDNA probes 18
DNA restriction fragment length polymorphism 103
- typing 137-148
- - in narcolepsy 137
DOES, *see* disorders of excessive sleepiness
Domain 17
Dominant model 66
DP 82
DQ 82, 90
DQR1 61
DQR2, 6 61
DQR2-6 91
DQw1 89, 93, 104, 111
DR 82
DR1 111
DR2 12, 45, 62, 78, 91, 93, 95, 102, 104, 111, 113, 119-128, 134, 147, 197, 198
- allele 108
- haplotype 148
- in healthy subjects 67
- negative 6, 176, 179
- - narcolepsy 5, 72, 173, 180, 181-182
- - narcoleptic patients 72
- - narcoleptics 182
- positive 2, 6, 113, 176
DR2/DQw1 115
Drop attacks of the elderly 36, 59
DRw15 12
Dw2 12, 45, 62, 82, 121-128, 147
Dw12 2, 12, 45, 62, 82, 104, 121-128, 147

EcoR1-digested DQ beta DNA 22
EcoRI 82
EcoRV 82
EDS, *see* excessive daytime sleepiness
EHS, *see* essential hypersomnia
Einschlafsucht 5
Encephalitis lethargica 164
Endonuclease 19
Enteric bacteria 21
Environmental agents 86
- stress factor 45
Eosin Y solution 14
Epidemiology 41
Epilepsy 3, 36, 59, 100
Epileptoid personality 33
ESD, *see* esterase D
Essential hypersomnia (EHS) 42, 43, 59, 172, 183-185
- -, abnormal REM manifestations 181
- -, aborted forms of narcolepsy 176-179, 183
- -, attitudes toward sleepiness 182
- -, diagnostic criteria 59, 172
- -, mild hypersomnia with neurotic attitudes 179
- -, subtypes 172, 173
- narcolepsy 3
Esterase D (ESD) 42
Excessive daytime sleepiness (EDS) 1, 34, 36, 98, 102, 105, 109, 112
- - somnolence (EDS) 36, 43, 59, 90, 93, 185
- - -, HLA in 184-185
Exogenous factors 71-72

Factor B 130
Family studies 42, 62-64, 93, 95, 119
Ficoll-Hypaque solution 14
Ficoll-mitrizoate 90
FJO 82

GC, *see* Group-specific component
1D-IEF Gel 17
Gelineau-Redlich's syndrome 5
Gelineau's syndrome 5

Gene library 146
Genetic marker(s) 42, 191, 197
- model 42, 45, 65, 66
- -, dominant 66
- -, heritability 65
- -, single mutation hypothesis 73
- -, two-threshold multifactorial 42, 45, 65-67
- -, - - with dominant Dw2 45
- study 4, 42-44
genomic clone 146
- DNAs 18
Glycoprotein 16, 17
GOT, *see* soluble glutamate-oxalate transaminase
Graft survival rate 19
Group-specific component (GC) 42
Growth hormone 39
- - secretion 40
Guidance for living 52
Guillain-Barré syndrome 86

H-2 10
Hallucinatory paranoid state 52
Haplotype 16, 62
- frequencies 62
Haptoglobin (HP) 42
Heavy chains 16, 17
Heritability 65
- of liability to narcolepsy 44
Heterodimetric 17
History 3
HLA (human leukocyte antigen system A) 1, 10-19, 86, 100, 176, 184
HLA-A 197
- antigen 11
-, B, C 97, 101, 112
-, -, - antigens 99
HLA antigen 97, 167, 191
- - on platelet 20
HLA-B 197
- antigen 11
HLA-B27 20, 21
- with ankylosing spondylitis 20
HLA-C 197
- antigen 11
HLA class I (HLA-A, B, C) antigens 11, 15, 16, 17
- - - heavy chain 17
- - II alloantigen molecule 17
- - - (HLA-D, DR, DQ, DP) antigens 11, 15, 16, 17
- - III HLA system 21
- compatible platelet 20
HLA-D 112, 137
- determinant(s) 121-122
HLA and disease 20, 108
- disorders of excessive daytime somnolence 184-185
HLA-DP 128
HLA-DQw1 93, 142
HLA-DR 11, 90, 97, 101, 102, 110, 197
HLA DR2 2, 7, 45, 86, 89, 94, 98, 101, 103, 104, 105, 108, 112, 115, 135, 142, 159, 176, 187, 189, 191, 199, 201
HLA DR2 DNA 103
HLA DR2/DQ 158
HLA DR2 DQw1 93
HLA DR2-Dw2 45
- susceptibility to narcolepsy 142
HLA-DR antigens 100
- typing 110
HLA-D region 121, 122, 128, 138
- specifities 121-124
- subregion 128
- typing 91
HLA-Dw2 102, 121
HLA-Dw2 HTC 124
HLA in essential Hypersomnia 183-184
- excessive daytime somnolence 184-185
- identical sibling 19
- in Kleine-Levin syndrome 184
- in narcolepsy 191
- Nomenclature Committee 11
- system 1, 11, 20
- typing 2, 20, 97, 110, 124, 186, 187, 190
Homozygous B lymphoblastoid 140
- - - cell lines 138, 140
- typing cell (HTC) 11, 15, 122-127
Hormone receptor 20
HP, *see* haptoglobin
HTC, *see* homozygous typing cell
Human leukocyte antigen, *see* HLA
Hydrophobic transmembrane segment 17
Hypersomnolence 104
Hypervariable region 17
Hypnagogic hallucination 4, 29, 31, 38, 90, 100, 102, 111, 112, 115, 159, 166, 174, 175, 176
Hypnolepsy 5

Idiopathic 197
- CNS hypersomnolence 173-176
- hypersomnia 172-176
- -, essential features 172-173, 176
- -, monosymptomatic form 173
- -, polysymptomatic form 173, 175, 176
- narcolepsy 69
1D-IEF 18
IEF banding pattern 18
Imipramine 6, 41, 52, 177
Immune basis 77
- responses 10, 11, 21, 146, 148
Immunogenetics 1

Immunoglobulin constant region domain 17
Immunological features 150-157, 158, 160
Immunosuppressive drug 19
Inclusion of HLA-B specificities into Bw4 and Bw6 13
Independent narcolepsy 5
Inemuribyo 5
Insulin-induced hypoglycemia 40
International Histocompatibility Workshop 11, 15
Intradomain disulfide bond 17
Inverted phase contrast microscope 14
Isoelectric points (pI) 18
Isolated EDS-CNS hypersomnia 109

Japan Narcolepsy Association (JNA, Narco-Kai) 6, 53
- - -, activities of 53
- - -, contributions of 53
- - -, social impact of 54
Japanese Experience 24
JNA, *see* Japan Narcolepsy Association
Juvenile onset diabetes (JOD) 86, 108
- type 1 diabetes mellitus 160

Kidney transplantation 19
- -, from cadavers 19
Kleine-Levin syndrome 184

LCT, *see* lymphocytoxicity test
LD-MN2 82
Leukoagglutinin 10
Light chains 16, 17
Linkage disequilibrium 16, 20, 77, 89, 115, 121
Lupus erythematosus 112, 165
Lymphocyte subsets 150-156
Lymphocytotoxity test (LCT) 10, 11

Macrophage 17, 21
Major histocompatibility complex (MHC) 10, 11, 94, 108, 130, 159
- - -, class I 21, 108, 114
- - -, class II 21, 108, 114
- - -, class III 130
- - -, DP 137
- - -, DQ 137
- - -, DR 137
- - -, enclosed complement 79
- - -, haplotype 134, 140, 142, 146
Mechanism for narcolepsy-DR2 association 72-73, 156-157
Mendelian codominant traits 16
- inheritance model 44
Methamphetamine 41, 52
Methylphenidate 41, 52, 102, 152-153, 155, 177
MHC, *see* major histocompatibility complex
Mixed lymphocyte culture (MLC) 11, 15
- - reaction (MLR) 82, 121-123, 125-128
MLC, *see* mixed lymphocyte culture
MLR, *see* mixed lymphocyte reaction
Mode of inheritance 198
Monocyte 17
Monosymptomatic form 173
- narcolepsy 80, 179, 181
Monozygotic twins 10, 197
Mouse monoclonal antibody 14, 17
MSLT, *see* multiple sleep latency test
Multifactorial inheritance model 44, 197, 198
Multiparous women's sera 10, 14
Multiple discriminant function analysis 192
- sclerosis 59, 86, 94, 102, 156, 160, 166
- sleep latency test (MSLT) 34, 37, 38, 98, 100, 101, 105, 108-109, 111, 112, 113, 152-153, 155, 186, 187, 190
Muscle weakness 109, 181, 182
Myotonic dystrophy 185
Mysthenia gravis 36, 86, 156, 160

Narco-Kai, *see* Japan Narcolepsy Association
Narcolepsy 2, 3, 22, 90, 93, 94, 100-105, 108, 112, 132, 159, 164, 181, 186, 189, 197, 201
-, aborted forms of 172, 176-179, 182, 183
-, age of oneset 46
-, associations 6
-, attitude toward sleepiness 182
-, canine model 156
-, cataplexy 85, 158
-, without cataplexy 111
-, clinical features 24
-, concept 33
-, definition 34
-, diagnostic criteria 2, 58, 72, 181
-, differential diagnosis 36
-, disease 104
-, DR2-negative 5, 72, 173, 180, 181-182
-, essential 3
-, family study 62-64
-, genetic study 4
-, history 3
-, idiopathic 69
-, independent 5
-, Japanese experiences 24, 58-75
-, monosymptomatic 179, 181
-, other complications 32
-, polysomnographic findings 38
-, prevalence 50
-, prevention 67
-, psychogenic 71
-, psychological factors 4
-, secondary 3
-, symptomatic 4, 69

-, syndrome 108
-, tetrad 4
-, treatment 51
Narcoleptic DR2/Dw2 haplotype 156
- patients 69
- symptoms 101
- syndrome 158
- tetrad 5, 98
Narcoleptoid personality 32, 33, 182
Naturally occurring antibodies 14
Neuroendocrine findings 39
Neuropharmacological findings 41
Neurotransmitter 159
Neutralized formalin 14
NH2-terminal domains 17
Noctural myoclonus 174
- - DOES syndrome 36
- sleep-apnea DOES syndrome 36
Nonspecific toxicity 14
NWC 110

One-way MLC 15
Orthostatic hypotension 36, 59
Other complications 32

Paternity testing 21
Pemoline 41, 52, 152-153, 155, 178
Penetrance 66, 89, 95
Periodic somnolence 36, 184, 185
Pharmacotherapy 51
Phenothiazine derivate 52
PI, *see* serum alpha-1-trypsin inhibitor
Pipradol 41
Platelet apheresis 20
- increment 19
- random donor 19
- specific alloantigen 20
- transfusion 19
PLT, *see* primed lymphocyte test *and* primed lymphocyte typing
Poemoline 153
Polygraphic 102, 109, 111, 113, 187
Polymorphism 1, 19, 20, 21, 138
Polysomnogram 38, 39
Polysomnography 38, 90
Polysymptomatic form 173
- idiopathic hypersomnia 174, 175, 176
- narcolepsy 180
Poor sleep hygiene 36, 184
Postencephalitic parkinsonism 164
Predisposition 45
Pretransplant transfusion 19
Prevalence 50
Prevention 67
Primed lymphocyte test (PLT) 15
- - typing (PLT) 128
Prognosis 50
Psychogenic narcolepsy 4, 45, 71
Psychotic state 52
Purified B lymphocytes 114

RA 112
Rabbit complement 14
Ragweed pollen antigen (RPA) 86
Rapid eye movement (REM) 5, 38-39, 89, 109, 112, 113, 152-153, 158, 173-175, 177, 178, 186, 187
- - -, abnormalities 181
- - -, hypersomniacs 187
- - -, period 4
- - -, sleep 5, 166, 167
Receptor for pathogenic organism 20-21
Recombinant 15
Recombination 15, 16, 94
Recurrent daytime naps 24
Red blood cell types 199-201
Refractoriness 19
Refractory patient 20
Relative frequency (K value of Penrose) 41, 44
- risk 58, 59
REM, *see* rapid eye movement
Responder lymphocytes 15
Restless legs syndrome 172, 175
Restriction endonucleases 18, 90, 93
- enzyme 91
- fragment 148
- - length 85
- - - polymorphisms (RFLP) 18, 19, 81, 82, 110, 146
- molecule 146, 148
RFLP, *see* restriction fragment length polymorphisms

Sacroiliac joints 21
SB, *see* secondary B-cell antigen system
SDS-polyacrylamide gel electrophoresis 17
Secondary B-cell antigen system (SB) 15
- narcolepsy 3, 4
Segregation ratio 41, 43
Self/nonself recognition systems 11
Serological typing 14
Serum alpha-1-trypsin inhibitor (PI) 42
Sex difference 48
Single gene model 198
- mutation hypothesis 73
Sixth chromosome 11
Sleep apnea 102, 166
- - syndrome 36, 100, 112, 172, 175, 189
- - -, HLA antigens 184
- attacks 4, 25, 26, 98, 100, 102, 104, 111, 112, 115
- disorders 1, 22, 76, 80
- gene 156
- latency 166

Sleep log 51
- oneset REM (SOREM) 90, 93, 111, 115
- - - period (SOREMP) 4, 34, 99, 100, 101, 105
- paralysis 4, 31, 38, 90, 100, 102, 111, 112, 115, 159, 174-177
Social impact 53
Soluble glutamate-oxalate transaminase (GOT) 42
Somatogenic narcolepsy 45, 70-71
Somnolence 184
Somnosis 5
SOREM, *see* sleep onset REM
SOREMP, *see* sleep onset REM period
Southern blot technique 18
- blotting 81
- hybridization analysis of DNA polymorphisms 138
Split antigens 13
Stimulation cells 15
Strongest barrier for allografts 10
Subtypes 173
Subwakefulness syndrome 36
Supertypic antigens 13
Susceptibility 146
- to disease 138, 142, 145, 146, 148
- gene 20, 21
Symptomatic 197
- narcolepsy 4, 45, 69-70

Taijin-kyofu 175
Tag-1-digested DQ alpha DNA 22
TB22 61
TB23 60-61
T cell antigen receptor 146-148
Tissue typing 142
T lymphocytes 21, 90
- -, cytotoxic 21
Transfusion 19
Treatment 51
Tricyclic antidepressant 4, 37, 41
Tricyclics 115
Trifluoperazine 53
Twenty-one-hydroxylase deficiency 21
Two-dimensional gel electrophoreses 17
- nonequilibrium pH 17
Two-threshold multifactorial model 42
- - - with dominant HLA-Dw2 inheritance 45
Types of narcolepsy 162
Typing tray 14

Vertigo 36

Westphal-Gelineau's syndrome 5
WHO, *see* World Health Organization
World Health Organization (WHO) 11

MIX
Papier aus verantwortungsvollen Quellen
Paper from responsible sources
FSC® C105338

If you have any concerns about our products,
you can contact us on
ProductSafety@springernature.com

In case Publisher is established outside the EU,
the EU authorized representative is:
Springer Nature Customer Service Center GmbH
Europaplatz 3, 69115 Heidelberg, Germany

Printed by Libri Plureos GmbH
in Hamburg, Germany